POCKET ATLAS OF EMERGENCY MEDICINE

NOTICE

POCKET ATLAS OF EMERGENCY MEDICINE

Kevin J. Knoop
Program Director
Emergency Medicine Residency, Naval Medical Center
Portsmouth, Virginia

Lawrence B. Stack
Assistant Professor of Emergency Medicine
Vanderbilt University Medical Center
Nashville, Tennessee

Alan B. Storrow
Assistant Professor of Emergency Medicine
University of Cincinnati Medical Center
Cincinnati, Ohio

McGraw-Hill
HEALTH PROFESSIONS DIVISION

New York St. Louis San Francisco Auckland Bogota Caracas Lisbon London Madrid Mexico City Milan Montreal New Delhi San Juan Singapore Sydney Tokyo Toronto

McGraw-Hill

A Division of The ***McGraw-Hill*** *Companies*

POCKET ATLAS OF EMERGENCY MEDICINE

The views expressed in this work are those of the individual authors and do not reflect the official policy or position of the Departments of the Navy, Army, or Air Force, the Department of Defense, or the U.S. Government.

1 2 3 4 5 6 7 8 9 0 KGP/KGP 9 9

ISBN 0-07-135807-2

This book was set in Friz Quadrata by York Production Services. The editors were John Dolan and Pamela Touboul; the production supervisor was Rick Ruzycka. Quebecor Printing/Kingsport was printer and binder.

Cataloging-in-publication data is on file for this title at the Library of Congress.

DEDICATION

To the outstanding Emergency Medicine residents
of the Naval Medical Center Portsmouth,
Joint Military Medical Centers, University of Cincinnati,
and Vanderbilt University Medical Center,
who teach us something new every day.
Kevin J. Knoop
Lawrence B. Stack
Alan B. Storrow

To my children, Amelia and Stephen,
who are my greatest joy,
and
To my wife, Mary Jo,
for her unending support, love, and friendship.
Kevin J. Knoop

To my children, Laura, Andrew, and Emily,
God's greatest blessing to me,
and
To my wife Venette,
God's gift to me, for her patience and support
during the development of this project.
Lawrence B. Stack

To my children, Robert, Leslie, and Allison Marie,
who are the highlight of my life,
and, most importantly,
To my wife, Julia Ann,
for her cheerful spirit, encouragement, and devotion to a loving family.
Without her patience and many sacrifices this work
would never have been completed.
Alan B. Storrow

CHAPTER 13 CUTANEOUS CONDITIONS

Christopher R. Sartori | Michael B. Brooks

Part II
SPECIALTY AREAS

CHAPTER 14 PEDIATRIC CONDITIONS

Javier A. Gonzalez del Rey | Richard M. Ruddy

CONTRIBUTORS

Frank Birinyi, M.D., FACEP
Clinical Assistant Professor of Emergency Medicine
The Ohio State University
Attending Physician
Mount Carmel Medical Center
Mount Carmel East Hospital
Columbus, Ohio (2)

Diane M. Birnbaumer, M.D., FACEP
Associate Residency Director
Department of Emergency Medicine
Harbor-UCLA Medical Center
Torrence, California (9, 17)

Jeffery D. Bondesson, M.D.
Attending Physician
Kaiser Permanente Medical Center
San Diego, California (8)

Michael B. Brooks, M.D.
Attending Physician
Joint Military Medical Centers Emergency Medicine Residency
Brooke Army Medical Center
San Antonio, Texas (13)

Robert G. Buckley, M.D., FACEP
CDR, MC, USNR
Head
Department of Emergency Medicine
Naval Hospital
Rota, Spain (10)

Carey D. Chisholm, M.D., FACEP
Emergency Medicine Residency Director
Clinical Associate Professor of Emergency Medicine
Methodist-Indiana University
Indianapolis, Indiana (4)

Stephen Corbett, M.D.
Department of Emergency Medicine
Loma Linda University Medical Center
Loma Linda, California (7)

David Effron, M.D., FACEP
Department of Emergency Medicine
MetroHealth Medical Center
Cleveland, Ohio (3)

Lynn K. Flowers, M.D.
LCDR, MC, USNR
Attending Physician
Naval Hospital
Rota, Spain
Assistant Professor of Emergency Medicine
Eastern Virginia Medical School
Norfolk, Virginia (9)

Beverly C. Forcier, M.D.
Department of Emergency Medicine
MetroHealth Medical Center
Cleveland, Ohio (3)

Sarah J. Gahm, M.D.
Resident
Department of Emergency Medicine
Medical College of Pennsylvania
Philadelphia, Pennsylvania (6)

Javier A. Gonzalez del Rey, M.D., FAAP
Assistant Professor of Clinical Pediatrics and Emergency Medicine
University of Cincinnati College of Medicine
Attending Physician, Division of Emergency Medicine
Children's Hospital Medical Center, Cincinnati, Ohio (14)

Edward C. Jauch, M.D., M.S.
Assistant Professor
Department of Emergency Medicine
University of Cincinnati Medical Center
Cincinnati, Ohio (5, 6)

Kevin J. Knoop, M.D., M.S., FACEP
CAPT, MC, USN
Program Director
Emergency Medicine Residency
Naval Medical Center
Portsmouth, Virginia (4, 5, 7, 10)

Thomas F. Mauger, M.D.
Associate Professor of Ophthalmology
Department of Ophthalmology
William H. Havener Eye Center
The Ohio State University
Columbus, Ohio (2)

Timothy D. McGuirk, D.O., FACEP
CDR, MC, USN
Head, Clinical Investigation and Research Department
Naval Medical Center
Portsmouth, Virginia (1)

David W. Munter, M.D., FACEP
CAPT, MC, USN
Director, Medical Services
Naval Medical Center
Portsmouth, Virginia (1)

Dallas E. Peak, M.D.
Attending Physician
Department of Emergency Medicine
Methodist Hospital of Indiana
Indianapolis, Indiana (4)

Richard M. Ruddy, M.D., FAAP
Professor of Clinical Pediatrics and Emergency Medicine
University of Cincinnati College of Medicine
Director, Division of Emergency Medicine
Children's Hospital Medical Center
Cincinnati, Ohio (14)

Christopher R. Sartori, M.D.
Chief, Outpatient Dermatology
Wilford Hall Medical Center
San Antonio, Texas (13)

Daniel L. Savitt, M.D.
Attending Physician and Residency Director
Department of Emergency Medicine
Rhode Island Hospital
Assistant Professor of Medicine
Brown University
Providence, Rhode Island (11, 12)

Joseph C. Schmidt, M.D.
Chief Resident
Joint Military Medical Centers Emergency Medicine Residency
Wilford Hall Medical Center
San Antonio, Texas (16)

Charles J. Schubert, M.D., FAAP
Assistant Professor of Pediatrics
University of Cincinnati College of Medicine
Attending Physician, Division of Emergency Medicine
Children's Hospital Medical Center
Cincinnati, Ohio (14)

Robert A. Shapiro, M.D., FAAP
Associate Professor of Pediatrics
University of Cincinnati College of Medicine
Medical Director, Child Abuse Program
Attending Physician, Division of Emergency Medicine
Children's Hospital Medical Center
Cincinnati, Ohio (14)

Lawrence B. Stack, M.D., FACEP
Assistant Professor
Department of Emergency Medicine
Vanderbilt University Medical Center
Nashville, Tennessee (7, 16)

Alan B. Storrow, M.D., FACEP
Assistant Professor
Department of Emergency Medicine
University of Cincinnati Medical Center
Cincinnati, Ohio (11, 16)

Selim Suner, M.D., M.S.
Attending Physician
Department of Emergency Medicine
Rhode Island Hospital and Brown University
Providence, Rhode Island (12)

Alexander T. Trott, M.D.
Professor of Emergency Medicine
University of Cincinnati
College of Medicine
Cincinnati, Ohio (5)

Edwin Turner, M.D.
LCDR, MC, USNR
Attending Physician
Emergency Medicine Department
Naval Hospital
Great Lakes, Illinois (6)

Cathleen M. Vossler, M.D.
Resident
Department of Emergency Medicine
Rhode Island Hospital and Brown University
Providence, Rhode Island (11)

Richard E. Wyszynski, M.D.
Department of Emergency Medicine
MetroHealth Medical Center
Cleveland, Ohio (3)

Ken Zafren, M.D., FACEP, FAAEM
Alaska Regional Hospital
Anchorage, Alaska
Medical Director
Denali National Park Mountaineering Rangers and Lake Clark National Park, Alaska
Associate Medical Director (USA), Himalayan Rescue Association (16)

PHOTOGRAPHY CREDITS

Armed Forces Institute of Pathology
Bethesda, Maryland

Matthew Backer Jr., M.D.
RADM, MC, USNR (ret)
Attending Physician
Department of Obstetrics and Gynecology
Naval Medical Center
San Diego, California

Raymond C. Baker, M.D.
Professor of Pediatrics
University of Cincinnati College of Medicine
Pediatrician, Division of Pediatrics
Children's Hospital Medical Center
Cincinnati, Ohio

Judith C. Bausher, M.D.
Associate Professor of Pediatrics and Emergency Medicine
University of Cincinnati College of Medicine
Attending Physician, Division of Emergency Medicine
Children's Hospital Medical Center
Cincinnati, Ohio

Bill Beck, CRA
Clinic Photographer, Florida Eye Clinic
Altamonte Springs, FL

Frank Birinyi, M.D., FACEP
Clinical Assistant Professor of Emergency Medicine
The Ohio State University
Attending Physician
Mount Carmel Medical Center
Mount Carmel East Hospital
Columbus, Ohio

Centers for Disease Control and Prevention
Atlanta, Georgia

Richard A. Chole, M.D., PhD
Professor and Chair, Department of Otolaryngology
School of Medicine, University of California, Davis, Medical Center

Stephen Corbett, M.D.
Department of Emergency Medicine
Loma Linda University Medical Center
Loma Linda, California

Robin T. Cotton, M.D.
Professor
Department of Otolaryngology and Maxillofacial Surgery
Children's Hospital Medical Center
Cincinnati, Ohio

Richard A. Clinchy III, PhD, NREMT-P
American College of Prehospital Medicine
Ft. Walton Beach, FL

Barbara R. Craig, M.D.
CAPT, MC, USN
Medical Consultant for Child Abuse and Neglect
National Naval Medical Center
Bethesda, Maryland

Curatek Pharmaceuticals
Elk Grove Village, Illinois

Departments of Dermatology Collective Files,
Brooke Army Medical Center
Wilford Hall USAF Medical Center
San Antonio, Texas

Department of Dermatology
Naval Medical Center
Portsmouth, Virginia

Department of Medical Photography
Naval Medical Center
San Diego, California

Department of Ophthalmology
Naval Medical Center
Portsmouth, Virginia

Herbert L. DuPont, M.D.
Chief, Internal Medicine Service
St. Luke's Episcopal Hospital
Houston, Texas

Lee E. Edstrom, M.D.
Surgeon in Chief
Division of Plastic Surgery
Rhode Island Hospital
Assistant Professor of Surgery
Brown University
Providence, Rhode Island

Eric Einfalt, M.D.
LCDR, MC, USNR
Staff Physician
Emergency Medicine Department
Naval Medical Center
Jacksonville, Florida

Beverly C. Forcier, M.D.
Department of Emergency Medicine
MetroHealth Medical Center
Cleveland, Ohio

Geisinger Medical Center
Department of Emergency Medicine
Danville, Pennsylvania

Jeffrey S. Gibson, M.D.
LCDR, MC, USNR
Staff Physician
Emergency Medicine Department
Naval Medical Center
Jacksonville, Florida

Javier A. Gonzalez del Rey, M.D., FAAP
Assistant Professor of Clinical Pediatrics and Emergency Medicine
University of Cincinnati College of Medicine
Attending Physician, Division of Emergency Medicine
Children's Hospital Medical Center, Cincinnati, Ohio

Ralph A. Gruppo, M.D.
Professor of Pediatrics
University of Cincinnati College of Medicine
Director, Hemophilia Treatment Center
Children's Hospital Medical Center
Cincinnati, Ohio

H. Hunter Handsfield, M.D.
Professor of Medicine
University of Washington
Director, STD Control Program
Seattle-King County Department of Public Health
Seattle, Washington

Curtis Hunter, M.D.
Chief, Emergency Medical Services
General Leonard Wood Army Community Hospital
Fort Leonard Wood, Missouri

Liudvikas Jagminas, M.D.
Attending Physician
Department of Emergency Medicine
Rhode Island Hospital
Assistant Professor of Medicine
Brown University
Providence, Rhode Island

Edward C. Jauch, M.D. M.S.
Assistant Professor
Department of Emergency Medicine
University of Cincinnati Medical Center
Cincinnati, Ohio

Lee Kaplan, M.D.
Chief of Dermatology
VA Medical Center; San Diego, California
Associate Clinical Professor of Medicine and Dermatology
University of California, San Diego

Kevin J. Knoop, M.D., M.S., FACEP
CAPT, MC, USN
Program Director
Emergency Medicine Residency
Naval Medical Center
Portsmouth, Virginia

Paul J. Kovalchik, M.D., FACS
Colorectal Surgeon
Chesapeake, Virginia

David P. Kretzschmar, D.D.S., M.S.
Chief, Department of Oral and Maxillofacial Surgery
2nd Medical Group
Barksdale AFB, Louisiana
Assisant Professor
Department of Surgery
Louisiana State University Medical Center

Douglas R. Landry, M.D.
LCDR, MC, USNR
Emergency Medicine Department
Naval Medical Center
Portsmouth, Virginia

Louis LaVopa, M.D.
Attending Physician
Emergency Medicine Department
Naval Hospital
Agana, Guam

Lorenz F. Lassen, M.D.
CAPT, MC, USN
Assistant Professor of Otolaryngology—Head and Neck Surgery
Eastern Virginia Medical School
Director, Surgical Services
Naval Medical Center
Portsmouth, Virginia

Anne W. Lucky, M.D.
Volunteer Professor of Dermatology and Pediatrics
University of Cincinnati College of Medicine
Director, Dermatology Clinic
Children's Hospital Medical Center, Cincinnati, Ohio

C. Bruce MacDonald, M.D.
Assistant Professor, Department of Otolaryngology
Boston University School of Medicine
Boston, Massachusetts

Timothy D. McGuirk, D.O., FACEP
CDR, MC, USN
Head, Clinical Investigation and Research Department
Naval Medical Center
Portsmouth, Virginia

Patrick H. McKenna, M.D., FACS, FAAP
Assistant Clinical Professor of Urology and Pediatrics
University of Connecticut Health Center
Hartford, Connecticut

James Mensching, M.D.
LCDR, MC, USN
Attending Physician
Emergency Medicine Department
Naval Medical Center
Portsmouth, Virginia

Sherman Minton, M.D.
Professor Emeritus
Department of Microbiology and Immunology
Indiana University School of Medicine
Indianapolis, Indiana

Margaret P. Mueller, M.D.
Department of Emergency Medicine
Rhode Island Hospital and Brown University
Providence, Rhode Island

David W. Munter, M.D., FACEP
CAPT, MC, USN
Director, Medical Services
Naval Medical Center
Portsmouth, Virginia

Anthony J. Musielewicz, M.D.
Staff Physician
Naval Hospital, Guam

George L. Murrell, M.D.
LCDR, MC, USN
Department of Otolaryngology—Head and Neck Surgery
Naval Medical Center
Portsmouth, Virginia
Assistant Professor of Clinical Otolaryngology—Head and Neck Surgery
Eastern Virginia Medical School
Norfolk, Virginia

Michael J. Nowicki, M.D.
CDR, MC, USN
Division of Pediatric Gastroenterology
Department of Pediatrics
Naval Medical Center
Portsmouth, Virginia

Alan E. Oestreich, M.D.
Professor of Radiology and Pediatrics
University of Cincinnati College of Medicine
Chief, Section of Diagnostic Radiology
Staff Radiologist
Children's Hospital Medical Center
Cincinnati, Ohio

Dallas E. Peak, M.D.
Attending Physician
Methodist Hospital of Indiana
Indianapolis, Indiana

Michael P. Poirier, M.D.
Assistant Professor of Pediatrics
Eastern Virginia Medical School
Division of Pediatric Emergency Medicine
Children's Hospital of the King's Daughters
Norfolk, Virginia

Michael Redman, PA-C
Staff, Emergency Medicine
Fort Leonard Wood Army Community Hospital
Fort Leonard Wood, Missouri

Sue Rist, FNP
CAPT, NC, USN (ret)
Naval Training Center
San Diego, California

Roche Laboratories
Nutley, New Jersey

Warren K. Russell, M.D.
LCDR, MC, USNR
Head, Emergency Medicine Department
Naval Hospital
Roosevelt Roads, Puerto Rico

Katrina C. Santos, HM3, USN
Ocular Technician
Department of Ophthalmology
Naval Medical Center
Portsmouth, Virginia

Christopher R. Sartori, M.D.
Chief, Outpatient Dermatology
Wilford Hall Medical Center
San Antonio, Texas

Adam R. Saperston, M.D., M.S.
LCDR, MC, USN
Naval Medical Center
Portsmouth, Virginia

Daniel L. Savitt, M.D.
Attending Physician and Residency Director
Department of Emergency Medicine
Rhode Island Hospital
Assistant Professor of Medicine
Brown University
Providence, Rhode Island

Robert A. Shapiro, M.D.
Associate Professor of Pediatrics and Emergency Medicine
University of Cincinnati College of Medicine
Attending Physician, Division of Emergency Medicine
Children's Hospital Medical Center
Cincinnati, Ohio

Virender K. Sharman, M.D.
Fellow
Division of Digestive Disease and Nutrition
University of South Carolina School of Medicine
Columbia, South Carolina

D. J. Spalton, FRCS, MRCP
Consultant Ophthalmic Surgeon
Medical Eye Unit
St. Thomas's Hospital
London, UK

Lawrence B. Stack, M.D., FACEP
Assistant Professor
Department of Emergency Medicine
Vanderbilt University Medical Center
Nashville, Tennessee

Walter Stamm, M.D.
Professor of Medicine
Head, Infectious Diseases Division
Harborview Medical Center
Seattle, Washington

James F. Steiner, D.D.S.
Professor of Pediatrics
University of Cincinnati College of Medicine
Pediatric Dentistry
Children's Hospital Medical Center
Cincinnati, Ohio

Alan B. Storrow, M.D., FACEP
Assistant Professor
Department of Emergency Medicine
University of Cincinnati Medical Center
Cincinnati, Ohio

Selim Suner, M.D., M.S.
Attending Physician
Department of Emergency Medicine
Rhode Island Hospital and Brown University
Providence, Rhode Island

Alexander T. Trott, M.D.
Professor, Department of Emergency Medicine
University of Cincinnati College of Medicine
Cincinnati, Ohio

Edwin Turner, M.D.
LCDR, MC, USNR
Attending Physician
Emergency Medicine Department
Naval Hospital
Great Lakes, Illinois

Cathleen M. Vossler, M.D.
Resident
Department of Emergency Medicine
Rhode Island Hospital and Brown University
Providence, Rhode Island

Richard E. Wyszynski, M.D.
Department of Emergency Medicine
MetroHealth Medical Center
Cleveland, OH

The *Pocket Atlas of Emergency Medicine* was developed after the publication of the first edition of the *Atlas of Emergency Medicine.* The purpose of the *Pocket Atlas* is to provide a more compact presentation for the student, resident, and clinician.

We chose the photographs and accompanying text based on our experiences as emergency physicians and teachers. The *Pocket Atlas* does not replace the original *Atlas.* Rather, it provides the reader with a portable reference for some of the most common conditions presenting to emergency departments and urgent care centers.

As we are now preparing material for the next edition of our book, we welcome readers' comments on both the *Atlas* and the *Pocket Atlas.* It is our intention that both books evolve in response to changes in medicine and to the needs of students, residents, and practitioners.

The Editors

PART I

REGIONAL ANATOMY

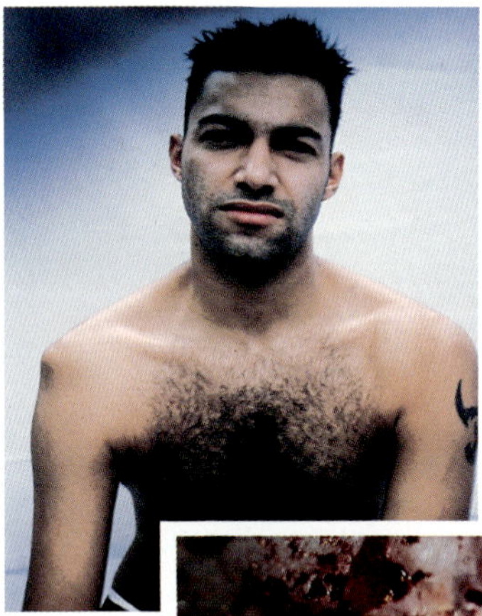

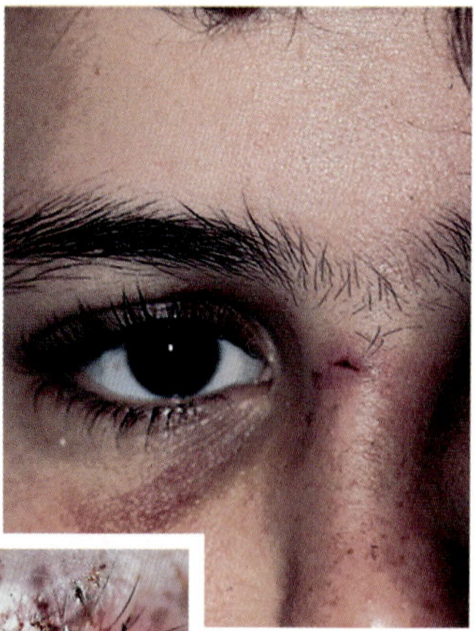

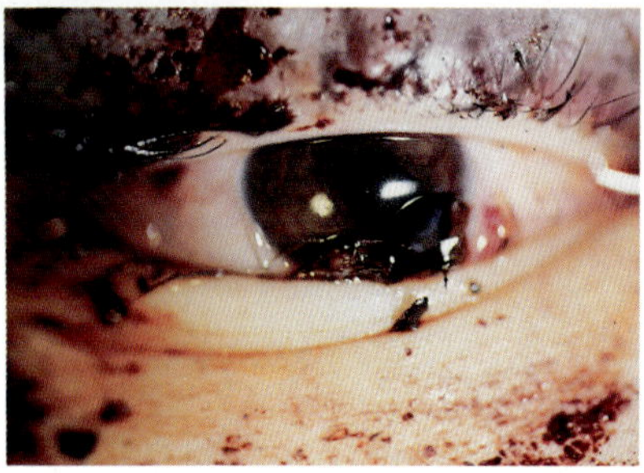

CHAPTER 1

HEAD AND FACIAL TRAUMA

David W. Munter
Timothy D. McGuirk

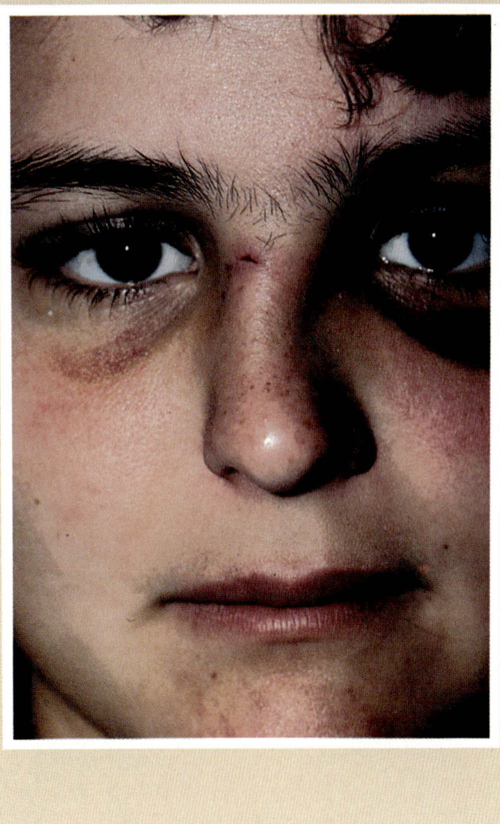

Associated Clinical Features

The skull base comprises the floors of the anterior, middle, and posterior cranial fossae. Trauma resulting in fractures to this basilar area typically do not have localizing symptoms. Plain skull radiographs are poor in identifying these fractures. Indirect signs of the injury may include visible evidence of bleeding from the fracture into surrounding soft tissue such as a Battle's sign or raccoon eyes (Figs. 1.1, 1.2). Bleeding into other structures including hemotympanum (Fig. 1.3) or blood in the sphenoid sinus seen as an air-fluid level may also be seen. Cerebrospinal fluid (CSF) leaks may also be evident and noted as clear or pink rhinorrhea. If CSF is present, a dextrose stick test may be positive. The fluid can be placed on filter paper and a "halo" or double ring may be seen (Fig. 1.4).

Differential Diagnosis

Direct trauma without skull fracture can result in external ecchymosis. Barotrauma can cause hemotympanum. Facial injuries and fractures can cause facial ecchymosis.

ED Treatment and Disposition

The mainstay of therapy is to identify underlying brain injury, which is best accomplished by CT. CT is also the best diagnostic tool for identifying the fracture site, but fractures may not always be evident. Evidence of open communication such as a CSF leak mandates neurosurgical consultation and admission. Otherwise, the decision for admission is based on the patient's clinical condition, other associated injuries, and evidence of underlying brain injury as seen on CT. The use of antibiotics in the presence of a CSF leak is controversial because of the possibility of selecting resistant organisms.

Clinical Pearls

1. The clinical manifestations of basilar skull fracture may take several hours to fully develop.
2. Since plain films are unhelpful, there should be a low threshold for head CT in any patient with head trauma, loss of consciousness, obtundation, severe headache, visual changes, or nausea or vomiting.
3. The use of filter paper or dextrose stick test to determine if CSF is present in rhinorrhea is not 100% reliable.

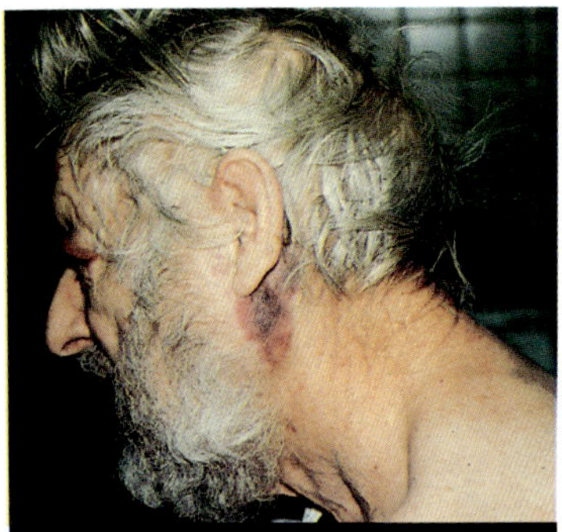

Figure 1.1
Battle's Sign

Ecchymosis in the postauricular area develops when the fracture line communicates with the mastoid air cells, resulting in blood accumulating in the cutaneous tissue. This sign may take several hours to fully develop. (Courtesy of Daniel L. Savitt, MD.)

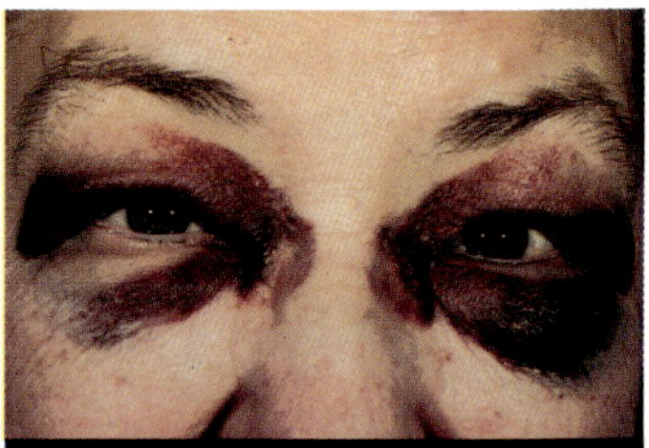

Figure 1.2
Raccoon Eyes

Ecchymosis in the periorbital area, resulting from bleeding from a fracture site in the anterior portion of the skull base. May also be caused by facial fractures. (Courtesy of Frank Birinyi, MD.)

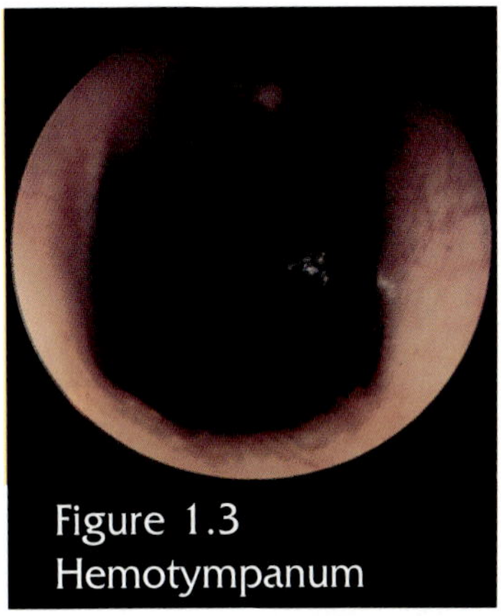

Figure 1.3
Hemotympanum

Seen in a basilar skull fracture when the fracture line communicates with the auditory canal, resulting in bleeding into the middle ear. Blood can be seen behind the tympanic membrane. (Courtesy of Richard A. Chole, MD, PhD.)

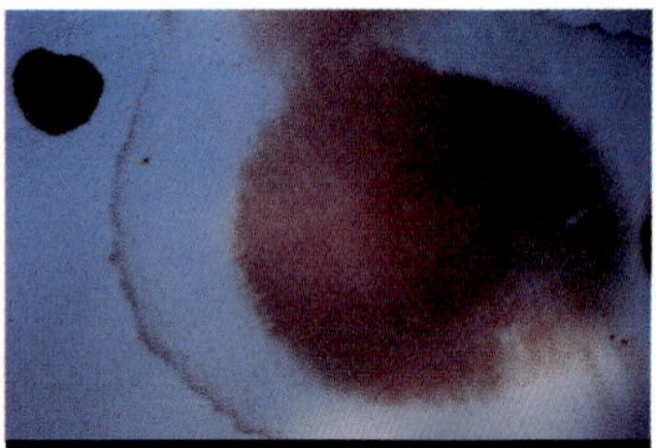

Figure 1.4 Cerebrospinal Fluid Leak

This example, from the nose, can be difficult to distinguish from blood or mucus. The distinctive double-ring sign, seen here, comprises blood (inner ring) and CSF (outer ring). The reliability of this test has been questioned. (Courtesy of David W. Munter, MD.

Associated Clinical Features

Clinically significant nasal fractures are almost always evident on examination, with deformity, swelling, and ecchymosis present (Fig. 1.5). Injuries may occur to other surrounding bony structures, including fractures of the orbit, frontal sinus, or cribriform plate. A history of a mechanism with significant force, loss of consciousness, or findings of facial bone injury or CSF leak should alert the clinician to look for these associated injuries. Epistaxis may be due to a septal or turbinate laceration, but can also be seen with fractures of surrounding bones including the cribriform plate. Septal hematoma (Fig. 1.6) is a rare but important complication that, if untreated, may result in necrosis of the septal cartilage and a resultant "saddlenose" deformity.

Differential Diagnosis

Nasal fractures may have associated facial injuries such as orbital, frontal sinus, or cribriform plate fractures, and these more serious injuries must be ruled out. A simple nasal contusion may present identically to a simple nasal fracture with pain, swelling, and ecchymosis. A frontonasoethmoid fracture has nasal or frontal crepitus and may have associated telecanthus or obstruction of the nasolacrimal duct.

ED Treatment and Disposition

Look for more serious injuries first. Patients with associated facial bone deformity or tenderness may require radiographs to rule out facial fractures. Nasal fractures rarely require radiographs (Fig. 1.7). Obvious deformities are referred within 2 to 5 days for reduction after the swelling has subsided. Nasal injuries without deformity need only conservative therapy with an analgesic and possibly a nasal decongestant. Septal hematomas must be immediately drained, with packing placed to prevent reaccumulation. In some cases, epistaxis may not be controlled by pressure alone and may require nasal packing. Lacerations overlying a simple nasal fracture should be vigorously irrigated and primarily closed with the patient placed on antibiotic coverage. Complex nasal lacerations with underlying fractures should be referred for closure. Nasal fractures with mild angulation and without displacement may be reduced in the ED by manipulating the nose with the examiner's thumbs into the correct alignment.

Clinical Pearls

1. Rule out any life threats or serious associated injuries.
2. Control epistaxis to perform a good intranasal examination. If there is no epistaxis or deformity, treat the patient with ice and analgesics. If obvious deformity is present, including a new septal deviation or deformity, treat with ice and analgesics and refer to ENT in 2 to 5 days for reduction.

3. Although the effectiveness of prophylactic antibiotics to prevent toxic shock syndrome is unproved, every patient discharged with nasal packing should be placed on antistaphylococcal antibiotics and referred to ENT in 2 to 3 days.
4. Consider cribriform plate fractures in patients with clear rhinorrhea after nasal injury, with the understanding that this finding may be delayed.
5. Check every patient for a septal hematoma.

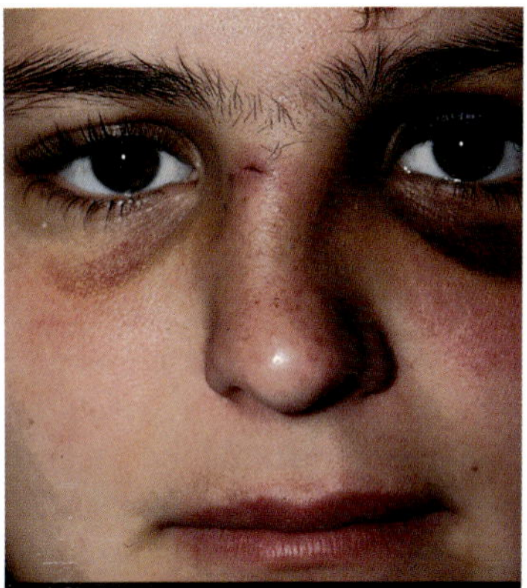

Figure 1.5
Nasal Fracture

Deformity is evident on examination. Note periocular ecchymosis indicating the possibility of other facial fractures (or injuries). The decision to obtain radiographs is based on clinical findings. A radiograph is not indicated for an isolated simple nasal fracture. (Courtesy of David W. Munter, MD.)

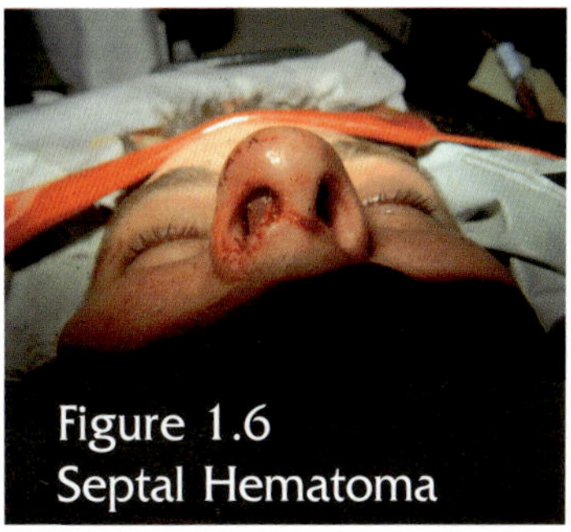

Figure 1.6
Septal Hematoma

A bluish, grapelike mass on the nasal septum. If untreated, this can result in septal necrosis and a saddle-nose deformity. An incision, drainage, and packing are indicated. (Courtesy of Lawrence B. Stack, MD.)

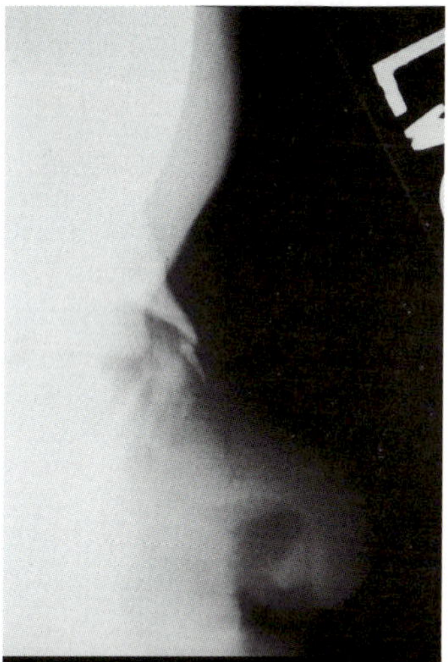

Figure 1.7
Nondisplaced Nasal Fracture

Radiograph of a fracture of the nasal spine, for which no treatment other than ice and analgesics is needed. This radiograph did not change the treatment or disposition of the patient. (Courtesy of Lorenz F. Lassen, MD.)

Associated Clinical Features

Blowout fractures occur when the globe sustains a direct blunt force. There are two mechanisms of injury. The first is a true blowout fracture where all energy is transmitted to the globe. The spherical globe is stronger than the thin orbital floor, and the force is transmitted to the thin orbital floor or medially through the ethmoid bones with the resultant fracture. The object causing the injury must be smaller than 5 to 6 cm, otherwise the globe is protected by the surrounding orbit. Fists or small balls are the typical causative agents. This mechanism of injury is more likely to cause entrapment and globe injury. The second mechanism of injury occurs when the energy from the blow is transmitted to the infraorbital rim causing a buckling of the orbital floor. Entrapment and globe injury is less likely with this mechanism of injury. Patients with blowout fractures have periorbital ecchymosis and lid edema (Figs. 1.8, 1.9), but may sustain eye injuries as well, including chemosis, subconjunctival hemorrhage, or infraorbital numbness from injury to the infraorbital nerve. Other eye injuries should be sought and ruled out with a careful physical examination and include corneal abrasion, hyphema, enophthalmos, proptosis, iridoplegia, dislocated lens, retinal tear, retinal detachment, and ruptured globe. If the inferior rectus muscle is extruded into the fracture, it may become entrapped, and upward gaze is limited with resultant diplopia (Figs. 1.10, 1.11). Due to the communication with the maxillary sinus, subcutaneous emphysema is common.

Differential Diagnosis

Orbital contusions present with similar physical findings. Orbital rim fractures are clinically similar to orbital blowout fractures. Other facial fractures (zygoma, tripod, LeFort) may involve the orbital floor, but involve more extensive injuries to the face outside of the orbit.

ED Treatment and Disposition

Plain radiography to include a Caldwell view (showing orbital rim and walls) and a Waters view (orbital floor and roof) demonstrates the fracture. Patients without eye injury or entrapment may be treated conservatively with ice and analgesics, and referred for follow-up in 2 to 3 days. Patients with blood in the maxillary sinus are usually treated with antibiotics. Strongly consider an ophthalmology consultation in patients with a true blowout fracture (all energy transmitted to the globe), since up to 30% of these patients sustain a globe injury. Patients with entrapment should receive a CT of the orbits and be referred on a same-day basis. Most specialists will observe fractures with entrapment for 10 to 14 days to allow for resolution of edema prior to operative repair.

Clinical Pearls

1. Enophthalmos, limited upward gaze, diplopia with upward gaze, or infraorbital anesthesia from entrapment or injury to the infraorbital nerve should heighten suspicion of a blowout fracture.
2. Compare the pupillary level on the affected side with the unaffected side, since it may be lower from prolapse of the orbital contents into the maxillary sinus. Subtle abnormalities may be appreciated as an asymmetric corneal light reflex (Hirschberg's reflex).
3. Subcutaneous emphysema on clinical examination, a soft-tissue teardrop along the roof of the maxillary sinus on plain film, or an air-fluid level in the maxillary sinus on plain film should also be interpreted as evidence of a blowout fracture.
4. Some patients present with unusual complaints, such as their eye swelling up after blowing their nose (from subcutaneous emphysema) or air bubbles emanating from the tear duct.
5. Carefully examine the eye for visual acuity, hyphema, or retinal detachment. Remember to assess the nose for a septal hematoma.

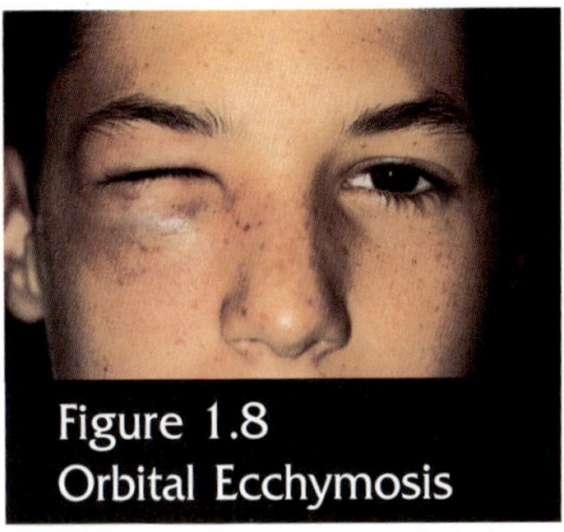

Figure 1.8
Orbital Ecchymosis

Sustained from blunt trauma to the globe, with some of the force directed to the inferior orbital rim. This patient presents with subtle signs only (ecchymosis and swelling with no entrapment or eye injury), yet has the classic signs on plain films (Figure 1.9). This patient demonstrates that orbital floor fractures can present with subtle physical findings. (Courtesy of Kevin J. Knoop, MD, MS.)

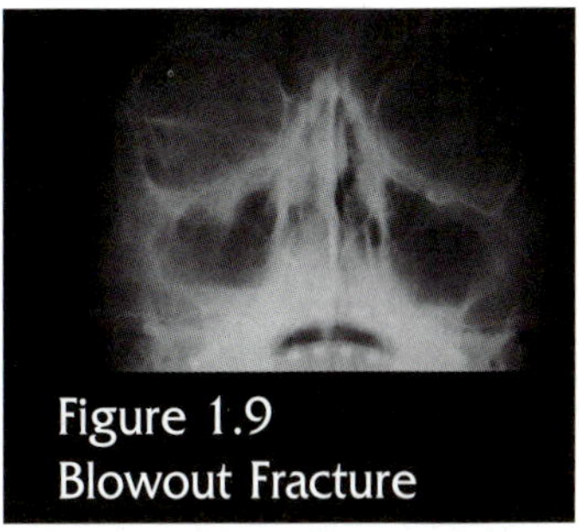

Figure 1.9
Blowout Fracture

Plain film demonstrating a fracture of the floor of the right orbit, with a teardrop sign due to extruded orbital contents. There is an associated air-fluid level in the maxillary sinus due to blood. Note the two lines seen at the inferior orbit: the infraorbital rim and inferior floor of the orbit. These are well visualized on the unaffected side, but disrupted on the affected side. (Courtesy of Kevin J. Knoop, MD, MS.)

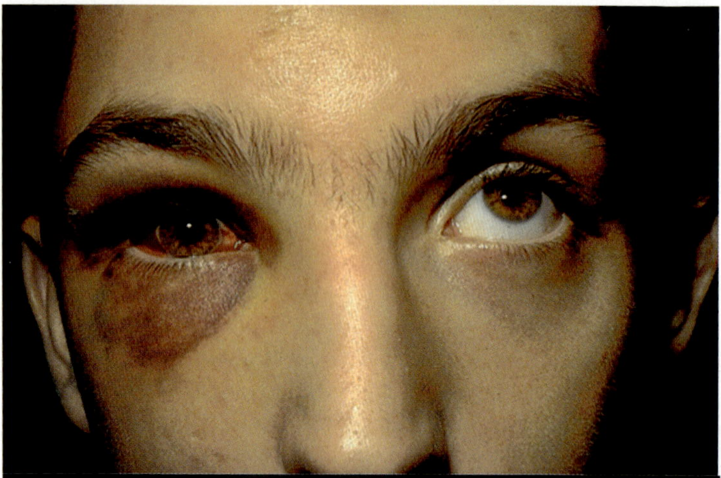

Figure 1.10 Inferior Rectus Entrapment

The inferior rectus muscle is entrapped within the blowout fracture. When the patient tries to look upward, the affected eye has limited upward gaze. The patient experiences diplopia with this maneuver. (Courtesy of Lawrence B. Stack, MD.)

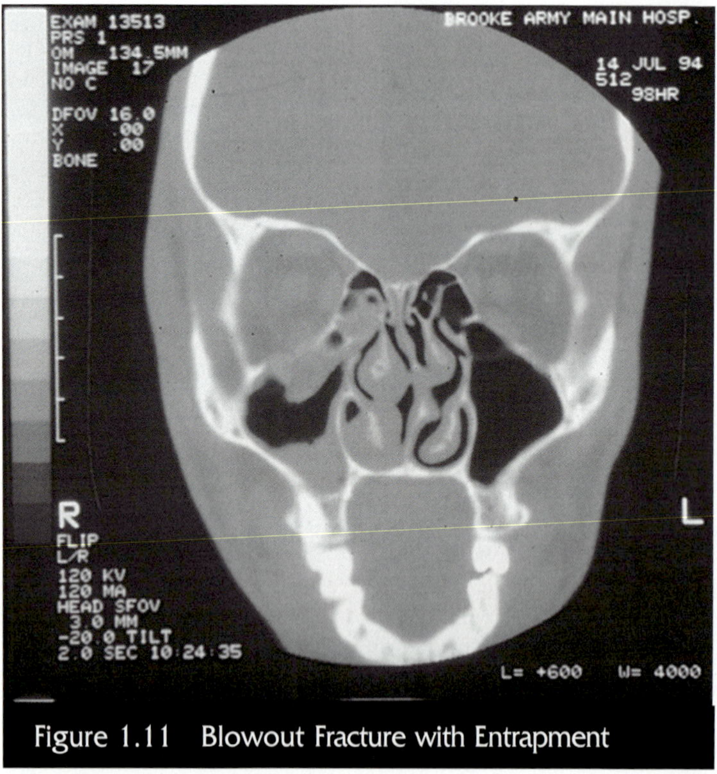

Figure 1.11 Blowout Fracture with Entrapment

CT of the patient demonstrating the entrapped muscle extruding into the maxillary sinus. (Courtesy of Lawrence B. Stack, MD.)

Associated Clinical Features

Injuries to the external ear may be open or closed. Blunt external ear trauma may cause a hematoma (otohematoma) of the pinna (Fig. 1.12), which if untreated, may result in cartilage necrosis and chronic scarring or further cartilage formation and permanent deformity ("cauliflower ear") (Fig. 1.13). Open injuries include lacerations (with and without cartilage exposure) and avulsions (Fig. 1.14).

Differential Diagnosis

These injuries are normally self-evident. Pinna hematomas and contusions can sometimes be difficult to distinguish, but flocculence is the hallmark of the hematoma.

ED Treatment and Disposition

Pinna hematomas must undergo incision and drainage or large needle aspiration using sterile technique, followed by a pressure dressing to prevent reaccumulation of the hematoma. This procedure may need to be repeated several times, hence, after emergency department drainage, the patient is treated with antistaphylococcal antibiotics and referred to ENT or plastic surgery for follow-up in 24 h. Lacerations must be carefully examined for cartilage involvement, and if present, copious irrigation, closure, and postrepair oral antibiotics covering skin flora are indicated. Simple skin lacerations may be repaired primarily with nonabsorbable 6-0 sutures. The dressing after laceration repair is just as important as the primary repair. If a compression dressing is not placed, hematoma formation can occur. Complex lacerations or avulsions normally require ENT or plastic surgery referral.

Clinical Pearls

1. Pinna hematomas may take hours to develop, so give patients with blunt ear trauma careful discharge instructions, with a follow-up in 12 to 24 h to check for hematoma development.
2. Failure to adequately drain a hematoma, reaccumulation of the hematoma owing to a faulty pressure dressing, or inadequate follow-up increases the risk of infection of the pinna (perichondritis) or of a disfiguring cauliflower ear.
3. Copiously irrigate injuries with lacerated cartilage, which are usually able to be managed by primary closure of the overlying skin. Direct closure of the cartilage is rarely necessary and is indicated only for proper alignment, which helps lessen later distortion. Use a minimal number of absorbable 5-0 or 6-0 sutures through the perichondrium.
4. Lacerations to the lateral aspect of the pinna should be minimally debrided because of the lack of tissue at this site to cover the exposed cartilage.

5. In the case of an avulsion injury, the avulsed part should be cleansed, wrapped in saline-moistened gauze, placed in a sterile container, then placed on ice to await reimplantation by ENT.

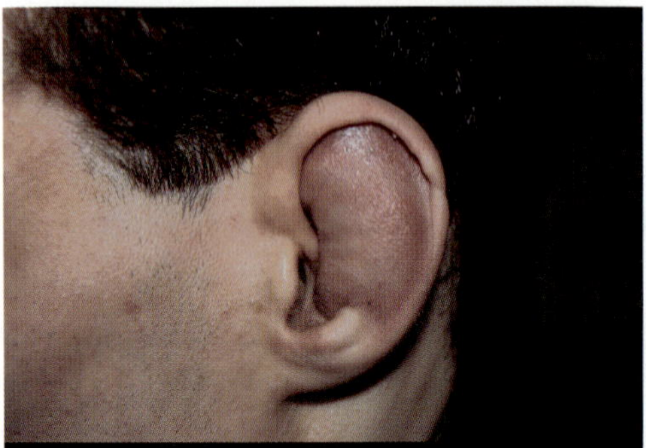

Figure 1.12 Pinna Hematoma

A hematoma has developed and is characterized by swelling, discoloration, ecchymosis, and flocculence. Immediate incision and drainage or aspiration is indicated, followed by an ear compression dressing. (Courtesy of C. Bruce MacDonald, MD.)

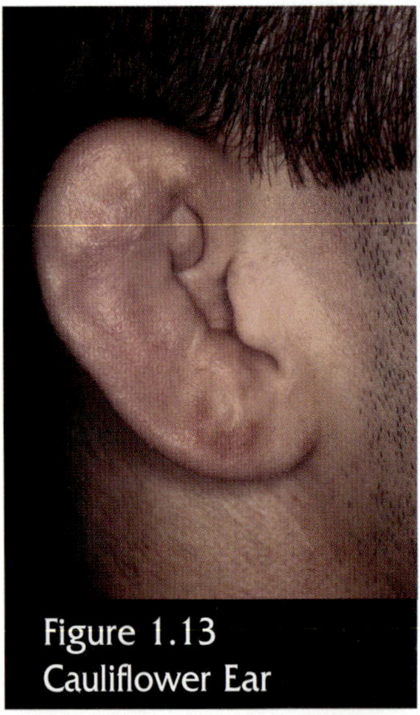

Figure 1.13
Cauliflower Ear

Repeated pinna trauma or undrained hematomas can result in cartilage necrosis and subsequent deforming scar formation. (Courtesy of Timothy D. McGuirk, DO.)

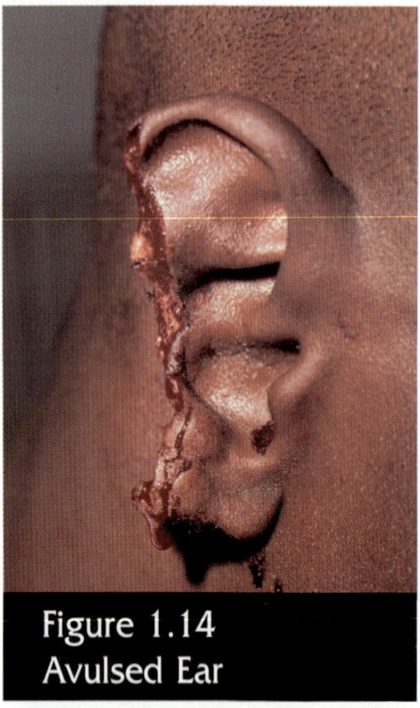

Figure 1.14
Avulsed Ear

This ear injury, sustained in a fight, resulted when the pinna was bitten off. Plastic repair is needed. Wrap the avulsed part in sterile gauze soaked with saline, and place in a sterile container on ice. (Courtesy of David W. Munter, MD.)

CHAPTER 2

OPHTHALMOLOGIC CONDITIONS

Frank Birinyi
Thomas F. Mauger

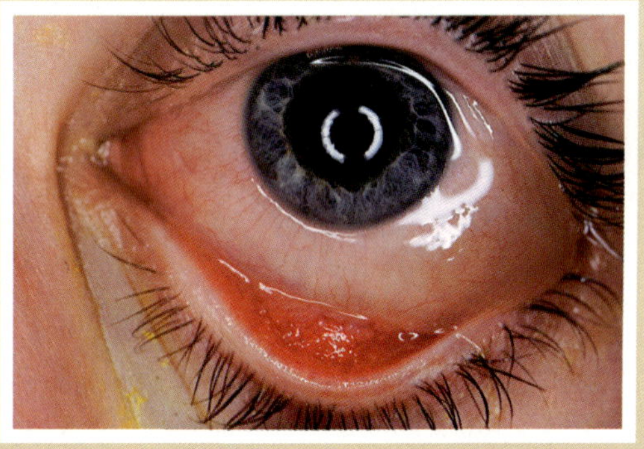

Associated Clinical Features

Bacterial conjunctivitis is characterized by the acute onset of conjunctival infection and purulent drainage. *Staphylococcus aureus* is the most common cause in adults and children. Typically symptoms begin in one eye and spread to the other. Mucopurulent discharge (Fig. 2.1) results in sticking together of the eyelids on awakening. In some cases, lid edema and erythema, chemosis, and superficial punctate keratitis may develop.

The most severe form of acute purulent conjunctivitis is associated with *Neisseria gonorrhoeae.* Neisseriae are capable of invading an intact corneal epithelium, and infection can be seen at any age. Clinically symptoms are hyperacute in onset and include marked eyelid swelling along with tenderness, marked conjunctival hyperemia, pain, chemosis, and preauricular adenopathy. The discharge is prominent, thick, copious, and purulent. Corneal findings include a diffuse epithelial haze, epithelial defects, marginal infiltrates, and peripheral ulcerative keratitis that can rapidly progress to perforation.

Neonatal conjunctivitis is discussed separately.

Differential Diagnosis

Other etiologies of conjunctivitis (viral, allergic), as well as iritis, glaucoma, scleritis, and foreign body also present as a red eye.

ED Treatment and Disposition

Treatment involves local hygiene (warm moist compresses, frequent hand washing) and broad spectrum antibiotic drops (sulfacetamide, gentamicin). One drop every 3 h for 7 to 10 days is adequate and usually results in rapid resolution. If there is no response after 48 to 72 h, cultures and ophthalmologic consultation should be considered. Cultures should also be taken in cases of severe acute (hyperacute), persistent, refractory, or chronic conjunctivitis.

The treatment of gonococcal conjunctivitis is both systemic (ceftriaxone 1 g IM) and topical (penicillin G 100,000 U/mL every 2 h or bacitracin ophthalmic ointment 500 U/g every 2 h, tapering over 48 h to five times a day). Because of the frequent coexistence of chlamydia with gonococcal infections, patients should also receive treatment for *Chlamydia* (doxycycline 100 mg twice a day for 7 to 10 days in nonpregnant patients, azithromycin 1 g orally for pregnant patients). Patients with corneal involvement should be hospitalized to receive additional IV ceftriaxone (1 g every 12 h). Sexual partners should be advised and evaluated.

Clinical Pearls

1. Worsening symptoms during topical treatment with any antibiotic, especially Neosporin or a sulfonamide (e.g., Sodium Sulamyd), may represent a contact allergic reaction.
2. *N. gonorrhoeae* conjunctivitis must be considered in the sexually active adult with a purulent eye discharge.
3. Topical corticosteroids are contraindicated for conjunctivitis treatment because a herpetic cause would be greatly exacerbated.
4. In early or mild cases of bacterial conjunctivitis, symptoms may be limited to mild conjunctival infection without frankly purulent drainage evident to the physician. Thus, empiric antibiotic therapy is warranted in most cases of conjunctivitis.

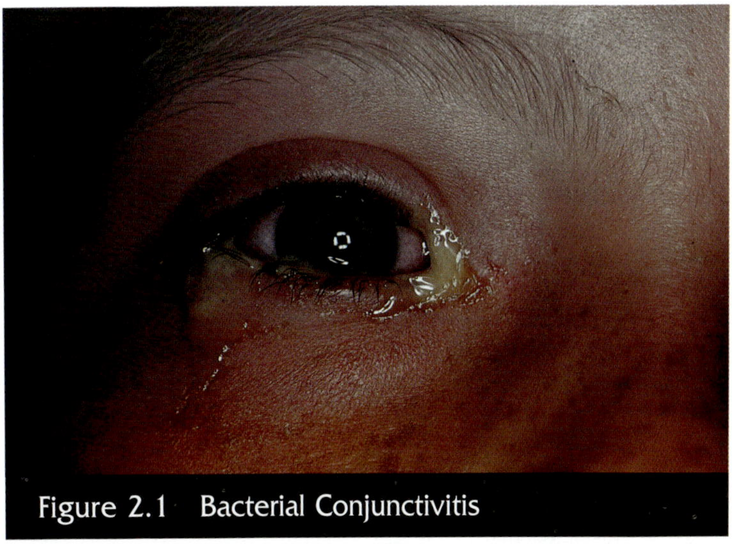

Figure 2.1 Bacterial Conjunctivitis

Mucopurulent discharge, conjunctival injection, and lid swelling, in a 10-year-old with *Haemophilus influenzae* conjunctivitis. (Courtesy of Frank Birinyi, MD.)

Associated Clinical Features

Viral conjunctivitis is a conjunctival infection caused most commonly by adenoviruses. Clinical features range in severity but usually are mild and typically include burning or irritation, conjunctival injection, lid edema, chemosis, and a thin, watery discharge. The infection usually begins in one eye; however, both eyes usually become involved because of autoinoculation (Fig. 2.2). The palpebral conjunctiva may demonstrate hyperemia and follicles. A punctate keratitis may appear several days after the onset of symptoms, followed several weeks later by subepithelial infiltrates. The visual acuity and pupillary reactivity are normal.

Pharyngoconjunctival fever, usually caused by adenovirus type 3, is highly infectious and should be considered if there is fever, upper respiratory tract infection (cold, flu, or sore throat), and preauricular adenopathy. It is seen predominantly in the young and institutionalized, with epidemics occurring in families, schools, and military camps.

Epidemic keratoconjunctivitis is discussed in the following section.

Differential Diagnosis

Similar symptoms are seen in allergic and bacterial conjunctivitis and other causes of a red eye (scleritis, glaucoma, iritis). Less common diagnoses include preseptal cellulitis and dacryoadenitis.

ED Treatment and Disposition

Many cases are self-limited and mild. Cool compresses are helpful. Meticulous hygiene (hand washing by the family and instrument cleaning by medical personnel) is necessary to prevent spread. Because the signs and symptoms of viral conjunctivitis are not always adequate in distinguishing it from bacterial conjunctivitis, antibacterial eyedrops are usually prescribed. Antivirals are ineffective against adenovirus. Symptoms may persist for several weeks, and follow-up is indicated if symptoms are not beginning to resolve in 4 to 7 days.

Clinical Pearls

1. Adenoviruses are the most common cause of acute conjunctivitis.
2. A complete eye examination is necessary to rule out other more serious causes of a red eye before the diagnosis of viral conjunctivitis is made.

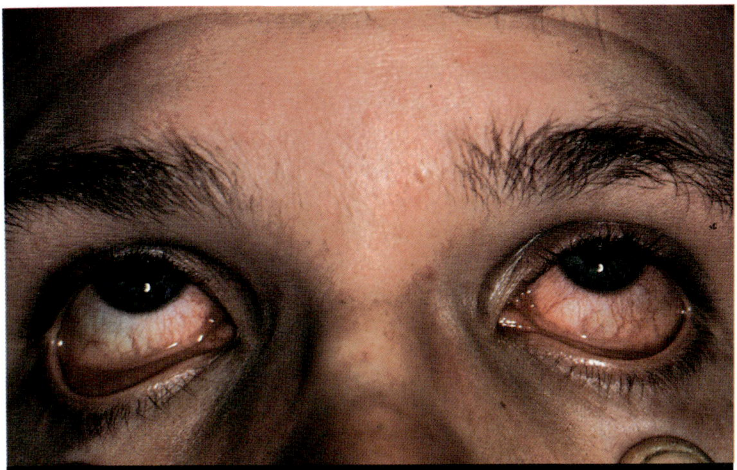

Figure 2.2 Viral Conjunctivitis

Note the classic asymmetric conjunctival injection. Symptoms first developed in the left eye, with symptoms spreading to the other eye a few days later. A thin, watery discharge is also seen. (Courtesy of Kevin J. Knoop, MD, MS.)

Associated Clinical Features

Epidemic keratoconjunctivitis (EKC) is a severe and highly contagious adenovirus infection involving the conjunctiva and cornea. Viral transmission usually occurs through direct or indirect contact with the ocular secretions of infected individuals. The incubation period after exposure is about 8 days. Initial symptoms include watery or mucopurulent discharge, foreign body sensation, and mild photophobia. Clinical findings include edema of the eyelids, chemosis, marked diffuse conjunctival hyperemia, subconjunctival hemorrhage, and a follicular and papillary conjunctival reaction (Fig. 2.3). Pseudomembranes overlying the palpebral conjunctiva and tender preauricular nodes may be present. A painful keratitis may develop (usually after 5 to 7 days) and initially appears as a fine punctate epithelial keratitis that stains with fluorescein (Figs. 2.4 and 2.5). These punctate lesions gradually coalesce to form coarse spots. Subepithelial infiltrates may develop centrally by the end of the second week. These lesions resolve and are replaced by small circular white subepithelial opacities (that do not stain with fluorescein) that may last months or even years. These are believed to result from host immune response rather than from active viral replication.

Symptoms usually begin unilaterally in young adults during the fall and winter months. Bilateral involvement may develop 4 to 5 days later, with less severe symptoms in the second eye, probably due to partial immune protection of the host. There are few to no systemic complaints. Thus in patients with systemic complaints and associated fever, upper respiratory tract infection, pharyngitis, otitis media, and diarrhea, the diagnosis is more likely to be pharyngoconjunctival fever (also caused by adenovirus).

Differential Diagnosis

Other viruses and causes of red eye (bacterial conjunctivitis, iritis, scleritis, glaucoma, herpetic infection) need to be considered.

ED Treatment and Disposition

Although EKC may be severe, the condition is self-limited and therapy is mainly palliative. Cool compresses, antipyretics, topical vasoconstrictors (Vasocon), and dark sunglasses provide symptomatic relief. Antibiotics and antivirals are ineffective. Topical broad spectrum antibiotic drops are usually prescribed, since it is difficult to distinguish viral causes from bacterial causes. In the presence of membrane formation, topical broad spectrum antibiotic ointments may be prescribed to lubricate and protect the cornea. The use of topical corticosteroids is controversial. They may have a role in those patients with marked symptoms (severe conjunctival pseudomembrane formation, severe foreign body sensation, reduced visual acuity secondary to epithelial or subepithelial keratitis). Although topical steroids do provide dramatic symptomatic relief, they have no beneficial therapeutic effect on the ultimate clinical outcome. Patients with EKC should limit their exposure to others for 2 weeks after the onset of the disease and use separate linens.

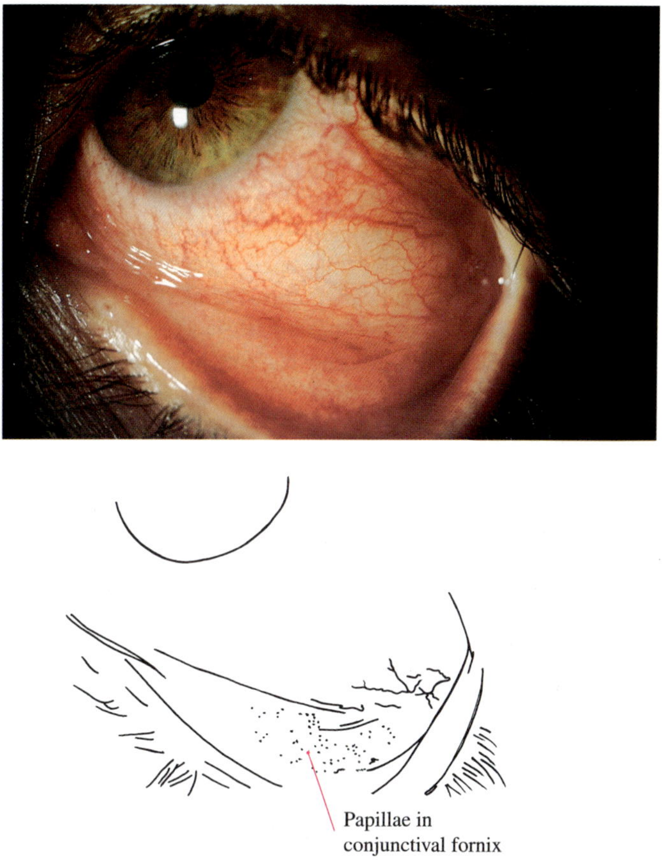

Figure 2.3 Epidemic Keratoconjunctivitis (EKC)

Diffuse injection of the bulbar conjunctiva is seen in addition to a papillary reaction of the palpebral conjunctiva—a classic finding in EKC. (Courtesy of Katrina C. Santos.)

Clinical Pearls

1. A nonspecific adenovirus conjunctivitis will resolve in 10 to 14 days; a virulent adenovirus causing EKC will peak in 5 to 7 days, and may last 3 to 4 weeks.
2. Frequent hand washing and use of separate linens is advised for patients and family members to reduce exposure.
3. Pharyngoconjunctival fever should be considered if there is an associated fever, pharyngitis, and upper respiratory tract infection.
4. EKC may be nosocomially transmitted by tonometry (the footplate of the Schiøtz tonometer, the prism of the applanation tonometer), contaminated solutions (topical anesthetics), and the physician's fingers. Regular hand washing by the physician (and patient) and careful cleaning (using alcohol or Dakin's solution) and sterilization of instruments are therefore important. Adenovirus can be recovered for extended periods of time from these surfaces.

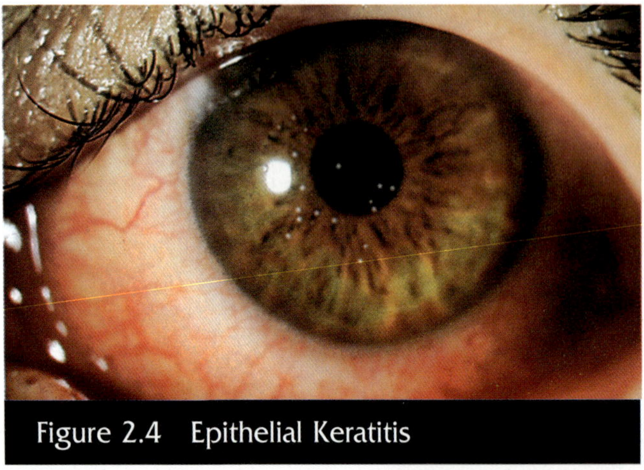

Figure 2.4 Epithelial Keratitis

This usually develops after 5 to 7 days and is seen as a fine punctate abrasion pattern over the cornea. (Courtesy of Katrina C. Santos.)

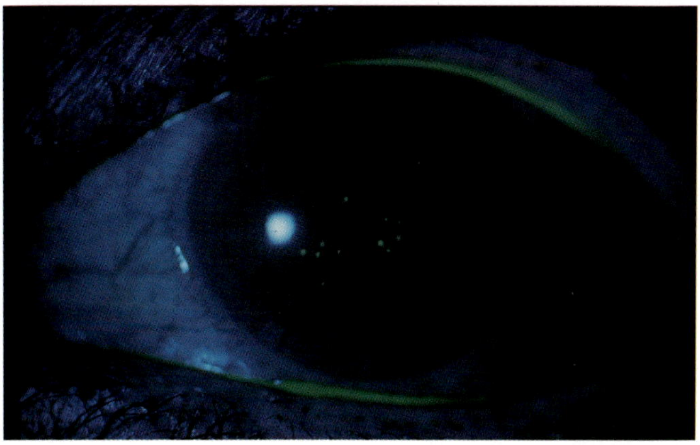

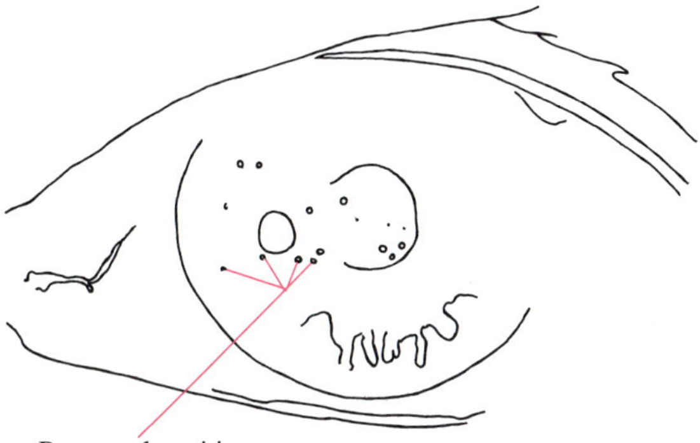

Figure 2.5 Fluorescein Stain

This demonstrates epithelial keratitis from the prior photo. (Courtesy of Katrina C. Santos.)

Associated Clinical Features

Allergic conjunctivitis is a recurrent condition whereby airborne allergens (pollen) precipitate hypersensitivity reactions in the conjunctiva. The hallmark symptom of itching is due to a host of allergens including pollens (ragweed, grasses, trees, weeds), as well as animal dander, mold, or dust. Allergic conjunctivitis is usually transient and self-limited, and is seasonal if it is due to pollens. Associated clinical features include conjunctival injection and edema, burning, discharge (clear, white, or mucopurulent), and chemosis (swelling of the bulbar conjunctiva). Chemosis may be marked. Small to medium-sized papillae or follicles may be seen on the palpebral conjunctiva (Fig. 2.6). The eyelids may be red and swollen. There may be a personal or family history of atopy, eczema, asthma, and allergic rhinitis (hay fever).

Vernal conjunctivitis is an infrequent but serious form of allergic conjunctivitis that mainly affects young males (4 to 16 years of age) during the warm months or in tropical climates. In addition to the symptoms seen in allergic conjunctivitis (intense itching, drainage that is characteristically tenacious and ropy, and mild chemosis and conjunctival injection), a diffuse papillary hypertrophy develops with giant (cobblestone) papillae over the upper tarsal plate (Fig. 2.7). Corneal findings include a sterile ulcer (well delineated with an oval or shield shape and no surrounding haze or iritis), limbal follicles (infiltrates), Horner-Trantas' dots (superficial cellular and eosinophil infiltrates that straddle the limbus and appear as raised white dots), and superficial punctate keratopathy.

Differential Diagnosis

Other etiologies of a red eye (scleritis, iritis, glaucoma, bacterial conjunctivitis) should be considered.

ED Treatment and Disposition

The initial therapy of allergic conjunctivitis should be primarily aimed at the identification of the allergen and its elimination, if possible. The severity of the allergic condition is directly proportional to the level and duration of the allergen exposure. Limiting time outdoors (to avoid pollen-bearing wind), wearing goggles or glasses outdoors, or using air conditioners with appropriate filters should be suggested to decrease airborne allergen contact.

Cool compresses are recommended four times a day, as are topical tear substitutes 4 to 8 times a day. Topical antihistamines (e.g., Levcoabastine, four times a day) are helpful. Vasoconstrictor eyedrops are indicated for moderate or severe cases. Naphcon-A (1 to 2 drops every 3 to 4 h), now available over the counter, is frequently used and contains both an antihistamine (pheniramine) and a vasoconstrictor (naphazoline). Antibacterial eyedrops are prescribed if it is difficult to distinguish the etiology of the conjunctivitis. Elective ophthalmology follow-up is appropriate.

Lodoxamine 0.1%, a mast cell stabilizer similar to cromolyn, has been shown to be effective. Topical steroids may be prescribed after consultation with an ophthalmologist in those cases when all other modalities have been explored.

In vernal conjunctivitis, additional therapeutic agents include cromolyn sodium solution 4% (1 to 2 drops every 4 to 6 h) and aspirin (650 mg four times a day orally).

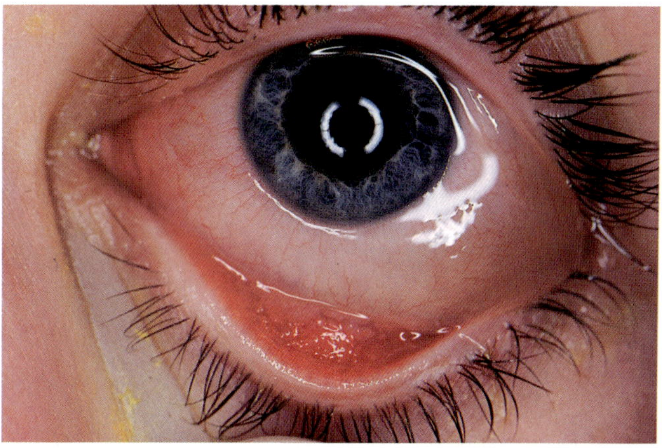

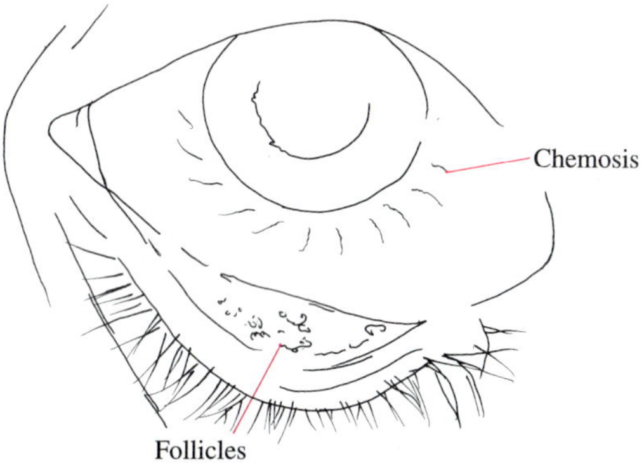

Figure 2.6 Allergic Conjunctivitis

Conjunctival injection, chemosis, and a follicular response in the inferior palpebral conjunctiva in this patient with allergic conjunctivitis secondary to cat fur. (Courtesy of Timothy D. McGuirk, DO.)

Clinical Pearls

1. Itching is the hallmark symptom of ocular allergy. Patients are usually the best source for identifying the allergen to which they are sensitive.
2. Topical corticosteroids may be used in severe cases but should not be prescribed by the ED physician without ophthalmology consultation. Complications of topical corticosteroid use include glaucoma, cataract formation, secondary infection, and corneal perforation.
3. Vernal conjunctivitis affects mainly children and adolescents and peaks in the warmer months.
4. Evert the upper lid to appreciate the large conjunctival papillae in vernal conjunctivitis. The cobblestone appearance is pathognomonic.

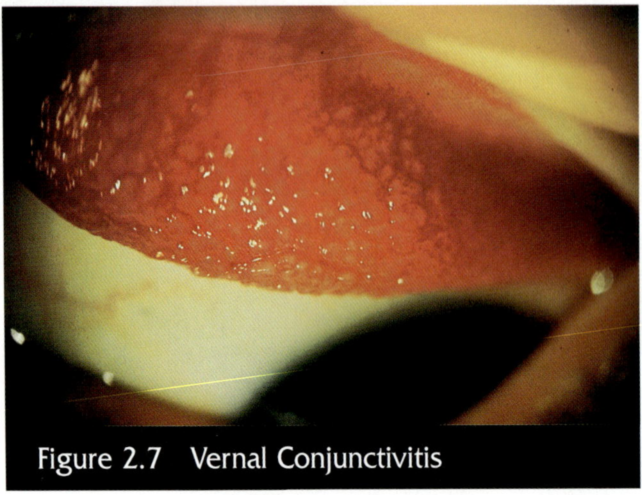

Figure 2.7 Vernal Conjunctivitis

The tarsal conjunctiva demonstrates giant papillae and a cobblestone appearance, pathognomonic for vernal conjunctivitis. (Courtesy of William Beck.)

Associated Clinical Features

A hordeolum is an acute infection and a localized abscess involving either the Meibomian glands, Zeis's glands, or Moll's glands. An internal hordeolum involves the Meibomian glands, and moderate swelling occurs. An external hordeolum (stye), involving glands of Zeis or Moll's glands, is smaller and more superficial (Fig. 2.8). A chalazion is a chronic granulomatous inflammation that develops as a foreign body reaction to sebum released into the surrounding tissue from the Meibomian glands. It may evolve from a hordeolum or may occur secondary to inspissation of sebum at the opening of the gland with subsequent gland rupture into the surrounding tissue. Chalazia are commonly seen in the ED (Fig. 2.9).

Common signs and symptoms include pain, focal swelling, erythema, and tenderness. If glands of Zeis are involved, the pathology is localized around the root of an eyelash. Focal inflammation around a chalazion may cause pointing of the lesion either anteriorly (toward the skin of the eyelid) or posteriorly (toward the tarsal conjunctiva) (Figs. 2.10 and 2.11). A chalazion may become sufficiently large as to press on the globe and cause astigmatism (corneal distortion that prevents focus). A chronic chalazion may appear as focal lid swelling without associated signs of inflammation.

There may be associated marginal blepharitis (a chronic low-grade inflammation of the lid margins with crusts around the lashes) or acne rosacea (a dermatologic condition with facial hyperemia, acneiform lesions, hypertrophy of sebaceous glands, and rhinophyma).

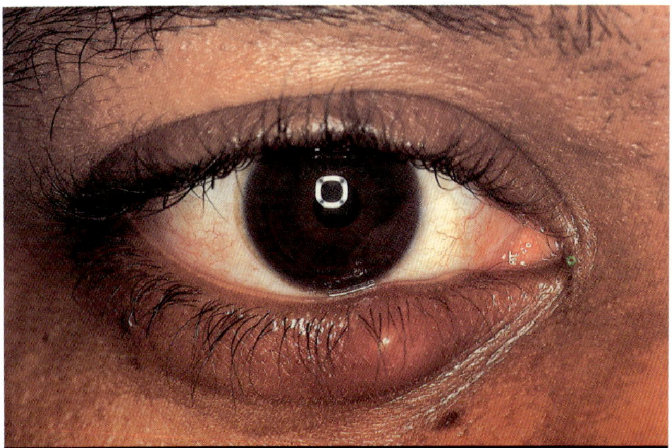

Figure 2.8 Hordeolum

Focal swelling and erythema at the lid margin are seen in this hordeolum. (Courtesy of Frank Birinyi, MD.)

Differential Diagnosis

Sebaceous cell or squamous cell carcinoma should be suspected in older patients with recurrent or persistent lesions. Preseptal cellulitis should be considered if the entire lid is erythematous and edematous. Pyogenic granuloma has a similar appearance, but it has hypertrophic tissue, a vascular core, and bleeds easily. Dacryocystitis should be considered if the lesion involves the medial aspect of the lower lid.

ED Treatment and Disposition

The process may be self-limited, with spontaneous drainage and resolution within 5 to 7 days. Warm compresses (two to four times a day for 5 to 15 min) and topical broad spectrum antibiotic ointment (bacitracin or erythromycin, every 3 h, applied to the conjunctival sac) are almost always effective. Systemic antibiotics are unnecessary unless there is a significant cellulitis. If the mass persists beyond 3 or 4 weeks, or if the lesion is sufficiently large to distort vision, referral to the ophthalmologist should be made for incision and curettage or intralesional corticosteroid injection. Gentle scrubbing of the eyelids and lashes may be indicated if marginal blepharitis is noted.

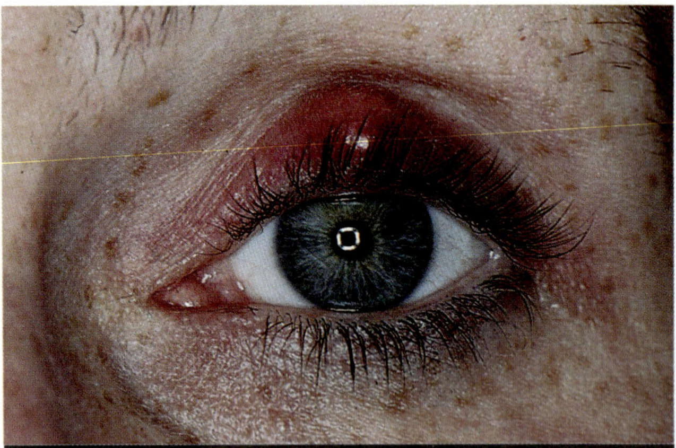

Figure 2.9 Chalazion

This chalazion shows nodular focal swelling and erythema. (Courtesy of Frank Birinyi, MD.)

Clinical Pearls

1. Excisional biopsy is indicated for recurrent chalazion to exclude malignancy.
2. *Staphylococcus aureus* is the most common bacterial pathogen.
3. Chalazia are often found in patients with marginal blepharitis, probably because the Meibomian gland orifices are blocked by the blepharitis infection.

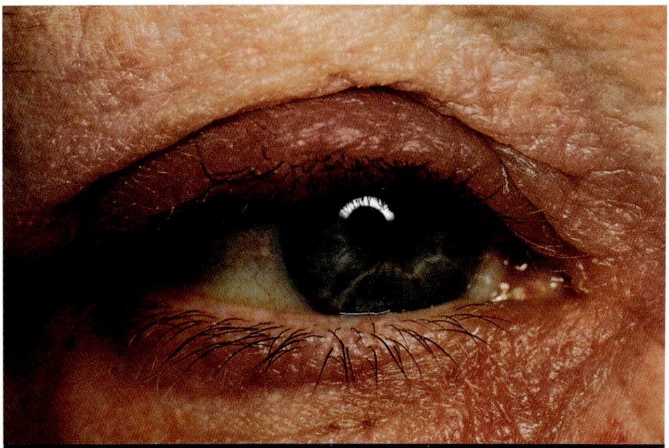

Figure 2.10 Chalazion

This chalazion is in an early stage. Lid swelling is evident with pointing of the chalazion to the inner tarsal conjunctiva. (Courtesy of Kevin J. Knoop, MD, MS.)

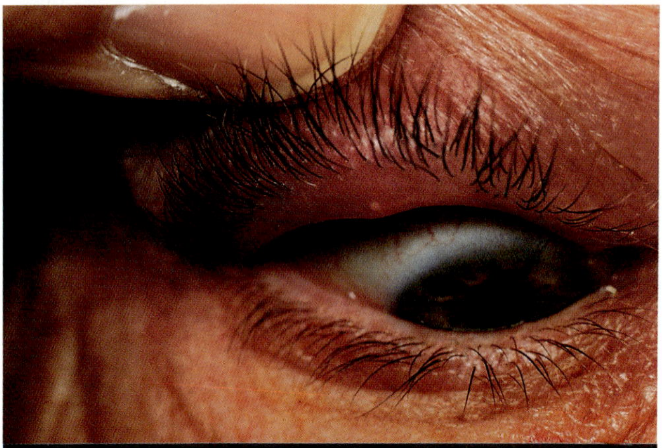

Figure 2.11 Chalazion

Pointing of the chalazion to the tarsal conjunctiva is more evident with slight lid eversion. (Courtesy of Kevin J. Knoop, MD, MS.)

Associated Clinical Features

Dacryocystitis, or inflammation of the lacrimal sac, is generally caused by a bacterial infection in the setting of an obstructed nasolacrimal duct. Hallmark findings are tearing (epiphora) and discharge. Acute dacryocystitis is associated with pain, swelling over the lacrimal sac (Fig. 2.12), and tenderness. Mucopurulent discharge may be expressed from the punctum when pressure is applied over the lacrimal sac. In adults, acute infection is due to *Staphylococcus aureus* or occasionally beta-hemolytic streptococci.

Dacryocystitis is usually seen in infants whose nasolacrimal passage remains closed (4 to 7% of newborns). In these cases, the duct normally opens spontaneously within the first month. Acute infection is uncommon in infants, but may develop secondary to *Haemophilus influenzae* and requires aggressive treatment to avoid orbital cellulitis. Organisms usually seen in chronic dacryocystitis include *Streptococcus pneumoniae* or, rarely, *Candida albicans.*

Dacryocystitis is uncommon in the intermediate age groups unless it follows chronic sinusitis, facial trauma, or (rarely) neoplasm.

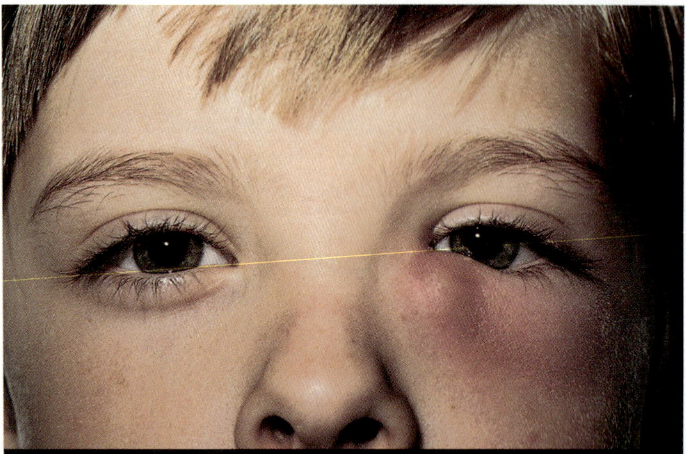

Figure 2.12 Dacryocystitis

Swelling and erythema over the medial lid and lacrimal sac developed in this 10-year-old patient with streptococcal pharyngitis. (Courtesy of Kevin J. Knoop, MD, MS.)

Differential Diagnosis

Chalazia, facial and orbital cellulitis, canaliculitis, canalicular stenosis, sinus tumors, ethmoid sinusitis, and mucoceles have similar features.

ED Treatment and Disposition

Acute dacryocystitis usually responds to oral antibiotics (amoxicillin-clavulanate), warm compresses, and gentle massage. Topical antibiotics may be used in chronic cases. Nonurgent ophthalmology or otolaryngology referral is required for definitive treatment—relief of the obstruction by dacryocystorhinostomy. In febrile and acutely ill cases of acute dacryocystitis, IV antibiotics (cefuroxime) are indicated.

In infants with chronic dacryocystitis, both topical and oral antibiotics may be used. Referral is indicated if signs do not regress by 6 to 9 months of age or if acute dacryocystitis develops.

Clinical Pearls

1. The swelling is localized to the extreme nasal aspect of the lower lid and is usually unilateral.
2. The diagnosis of acute dacryocystitis may be confirmed by pressure on the lacrimal sac and the expression of purulent material from the punctum. (The lacrimal sac and lacrimal fossa are situated in the inferior medial aspect of the orbit, not on the side of the nose.)
3. The incidence follows a bimodal distribution. Dacryocystitis usually occurs in infants or persons over 40 years of age.

Associated Clinical Features

A pinguecula (Latin, *pingueculus* meaning "fatty") is a degenerative lesion of the bulbar conjunctiva. It appears as a yellow-white amorphous subepithelial nodule adjacent to the limbus, usually nasally (Fig. 2.13). A pinguecula is usually asymptomatic. It may become episodically inflamed, gradually enlarge over time, or become a pterygium.

A pterygium is a benign proliferation of fibrovascular tissue within the bulbar conjunctiva that extends onto the peripheral cornea. Typically a pterygium assumes a triangular configuration with the apex of the lesion directed toward the pupil (Fig. 2.14). Growth occurs from this apex onto the limbal cornea. Pterygia are often preceded by pingueculae. Risk factors are exposure to ultraviolet light (sunlight), wind, and dust. Pterygia are more commonly bilateral and, like pingueculae, the nasal portion of the conjunctiva is more commonly involved than the temporal portion. Pterygia may be asymptomatic or become inflamed. They give rise to mild symptoms of irritation and foreign body sensation. Decreased visual acuity may develop if the visual axis is involved or the lesion induces astigmatism (irregular corneal curvature resulting in refractive error).

Differential Diagnosis

A pseudopterygium, a scar in the bulbar conjunctiva extending onto the cornea secondary to previous ocular inflammation (chemical burn, trauma, infection) may also have a similar appearance. Episcleritis, corneal ulcer, and conjunctival neoplasm should be considered in the differential diagnosis.

ED Treatment and Disposition

A patient with mild disease can be treated with artificial tears or a topical vasoconstrictor (naphazoline). In more severe cases, topical steroids may be prescribed after consultation. Nonemergent referral to an ophthalmologist is appropriate. Excision of a pinguecula (or pterygium) is indicated if the lesion interferes with contact lens wear, becomes chronically inflamed, or constitutes a cosmetic problem. Pterygia are excised if they cause persistent discomfort, encroach significantly on the cornea to involve the visual axis, or restrict extraocular muscle movement.

Clinical Pearls

1. Pterygia are a particular problem in sunny, hot, and dusty regions. Eye protection (goggles, sunglasses) helps to reduce the irritation.
2. Pterygia and pingueculae are usually found on the nasal conjunctiva, adjacent to the limbus. They are usually bilateral and always in the horizontal meridian.

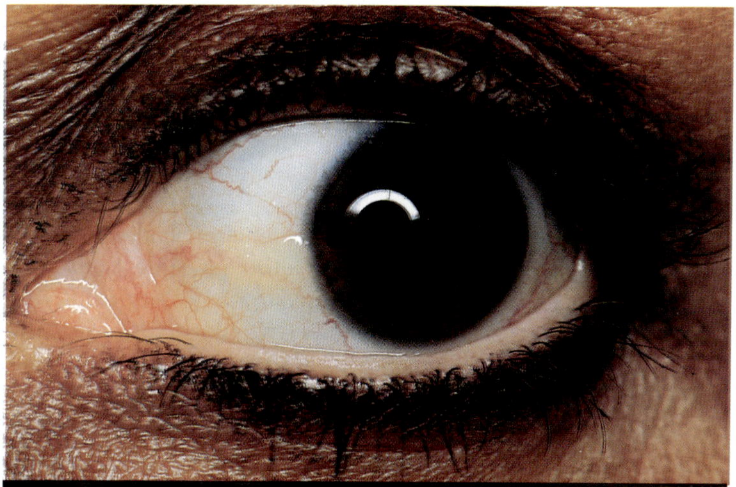

Figure 2.13 Pinguecula

A small area of yellowish "heaped up" conjunctival tissue is seen adjacent to the limbus on the nasal aspect. (Courtesy of Kevin J. Knoop, MD, MS.)

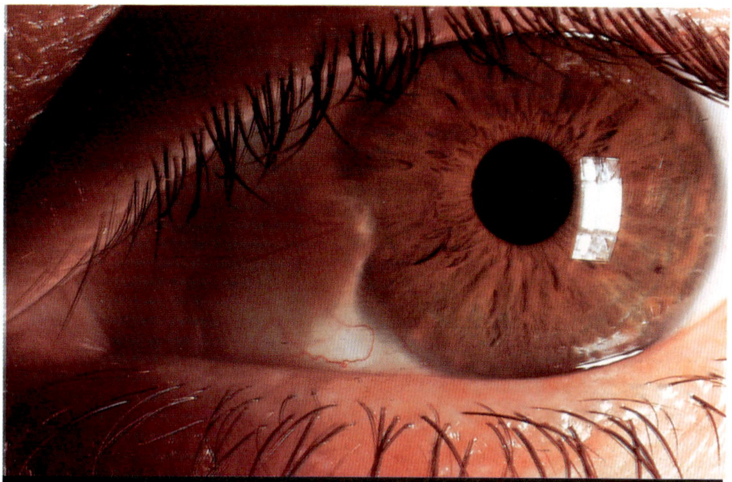

Figure 2.14 Pterygium

This pterygium appears as a raised vascular triangular area of bulbar conjunctiva that encroaches on the cornea. (Courtesy of the Department of Ophthalmology, Naval Medical Center, Portsmouth, VA.)

Associated Clinical Features

Herpes zoster ophthalmicus develops secondary to activation of latent varicella zoster virus within the trigeminal ganglion. Neuronal spread of the virus through the ophthalmic division of the trigeminal nerve results in crops of grouped vesicles in a dermatomal distribution (Fig. 2.15).

Herpes zoster keratitis is a common ophthalmic complication of herpes zoster ophthalmicus infection, although almost any ophthalmic abnormality in both anterior and posterior segments may be seen with herpes zoster ophthalmicus. Conjunctivitis, keratitis, and iritis are common. Common corneal lesions include a punctate epithelial keratitis (fine or coarse superficial defects), anterior stromal infiltrates, neurotrophic keratitis, and dendriform (pseudodendritic) keratitis. Pseudodendrites form from mucous deposition, are usually peripherally located, and stain only moderately with fluorescein. They may be differentiated from the dendrites of herpes simplex infection in that the pseudodendrites lack the rounded terminal bulbs at the end of the branches, and are broader and more plaquelike; when they are wiped from the cornea, an intact epithelium remains, unlike the epithelial defect seen with herpes simplex.

Corneal anesthesia or hypoesthesia is a frequent complication of herpes zoster keratitis. The majority, however, recover normal sensitivity within 2 to 3 months. With neurotrophic keratitis, however, corneal anesthesia is permanent.

Differential Diagnosis

Herpes simplex keratitis may similarly present with rash, red eye, and dendriform keratitis. Ocular complications of herpes zoster ophthalmicus may follow the rash by many months to years; they have a highly variable presentation that mimics almost any disease in the anterior pole of the eye.

ED Treatment and Disposition

Mild punctate epithelial keratitis and dendriform keratitis are self-limited and clear within a few days. For moderate or severe disease, however, debridement, warm compresses, lubricants (artificial tears), and topical broad spectrum antibiotics (to prevent secondary infection) may be recommended. Oral famciclovir (500 mg three times a day for 7 days) or acyclovir (800 mg five times a day for 10 days), if given within 72 h of onset, may ameliorate the course of the disease and the keratitis. (The effect on post-herpetic neuralgia is controversial.) Topical antivirals are generally not useful for herpes zoster. However, in those cases in which the diagnosis is not secure, it is probably advisable to add topical antivirals (trifluridine, 1%, 1 drop q 2 hrs. while awake) to assure coverage of herpes simplex. Cycloplegics (cyclopentolate) are used if an iritis is present. An ophthalmology consult is necessary.

The use of systemic steroids has been shown to reduce the incidence and severity of keratitis. Its effect on post-herpetic neuralgia is unclear. The use of oral steroids must be weighed against the risks, including systemic dissemination of the varicella zoster virus. Topical steroids have been shown to be effective in those cases with stromal infiltrates, since the infiltrates probably represent an immune response to soluble viral antigen.

Nonnarcotic and narcotic analgesics may be prescribed.

Clinical Pearls

1. A careful eye examination with corneal staining should be performed in patients with herpes zoster ophthalmicus to rule out corneal involvement.
2. Patients with skin lesions on the nose (Hutchinson's sign) are at higher risk for ocular involvement with herpes zoster since the sensory innervation to both the eye and the side of the tip of the nose is supplied by the nasociliary branch of the first division of the fifth cranial nerve. However, the eye may be involved without nasal involvement.
3. Corneal hypoesthesia and the appearance of dendrites with fluorescein staining are seen in both herpes zoster ophthalmicus and herpes simplex keratitis.
4. The severity of the cutaneous disease does not necessarily correlate with the severity of the ocular disease.
5. The prognosis is good and recurrences, unlike herpes simplex keratitis, are rare.

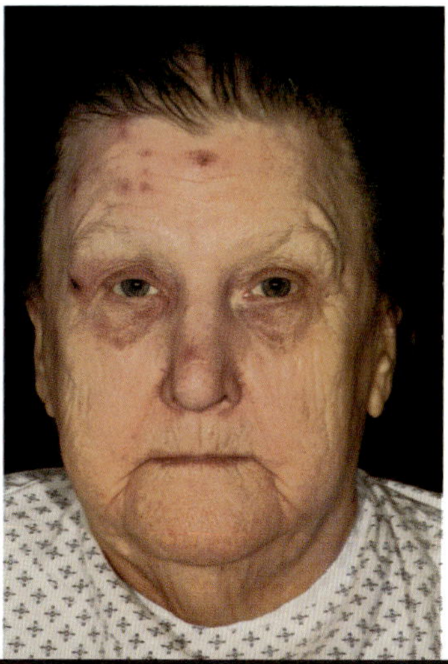

Figure 2.15 Herpes Zoster Ophthalmicus

A healing, vesicular rash in the distribution of the ophthalmic division (V1) of the trigeminal nerve is present in this 72-year-old diabetic patient. The presence of the lesion on the tip of the nose (Hutchinson's sign) increases the risk of ocular involvement. (Courtesy of Frank Birinyi, MD.)

Associated Clinical Features

A corneal ulcer is an inflammatory and ulcerative condition involving the cornea. Similar terms include infectious keratitis, bacterial keratitis, and ulcerative keratitis. Common etiologies include bacteria (*Staphylococcus, Streptococcus, Pseudomonas*) and viruses (herpes simplex). Keratitis secondary to herpes simplex is discussed separately. Corneal ulcers are commonly associated with extended wear soft contact lenses, whereby a minor corneal abrasion permits bacteria to penetrate the cornea. Infections secondary to fungi (*Aspergillus, Candida*) and protozoa (*Acanthamoeba*) are rare. However fungal infection should be suspected in cases of ocular trauma involving vegetable matter (a tree branch), chronic corneal disease (herpes keratitis), or cases involving steroid use. Contaminated contact lens solutions may contain bacteria or *Acanthamoeba.*

Symptoms associated with corneal ulcer include pain, photophobia, decreased vision, discharge, and a foreign body sensation. The ulcer appears as a corneal stromal infiltrate associated with conjunctival hyperemia (Fig. 2.16), a miotic pupil, chemosis, lid edema, and lid erythema. Slit-lamp biomicroscopy demonstrates an epithelial defect with fluorescein uptake. Findings in the anterior chamber include cells (inflammatory cells that appear as dust in a sunbeam) and flare (light scatter seen secondary to cells and proteins), keratic precipitates (inflammatory cells that have coalesced and adhered to the cornea), and hypopyon (a layer of white blood cells in the inferior or dependent portion of the anterior chamber).

Differential Diagnosis

Other possibilities include a sterile ulcer, residual corneal foreign body, rust ring, and sterile corneal infiltrate (secondary to an immune reaction to contact lens, solution, or *Staphylococcus*). Other causes of a red eye (conjunctivitis, glaucoma, scleritis) should also be considered.

ED Treatment and Disposition

Corneal ulcers should be treated as an ophthalmologic emergency and assumed to be bacterial until proved otherwise. An emergent ophthalmology consult is indicated, and stains and cultures should be obtained as expeditiously as possible before antibiotic treatment has commenced. Intensive topical treatment is the most effective route to treat corneal infections. Topical fluoroquinolone antibiotics (ciprofloxacin) may be given hourly. Fortified (concentrated) cefazolin and gentamicin may be used in combination, every 30 to 60 min. Subconjunctival injections of antibiotics (every 12 to 24 h) are used in very severe cases. Systemic antibiotics are not usually used except in cases in which the organism may have extended to the sclera (*Pseudomonas*) or if there is a high risk of concurrent systemic disease (*Neisseria, Haemophilus*). Cycloplegics are usually recommended for the accompanying iritis. Epithelial debridement may be beneficial. Steroids and an eye patch are contraindicated in the initial management. A contact lens wearer must discontinue contact lens wear.

Clinical Pearls

1. A bacterial corneal infection must be treated as an ophthalmologic emergency.
2. Corneal injury, including recent contact lens procedures, is a risk factor for the development of a corneal ulcer.
3. *Pseudomonas aeruginosa* is capable of destroying the cornea within 6 to 12 h. It should be suspected by its aggressive course, thick yellow-green or blue-green mucopurulent tenacious exudate, and ground-glass edema surrounding the ulcer.
4. *Acanthamoeba,* a ubiquitous protozoa, should be suspected in contact lens wearers with contaminated lens solutions or who swim wearing their contact lens. These patients characteristically have pain out of proportion to their clinical findings.
5. Infectious ulcers tend to develop centrally, away from the vascular supply (and immune system) of the limbus. A hypopyon is usually sterile, except in fungal ulcers.

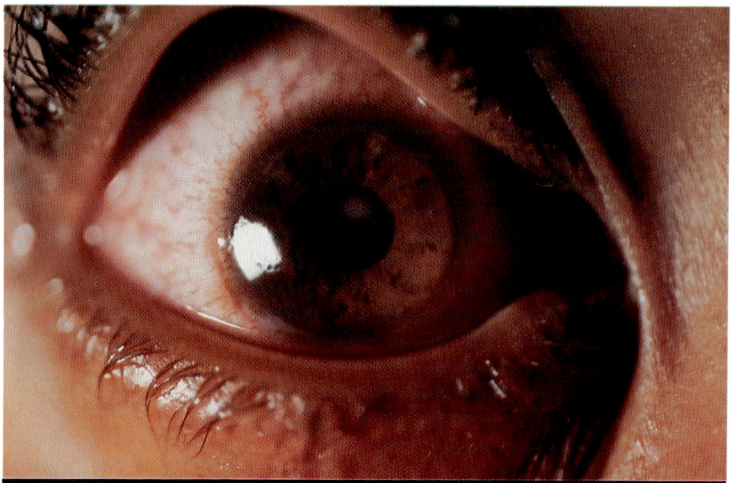

Figure 2.16 Corneal Ulcer

A circular corneal infiltrate is seen at 12 o'clock; conjunctival hyperemia is present. (A rectangular flash reflection is seen at 9 o'clock.) A mild limbal flush is noted superiorly. (Courtesy of Lawrence B. Stack, MD.)

Associated Clinical Features

Anisocoria is unequal pupil size. In room lighting the normal diameter of pupils is 3 to 5 mm. Pupil size is larger in childhood and smaller with age. Anisocoria of 1 to 2 mm may be a normal finding and is found in 5 to 20% of normal individuals. With normal (physiologic) anisocoria, the pupil size disparity is the same in light as in dark. In addition the pupils react normally to light and accommodation, are perfectly round, and no ptosis is present.

Differential Diagnosis

Associated redness, pain, or neurologic symptoms (ptosis, limited eye movements, abnormal reactivity) suggest that the anisocoria is secondary to underlying pathology. The most serious causes of anisocoria are neurogenic. In the setting of trauma, severe headache, or following intracranial surgery, anisocoria and a third-nerve palsy with ptosis and extraocular muscle palsies are early signs of an aneurysm or an expanding supratentorial mass with tentorial herniation.

In pathologic anisocoria, it may be difficult to ascertain which is the abnormal pupil. In this situation, pupil sizes in light and dark should be compared. Anisocoria that is greater in the dark suggests that the smaller pupil is abnormal; anisocoria that is greater in the light suggests that the larger is the abnormal pupil. Anisocoria with an abnormal small pupil may be secondary to Horner's syndrome, a long-standing Adie's pupil, iritis, or eyedrops (pilocarpine). Horner's syndrome causes ptosis and pupil miosis secondary to interruption of sympathetic fibers to the pupil. An Adie's pupil is initially dilated, but may become smaller than the unaffected pupil over time; etiologies of an Adie's pupil include orbit trauma, infection, zoster, diabetes, autonomic neuropathies, and Guillain-Barré syndrome. Anisocoria with an abnormal large pupil may be seen with an early Adie's pupil, ocular trauma (with iris sphincter damage) (Fig. 2.17), eyedrops (atropine, phenylephrine), or inadvertent contamination from a scopolamine patch.

ED Treatment and Disposition

The evaluation of anisocoria in the ED is dependent on the clinical presentation. A patient with the acute onset of anisocoria with an altered mental status or severe headache should be aggressively evaluated and treated as a neurosurgical emergency. A patient with long-standing anisocoria, on the other hand, may be discharged to follow-up with an ophthalmologist.

Pilocarpine may be helpful to the ED physician to differentiate nontraumatic causes of anisocoria where one pupil is abnormally dilated, for example, Adie's pupil, third-nerve palsy, or pharmacologic dilation. With low concentrations of pilocarpine (0.125%), an Adie's pupil will constrict significantly more than the unaffected pupil. With higher concentrations (1%), constriction occurs in those patients with third-nerve palsy but not with pharmacologic dilation.

Clinical Pearls

1. Compare pupil sizes in light and dark. In physiologic or normal anisocoria, the pupil size disparity is the same in light as in dark. Anisocoria that is greater in the dark suggests that the smaller pupil is abnormal; anisocoria greater in the light suggests that the larger pupil is abnormal.
2. An old photograph or driver's license viewed with an ophthalmoscope may be helpful to document the prior existence of anisocoria.
3. Some brands of eye makeup contain belladonna alkaloids, which can cause mydriasis.

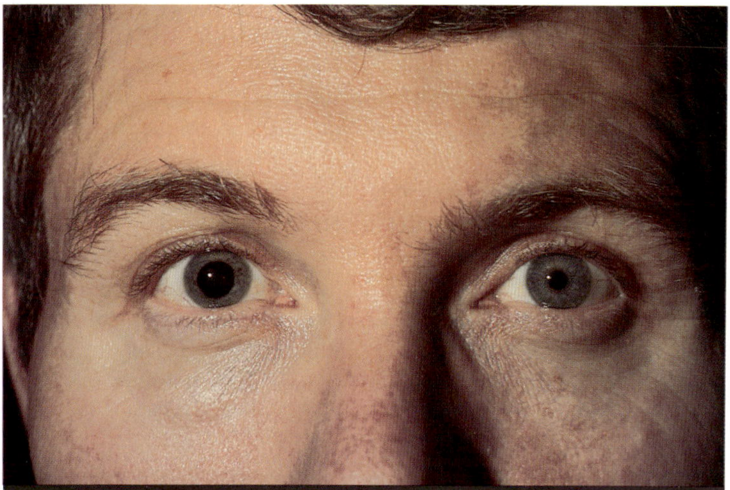

Figure 2.17 Normal Anisocoria

Marked chronic anisocoria secondary to prior trauma. (Courtesy of Kevin J. Knoop, MD, MS.)

Associated Clinical Features

An afferent pupillary defect (APD), also called a Marcus Gunn pupil, is indicative of a defect in the anterior visual pathway (retina, optic nerve, chiasm). It is best appreciated by the swinging flashlight test which discloses differences in afferent stimuli between the two eyes (Fig. 2.18). To perform this, a flashlight is directed onto one pupil and then the other. The critical observation to be made when evaluating the pupillary response is the initial response of the pupils when stimulated with light. The normal pupillary response to bright light is an initial constriction followed by a small amount of dilation. Normally the brief interval required to move the light from one eye to the other permits the pupils to begin to dilate. Under normal circumstances, when the light reaches the second eye, both pupils then initially constrict. In the abnormal situation, however, should the pupils instead dilate, the second pupil is said to have APD (Fig. 2.19). This positive finding indicates asymmetric function of the anterior visual pathway, that is, the eye with an APD perceives less light.

The swinging flashlight test is a useful screening technique and one of the most important assessments to make on the patient who complains of decreased vision. The test helps to differentiate whether the decreased vision is due to a media problem (cataract) or is due to optic nerve dysfunction. Although sensitive, the swinging flashlight test is not specific. Pathology may be anywhere anterior to the optic chiasm. Although a large retinal lesion may produce an APD, a positive finding almost always indicates a lesion in the optic nerve on the affected side.

In patients with an APD, associated findings might include decreased visual acuity and decreased visual fields. Funduscopic findings occasionally demonstrate the basis for the APD. These include a central retinal vein or artery occlusion, optic nerve pallor, optic nerve cupping, or severe vitreal hemorrhage.

An APD in the absence of gross ocular disease indicates a neurologic lesion in the anterior visual pathway. A Marcus Gunn pupil is best seen in conditions involving the optic nerve such as ischemic optic neuropathy, optic neuritis (including that seen with multiple sclerosis), retrobulbar optic neuritis, tumor, and glaucoma. Other conditions associated with an APD include central retinal artery or vein occlusion and a lesion of the optic chiasm or tract. Mild APD may be seen with vitreous hemorrhage, macular degeneration, retinal detachment, or other retinal disease. Small opacities do not produce an APD.

Differential Diagnosis

An Adie's pupil, seen predominately in young women, is unilaterally dilated. The reaction to light, both direct and consensual, is diminished or absent. An Argyll Robertson pupil (seen in neurosyphilis) is usually bilateral and miotic, and does not respond to light stimulation, but it does accommodate.

ED Treatment and Disposition

The finding of APD is nonspecific. A neurologic evaluation (history, physical examination, and CT scan) is important to assess for treatable conditions. In the absence of gross ocular or neurologic disease, a clinically stable patient may be discharged from the ED with ophthalmology follow-up.

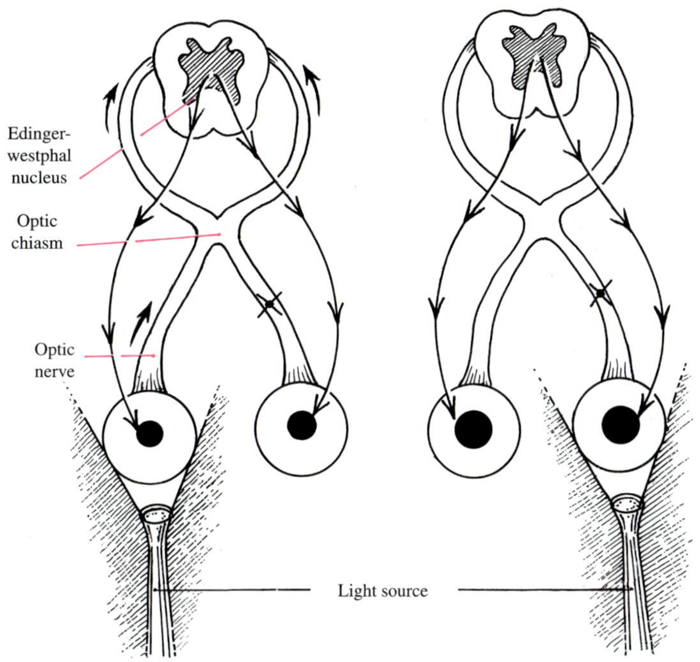

Figure 2.18 Afferent Pupillary Defect

Schematic representation of an afferent pupillary defect (APD) due to neurologic lesion in the anterior visual pathway.

Clinical Pearls

1. Ocular opacities such as a cataract do not result in APD. A dense vitreous hemorrhage, however, is capable of producing a mild defect.
2. Dim room illumination may be helpful when performing the swinging flashlight test. The patient should focus on an object 15 ft away to avoid the pupil constriction normally seen with accommodation.
3. The normal pupil response to bright light is an initial constriction followed by a small amount of dilation. In performing the swinging flashlight test, it is important to assess the initial reaction seen. In the APD, this initial reaction is dilation.
4. In the swinging flashlight test, *both* pupils will dilate when the flashlight moves from the normal eye to the affected eye, since pupil size is centrally mediated (midbrain).

5. If the affected eye is additionally damaged or paralyzed, an APD can still be assessed by observing the response of the normal pupil with light shined alternatively in each eye. That is, the swinging flashlight test is performed as before, but the physician maintains attention on the normal eye. As the light shines in the affected eye, the *normal* eye dilates due to the consensual response of the affected eye, which perceives less light than the normal eye.

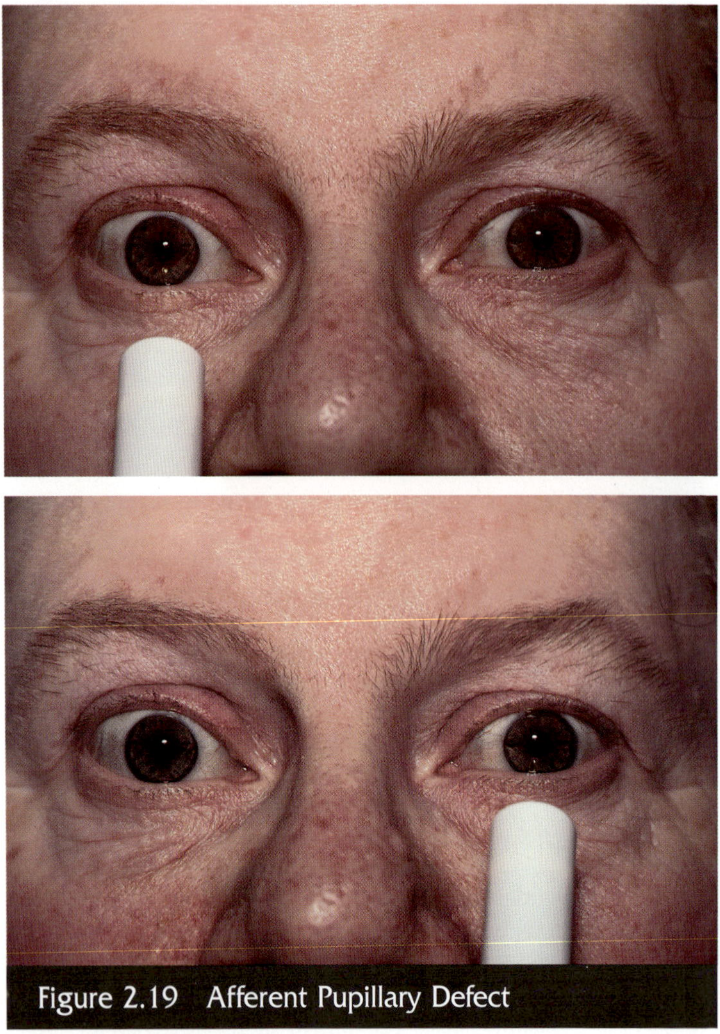

Figure 2.19 Afferent Pupillary Defect

These photographs demonstrate an APD of the left pupil. When the light shines in the affected left eye, the pupils are less constricted compared with when the light shines in the right eye. Thus, when swinging the light from the right pupil to the left, the pupils appear to dilate. The anisocoria here is subtle. (Courtesy of Frank Birinyi, MD.)

CHAPTER 3

FUNDUSCOPIC FINDINGS

David Effron
Beverly C. Forcier
Richard E. Wyszynski

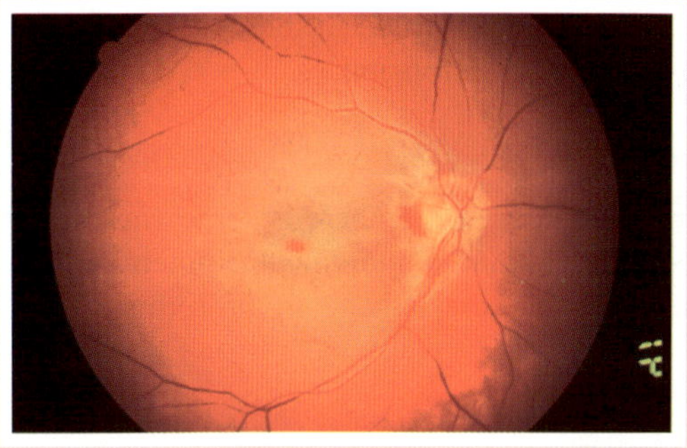

Associated Clinical Features

Disk

The disk is pale pink, approximately 1.5 mm in diameter, with sharp, flat margins (Fig. 3.1). The physiologic cup is located within the disk and usually measures less than six-tenths the disk diameter. The cups should be approximately equal in both eyes.

Vessels

The central retinal artery and central retinal vein travel within the optic nerve, branching near the surface into the inferior and superior branches of arterioles and venules, respectively. Normally the walls of the vessels are not visible; the column of blood within the walls is visualized. The venules are seen as branching, dark red lines. The arterioles are seen as bright red branching lines, approximately two-thirds or three-fourths the diameter of the venules.

Macula

An area of the retina located temporal to the disk; it is void of capillaries. The fovea is an area of depression, approximately 1.5 mm in diameter (similar to the optic disk) in the center of the macula. The foveola is a tiny pit located in the center of the fovea. These areas correspond to central vision.

Background

The background fundus is red; there is some variation in the color, depending on the amount of individual pigmentation and the visibility of the choroidal vessels beneath the retina.

Clinical Pearls

1. Fundal examination should be an integral part of any eye examination.
2. The cup/disk ratio is slightly larger in the African-American population.
3. The normal fundus should be void of any hemorrhages, exudates, or tortuous vasculature.

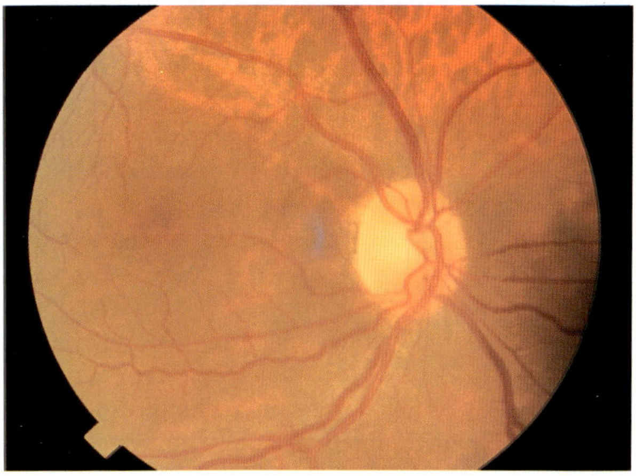

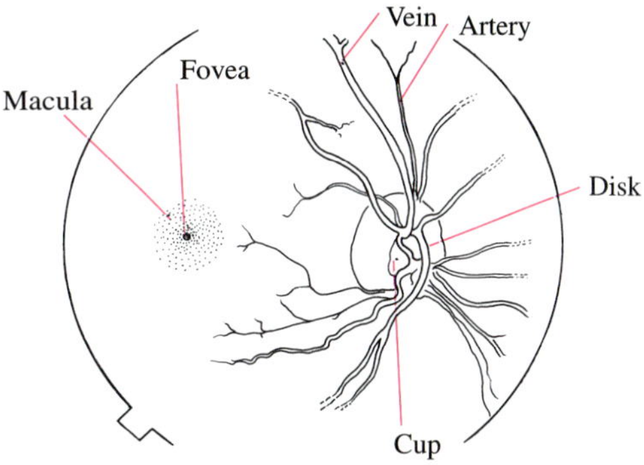

Figure 3.1 Normal Fundus

The disk has sharp margins and is normal color with a small central cup. Arterioles and venules have normal color, sheen, and course. Background is normal color. The macula is enclosed by arching temporal vessels. The fovea is located by a central pit. (Courtesy of Beverly C. Forcier, MD.)

Associated Clinical Features

Age-related macular degeneration, the leading cause of blindness in the elderly, increases in incidence with each decade over 50. Degeneration of the macula may be evidenced by accumulation of either drusen (small, discrete, round, punctate nodules), or soft drusen (larger, pale yellow or gray without discrete margins that may be confluent) (Fig. 3.2A and B). Most patients with drusen have good vision, although there may be decreased visual acuity and distortion of vision. There may be associated pigmentary changes and atrophy of the retina. Vision may slowly deteriorate if atrophy occurs.

Patients with early or late degenerative changes of their macula are at risk of developing subretinal neovascularization (SRNV), which is associated with distortion of vision, blind spots, and decreased visual acuity. Macular appearance may show dirty gray lesions, hemorrhage, retinal elevation, and exudation.

Differential Diagnosis

Hereditary macular degenerations, other acquired macular disorders, including toxicities, and retinal exudation may present similarly.

Hemorrhages and exudates can present from vascular disease, ocular disorders such as inflammations or infections, tumors, trauma, and hereditary disorders.

ED Treatment and Disposition

Patients with drusen need ophthalmologic evaluation every 6 to 12 months, or sooner if visual distortion or decreasing visual acuity develops. If a patient complains of deterioration of visual acuity or image distortion, prompt ophthalmic evaluation is warranted, probably including fluorescein angiography. If SRNV is present, laser treatment may be indicated.

Clinical Pearls

1. Age-related macular degeneration is the leading cause of blindness in the United States in patients older than 65 years of age.
2. Patient may have normal peripheral vision.
3. Untreated SRNV can lead to visual loss within a few days.
4. Patients frequently complain of distortion with SRNV.

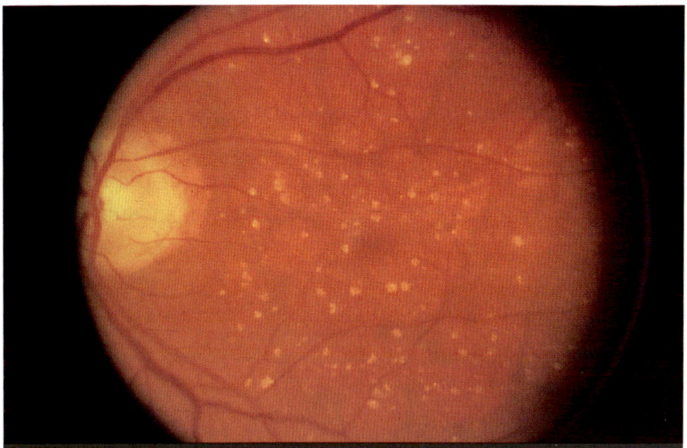

Figure 3.2A Age-Related Macular Degeneration, Drusen

Typical macular drusen and retinal pigment epithelial (RPE) atrophy (scalloped pigment loss) in age-related macular degeneration. (Courtesy of Richard E. Wyszynski, MD.)

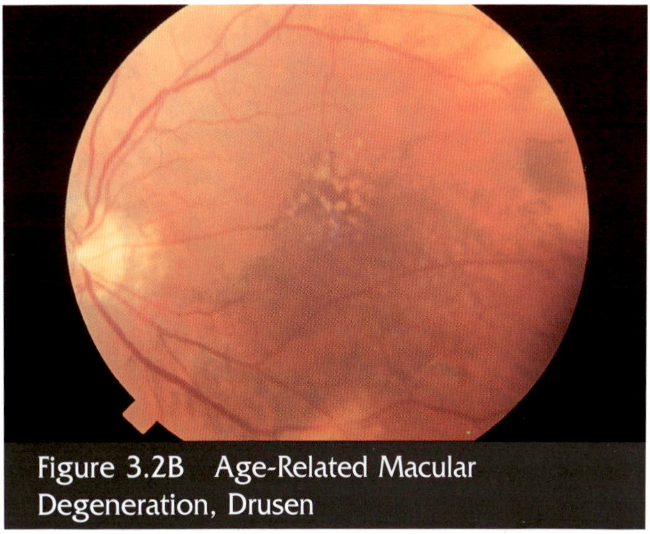

Figure 3.2B Age-Related Macular Degeneration, Drusen

Drusen are clustered in the center of the macula. (Courtesy of Richard E. Wyszynski, MD.)

Associated Clinical Features

Hard exudates (Figure 3.3*A*) are refractile, yellowish deposits with sharp margins composed of fat-laden macrophages and serum lipids. Occasionally the lipid deposits form a partial or complete ring (called a circinate ring) around the leaking area of pathology. If the lipid leakage is located near the fovea, a spoke, or star-type distribution of the hard exudates is seen.

Cotton wool spots, or soft "exudates," are actually microinfarctions of the retinal nerve-fiber layer, and appear white with soft or fuzzy edges (Fig. 3.3*B*).

Inflammatory exudates are secondary to retinal or chorioretinal inflammation.

Differential Diagnosis

Hard exudation and cotton wool spots are associated with vascular diseases such as diabetes mellitus, hypertension, and collagen vascular diseases, but can be seen with papilledema and other ocular conditions. Inflammatory exudates are seen in patients with such diseases as sarcoidosis and toxoplasmosis.

ED Treatment and Disposition

Routine referral for ophthalmologic and medical workup is appropriate.

Clinical Pearls

1. Hard exudates which are intraretinal may easily be confused with drusen that occur near Bruch's membrane, which separates the retina from the choroid.

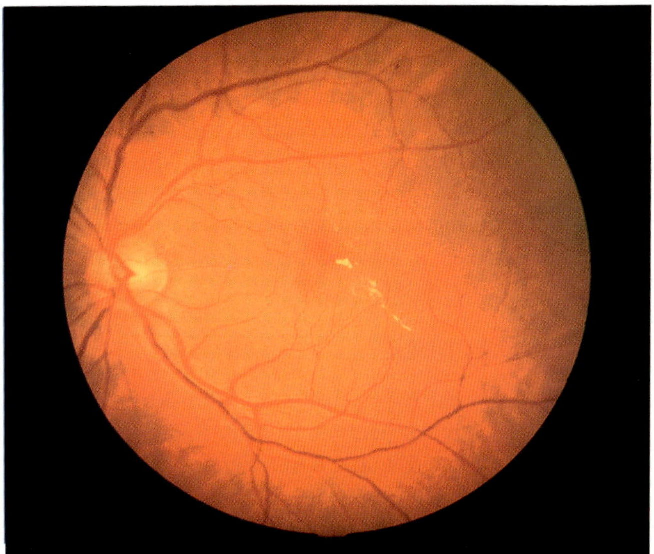

Figure 3.3A Hard Exudates

Linear collection of yellow lipid deposits with sharp margins in macula. (Courtesy of Beverly C. Forcier, MD.)

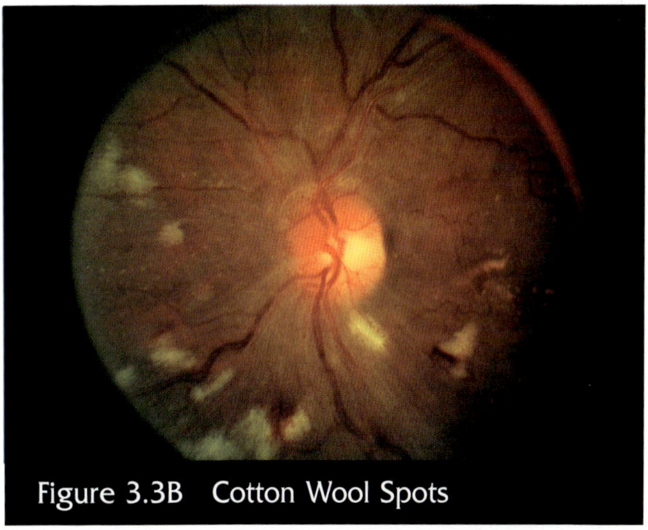

Figure 3.3B Cotton Wool Spots

White lesions with fuzzy margins, seen here approximately one-fifth to one-fourth disk diameter in size. Orientation of cotton wool spots generally follows the curvilinear arrangement of the nerve fiber layer. Intraretinal hemorrhages and intraretinal vascular abnormalities are also present. (Courtesy of Richard E. Wyszynski, MD.)

Associated Clinical Features

The typical patient experiences a sudden, painless monocular loss of vision, either segmental or complete. Visual acuity may range from finger counting or light perception to complete blindness. Fundal findings include these: most of the fundus is pale due to retinal edema; the fovea does not have the edema, and thus appears as a cherry red spot; the retinal arterioles are narrow and irregular; the retinal venules have a "boxcar" appearance (Fig. 3.4).

Differential Diagnosis

Arteriosclerosis, arterial hypertension, carotid artery disease, diabetes mellitus, and valvular heart disease are the most common systemic disorders associated with CRAO. Other associated disorders include vascular disorders, trauma, and coagulopathies. Temporal arteritis may present with similar visual complaints.

ED Treatment and Disposition

Attempts to restore retinal blood flow may be beneficial if performed in a very narrow time window after the acute event. This may be accomplished by (1) decreasing intraocular pressure with topical beta-blocker eyedrops or intravenous acetazolamide; (2) ocular massage, applied with cyclic pressure on the globe for 10 s, followed by release, then repeated. Urgent consultation with an ophthalmologist if the CRAO is less than a few hours old is indicated to determine if more aggressive acute therapy (paracentesis) is warranted. However, such aggressive treatment rarely alters the poor prognosis. Medical evaluation and treatment of associated findings may be warranted.

Clinical Pearls

1. History should focus on how long ago the episode occurred. If the loss of vision occurred recently, then the patient should be triaged and examined quickly so as to consult an ophthalmologist within the treatment window.
2. Sudden painless monocular vision loss is typical.
3. CRAO may be associated with temporal arteritis. This diagnosis should be strongly considered in all patients presenting with signs and symptoms of CRAO who are older than 55 years.

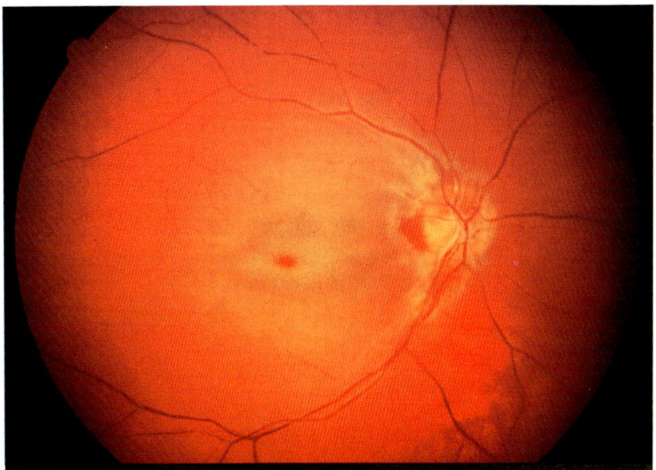

Figure 3.4 Central Retinal Artery Occlusion

The retinal pallor due to retinal edema is well demonstrated contrasting with the "cherry red spot" of the nonedematous fovea. Note the vascular narrowing and the "boxcar" appearance of the venules. (Courtesy of Richard E. Wyszynski, MD.)

Associated Clinical Features

Patients are usually older individuals and complain of sudden, painless visual loss in one eye. The vision loss is usually not as severe as CRAO and may vary from normal to hand motion. Funduscopy in a classic, ischemic CRVO shows a "blood and thunder" fundus: hemorrhages (including flame, dot or blot, preretinal, and vitreous) and dilation and tortuosity of the venous system. The arterial system often shows narrowing. The disk margin may be blurred. Cotton wool spots and edema may be seen (Fig. 3.5).

Differential Diagnosis

Retinal detachment, papilledema, and central retinal artery occlusion can have a similar appearance.

ED Treatment and Disposition

Treatment is rarely effective in preventing or reversing the damage done by the occlusion and is directed toward systemic evaluation to identify and treat contributing factors, hopefully decreasing the chance of contralateral CRVO. Ophthalmologic evaluation is necessary to confirm the diagnosis, estimate the amount of ischemia, and follow the patient so as to minimize sequelae of possible complications such as neovascularization and neovascular glaucoma.

Clinical Pearls

1. Sudden painless visual loss in one eye should be evaluated promptly to determine its etiology.
2. Look for the classic "blood and thunder" funduscopic findings.
3. Consider the differential diagnosis of acute *painful* (glaucoma, retrobulbar neuritis) versus *painless* vision loss (central retinal artery occlusion, anterior ischemic optic neuropathy, retinal detachment, subretinal neovascularization, and vitreous hemorrhage).

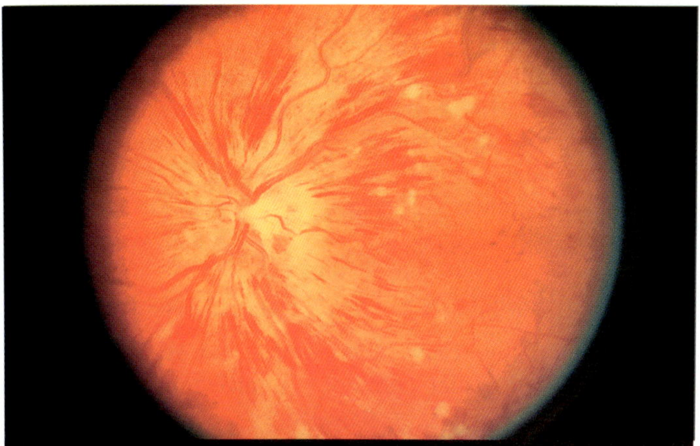

Figure 3.5 Central Retinal Vein Occlusion

The amount of hemorrhage is the most striking feature in this photograph. Also note the blurred disk margin, the dilation and tortuosity of the venules, and the cotton wool spots. Retinal edema is suggested by blurring of the retinal details. (Courtesy of Department of Ophthamology, Naval Medical Center, Portsmouth, VA.)

Associated Clinical Features

Fundus changes that may be seen with hypertension include generalized and focal narrowing of arterioles, generalized arteriolar sclerosis (copper or silver wiring), arteriovenous crossing changes, hemorrhages (usually flame-shaped), retinal edema and exudation, cotton wool spots, microaneurysms, and disk edema (Fig. 3.6).

Differential Diagnosis

Diabetic retinopathy, many hemopoietic and vascular diseases, traumas, localized ocular pathology, papilledema should all be considered.

ED Treatment and Disposition

Medical treatment of hypertension.

Clinical Pearls

1. Hypertensive arteriolar findings may be reversible if organic changes have not occurred in the vessel walls.
2. Always consider hypertensive retinopathy in the differential diagnosis of papilledema.

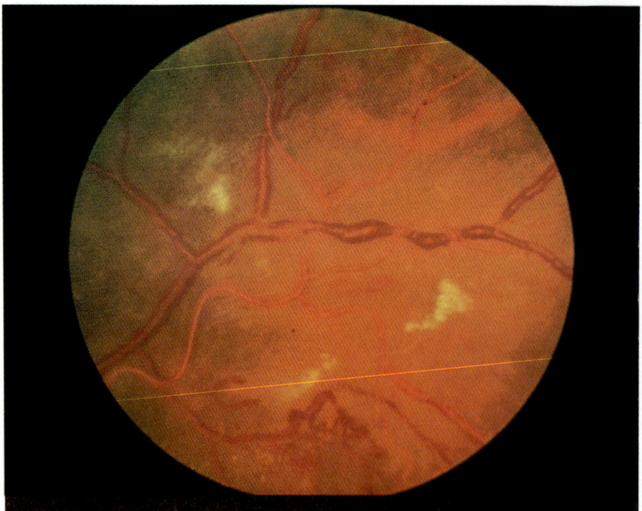

Figure 3.6 Hypertension

Chronic, severe systemic hypertensive changes are demonstrated by hard exudates, increased vessel light reflexes, and sausage-shaped veins. (Courtesy of Richard E. Wyszynski, MD.)

Associated Clinical Features

The early ocular manifestations of diabetes mellitus are referred to as background diabetic retinopathy (BDR). Fundus findings include flame or splinter hemorrhages (located in superficial nerve fiber layer) or dot and blot hemorrhages (located deeper in the retina), hard exudates, retinal edema, and microaneurysms (Fig. 3.7A and B). If these signs are located in the macula, the patient's visual acuity may be decreased or at risk of becoming compromised, requiring laser treatment. Preproliferative diabetic retinopathy can show BDR changes plus cotton wool spots, intraretinal microvascular abnormalities, and venous beading. Proliferative diabetic retinopathy is demonstrated by neovascularization at the disk (NVD) or elsewhere (NVE) (Fig. 3.7C). These require laser therapy owing to risk of severe visual loss from sequelae: vitreous hemorrhage, tractional retinal detachment, severe glaucoma.

Differential Diagnosis

Many vascular and hemopoietic diseases, such as collagen vascular disease, sickle cell trait, hypertension, hypotension, anemia, leukemia, inflammatory and infectious states, and ocular conditions can be associated with some of or all the above signs.

ED Treatment and Disposition

Routine ophthalmologic referral for laser or surgical treatment is indicated.

Clinical Pearls

1. Periodic ophthalmologic evaluations are recommended.
2. Microaneurysms typically appear 10 years after the initial onset of diabetes, although they may appear earlier in patients with juvenile diabetes.
3. Control of blood sugar alone does not prevent the development of vasculopathy.
4. Blurred vision can also occur from acute increases in serum glucose, causing lens swelling and a refractive shift even in the absence of retinopathy.

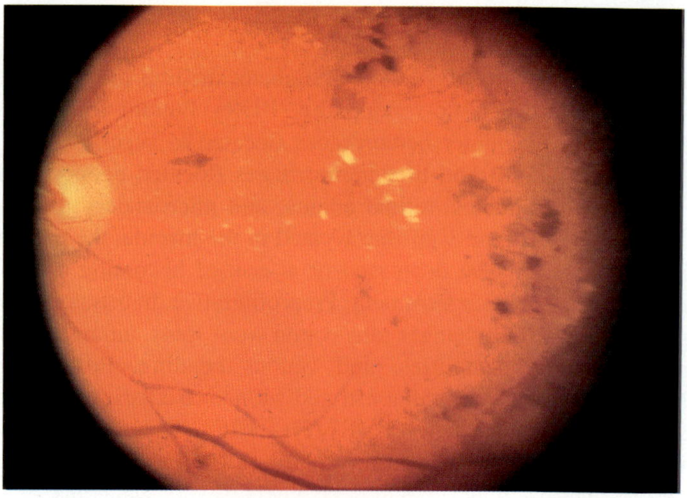

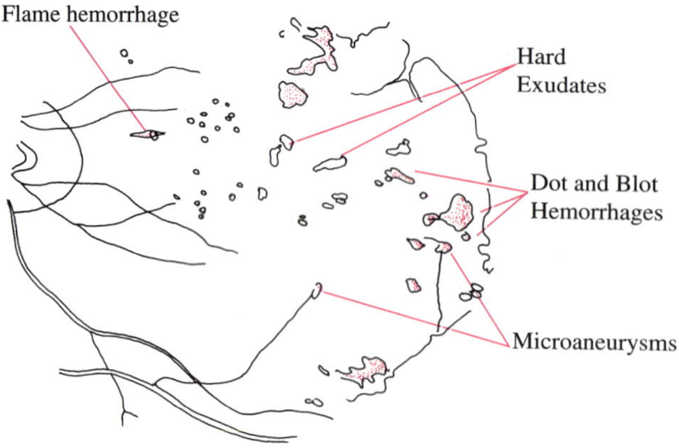

Figure 3.7A Background Diabetic Retinopathy

Hard exudates, dot hemorrhages, blot hemorrhages, flame hemorrhages, and microaneurysms are present. Because these changes are located within the macula, this is classified as diabetic maculopathy. (Courtesy of Richard E. Wyszynski, MD.)

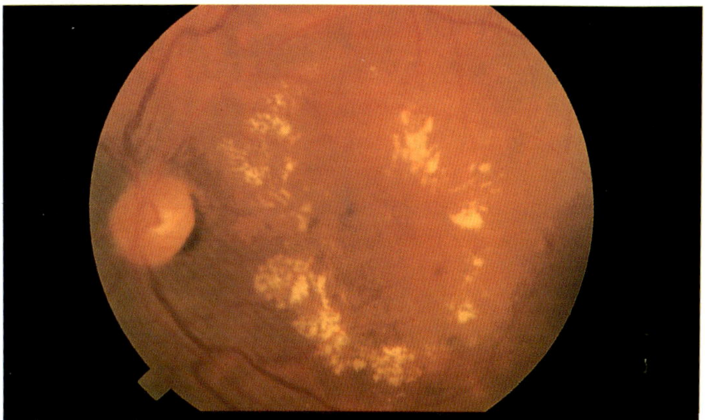

Figure 3.7B Background Diabetic Retinopathy

An example of diabetic maculopathy with a typical circinate lipid ring. (Courtesy of Richard E. Wyszynski, MD.)

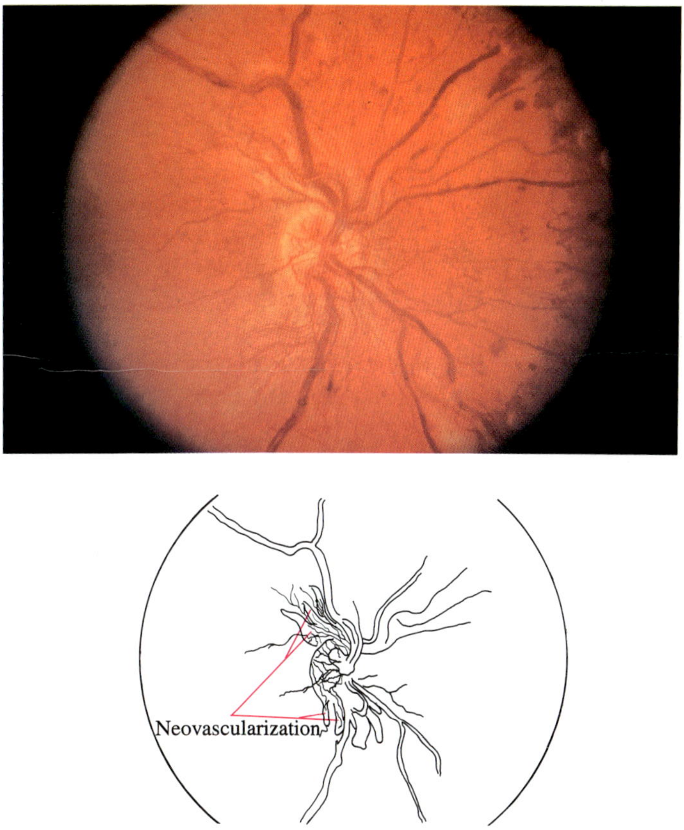

Figure 3.7C Proliferative Diabetic Retinopathy

In addition to the signs seen in background and preproliferative diabetic retinopathy, neovascularization is seen here coming off the disk. (Courtesy of Richard E. Wyszynski, MD.)

Associated Clinical Features

Papilledema refers to swelling of the optic nerve head, usually in association with elevated intracranial pressure. The optic disks are hyperemic with blurred disk margins; the venules are dilated and tortuous. The optic cup may be obscured by the swollen disk. There may be flame hemorrhages and infarctions (white indistinct cotton wool spots) in the nerve fiber layer and edema in the surrounding retina (Fig. 3.8).

Differential Diagnosis

Ocular inflammation (e.g., papillitis), tumors or trauma, central retinal artery or vein occlusion, optic nerve drusen, and marked hyperopia may present with similar findings.

ED Treatment and Disposition

Expeditious ophthalmologic and medical evaluation is warranted.

Clinical Pearls

1. The top of a swollen disk and the surrounding unaffected retina will not both be in focus on the same setting on direct ophthalmoscopy.
2. Papilledema is a bilateral process, though it may be slightly asymmetric. A unilateral swollen disk suggests a localized ocular or orbital process.
3. Vision is usually normal acutely, though the patient may complain of transient visual changes. The blind spot is usually enlarged.
4. Diplopia from a cranial nerve VI palsy can be associated with increased intracranial pressure and papilledema.

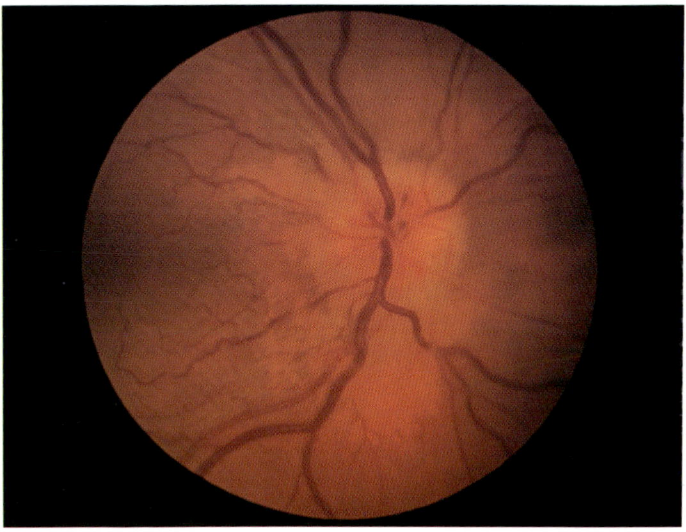

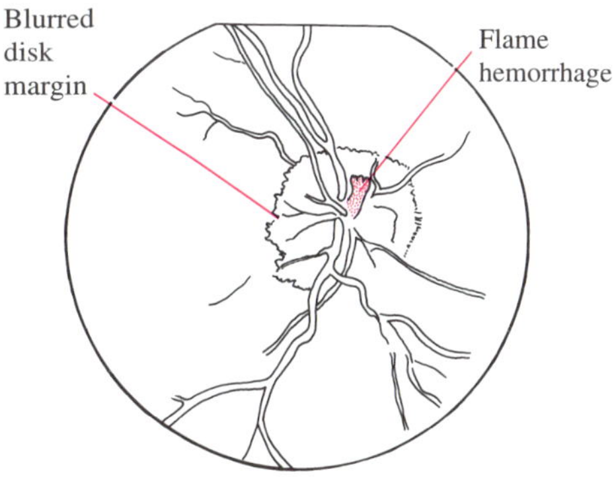

Figure 3.8 Papilledema

Disk is hyperemic and swollen with loss of sharp margins. The venules are dilated and tortuous. The cup is obscured. A small flame hemorrhage is seen at 12 to 1 o'clock on the disk margin. (Courtesy of Department of Ophthalmology, Naval Medical Center, Portsmouth, VA.)

Associated Clinical Features

Narrow or closed angle glaucoma results from a physical appositional impedence of aqueous humor outflow. Symptoms range from complaints of colored halos around lights and blurred vision to severe pain (may be described as a headache or brow ache) associated with nausea and vomiting. Intraocular pressures are markedly elevated. Perilimbal vessels are injected, the pupil middilated and poorly reactive to light, and the cornea may be hazy and edematous (see also Chapter 2 for external ocular images).

Two-thirds of glaucoma patients have open angle glaucoma due to an abnormality of primary tissues responsible for the outflow of fluid out of the eye. Often they are asymptomatic. They may have a family history of glaucoma. Funduscopy may show asymmetric cupping of the optic nerves (Fig. 3.9). The optic nerve may show notching, local thinning of tissue, or disk hemorrhage. Optic cups enlarge, especially vertically, with progressive damage. Tissue loss is associated with visual field abnormalities, usually in arcuate patterns. The intraocular pressure often, but not always, is greater than 21.

Differential Diagnosis

Acute Glaucoma

Painful visual loss (retrobulbar optic neuritis, iritis, endophthalmitis), referred pain from nonophthalmic source.

Chronic Glaucoma

Normal variants, ocular conditions like disk drusen or optic neuropathy.

ED Treatment and Disposition

Acute Narrow Angle Glaucoma

Emergent ophthalmologic consultation and administration of medications to decrease IOP (intraocular pressure). Beta-blocker drops (timolol), carbonic anhydrase inhibitors (acetazolamide), cholinergic stimulating drops (pilocarpine), hyperosmotic agents (osmoglyn), and alpha-adrenergic agonists (apraclonidine) may be employed prior to laser or surgical iridotomy (see also Chapter 2).

Open Angle Glaucoma

Long-term ophthalmic evaluation and treatment with medications and laser or surgery.

Clinical Pearls

1. A high index of suspicion must be maintained since associated complaints such as nausea, vomiting, and headache may obscure the diagnosis.
2. Open angle glaucoma usually causes no symptoms other than gradual loss of vision.
3. Congenital glaucoma is rare. However, because of prognosis if diagnosis is delayed, consider congenital glaucoma in infants and children with any of the following: tearing, photophobia, enlarged eyes, cloudy corneas.
4. Asymmetric cupping, enlarged cups, and elevated intraocular pressure are hallmarks of open angle glaucoma.

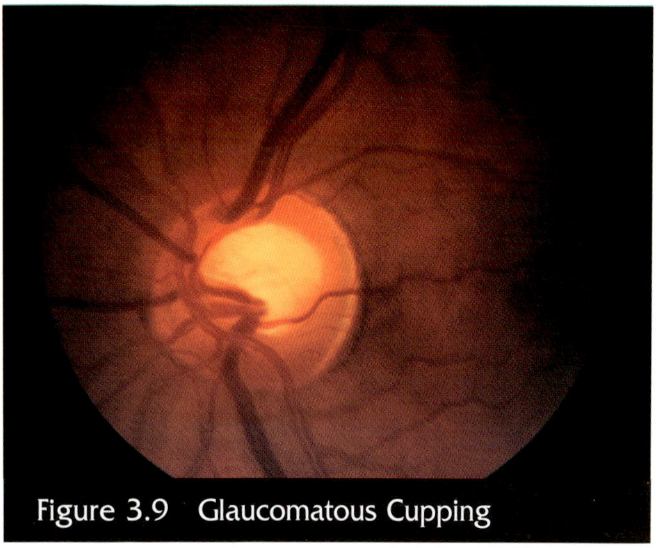

Figure 3.9 Glaucomatous Cupping

The cup is not central; it is elongated toward the rim supero temporally. (Courtesy of Department of Ophthalmology, Naval Medical Center, Portsmouth, VA.)

CHAPTER 4

OPHTHALMIC TRAUMA

Dallas E. Peak
Carey D. Chisholm
Kevin J. Knoop

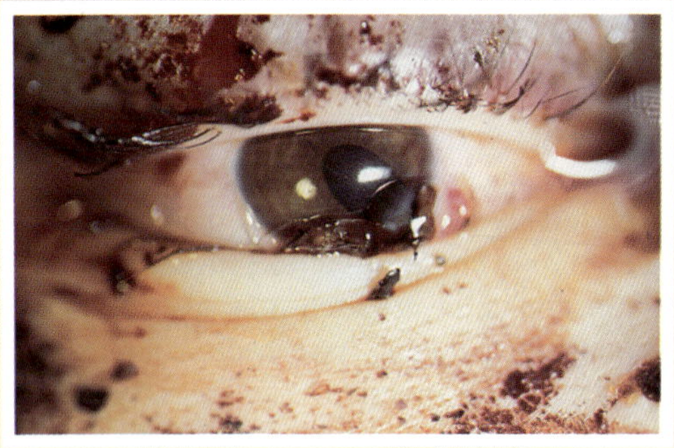

Associated Clinical Features

Corneal abrasions are heralded by the acute onset of eye discomfort accompanied by tearing and a foreign body sensation. Conjunctival injection may also be noted. If the area of abrasion is large or central, visual acuity may be affected. Large abrasions or delays in seeking care may be accompanied by photophobia and headache from ciliary muscle spasm. Associated findings or complications include traumatic iritis, hypopyon, or a corneal ulcer (described in Chap. 2). Examination before and after instillation of fluorescein, preferably with a slit lamp, usually reveals the defect (Figs. 4.1 and 4.2). Fluorescein pools and stains the area where corneal epithelium has been denuded.

Differential Diagnosis

Corneal foreign body, conjunctivitis, conjunctival foreign body, and corneal ulcer can present with similar complaints.

ED Treatment and Disposition

Instillation of topical anesthetic drops permits a better examination and relieves pain. A short-acting cycloplegic (e.g., cyclopentolate 0.5%, homatropine 5%) may reduce ciliary spasm and pain and should be considered in patients with larger abrasions or in those who complain of headache or photophobia. Topical antibiotic drops or ointment, preferably broad spectrum such as gentamicin, sulfacetamide, or erythromycin are used to prevent secondary bacterial infection. A soft double-layer patch may also be applied. Neither topical antibiotics nor patching have been scientifically validated, and routine use of these practices has recently been called into question. Follow-up is required for any patient who is still symptomatic after 12 h.

Clinical Pearls

1. Only sterile fluorescein strips should be used since the corneal epithelium, the primary barrier to infection, has been potentially disrupted.
2. Mucus may simulate the fluorescein uptake but its position changes with blinking.
3. Multiple linear corneal abrasions, the "ice-rink sign," may result from a foreign body adherent to the conjunctiva under the lid. The lid should always be everted to rule out a retained foreign body.
4. A high index of suspicion of a perforating injury should be maintained for any abrasion which occurs as a result of grinding or striking metal on metal.
5. Fluorescein streaming away from an "abrasion" (Seidel's test) may be an indication of a corneal perforation.

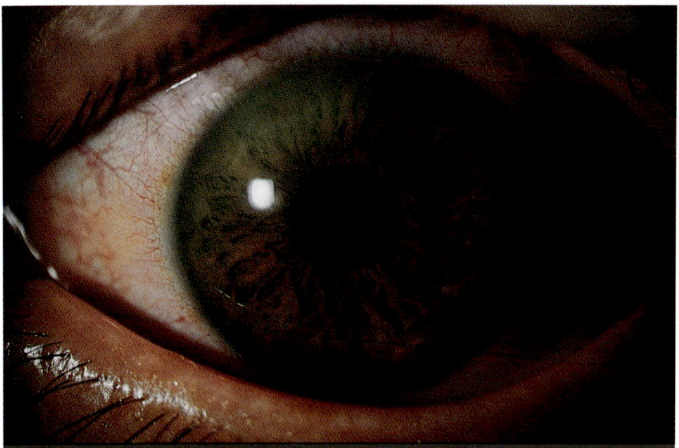

Figure 4.1 Corneal Abrasion

Seen under magnification from the slit lamp, corneal abrasion can sometimes be appreciated without fluorescein staining. This abrasion is seen without using the cobalt blue light. (Courtesy of Harold Rivera.)

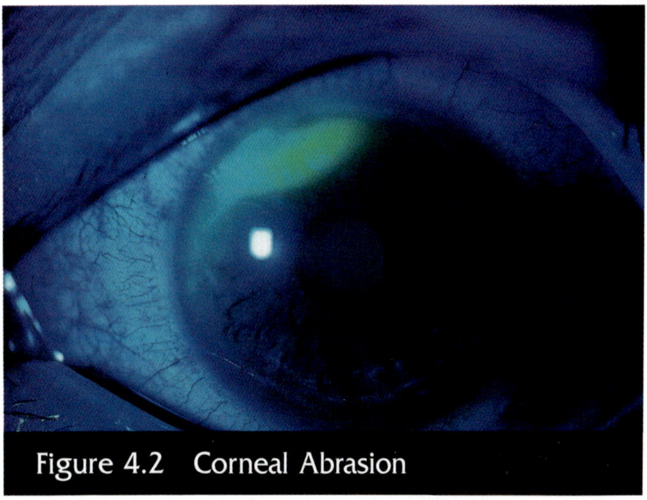

Figure 4.2 Corneal Abrasion

The same abrasion as Fig. 4.1 is seen under magnification from the slit lamp with fluorescein stain using the cobalt blue light. (Courtesy of Harold Rivera.)

Associated Clinical Features

Patients typically give a history of something in the eye or complain of foreign body sensation. If the foreign body overlies the cornea, the patient's vision may be affected. There may be tearing, conjunctival injection, and ciliary flush (Fig. 4.3). If several hours have elapsed since the occurrence of the injury, there may be headache and photophobia in addition to the above signs and symptoms.

Differential Diagnosis

The most important consideration in the differential is the possibility of a penetrating injury to the globe. A meticulous history about the mechanism of injury (grinding or metal on metal) must be elicited. Conjunctival foreign body, corneal abrasion, penetrating injury to the globe, intraocular foreign body, conjunctivitis, iritis, and glaucoma should also be considered.

ED Treatment and Disposition

If superficial, removal of the foreign body with a moist cotton-tipped applicator may be attempted; if unsuccessful, an eye spud, or small (25 gauge) needle may be used. After removal, if a residual corneal abrasion is present, instill an antibiotic solution or ointment. A "short-acting" cycloplegic (e.g., cyclopentolate 0.5%) should be considered in patients with complaints of headache or photophobia. Metallic foreign bodies are often accompanied by a "rust ring" discoloration of the surrounding corneal epithelium (Fig. 4.4). Removal of the rust ring can be attempted, either with a needle or preferably with a small burr drill device available commercially. Alternatively, the patient may be referred to an ophthalmologist the following day.

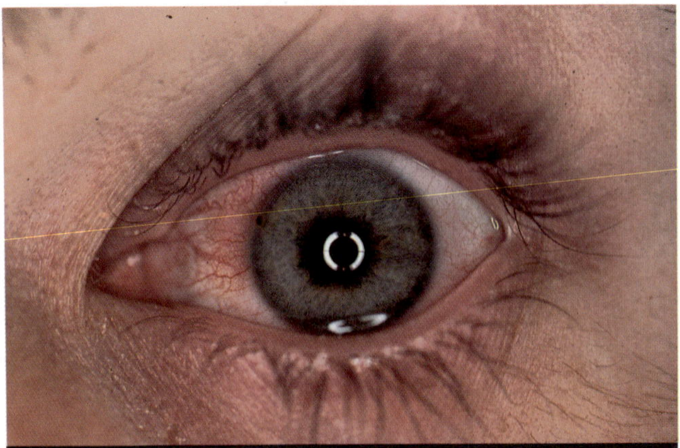

Figure 4.3 Foreign Body on the Cornea

A foreign body is lodged at 10 o'clock on the cornea. Note the localized ciliary flush in the surrounding conjunctiva at the limbus. (Courtesy of Kevin J. Knoop, MD, MS.)

Clinical Pearls

1. Treatment of a suspected penetrating injury to the globe includes immediate referral, eye rest, protective patching (Fig. 4.5), and elevating the head of the bed.
2. If history of ocular penetration is present, a diligent search for foreign body with either plain x-rays or CT scan is indicated (Fig. 4.6).
3. Be sure to evert the upper lid and search carefully for a foreign body. A foreign body adherent to the upper lid abrades the cornea producing the "ice-rink" sign, caused from multiple linear abrasions.
4. If a rust ring is present from a metallic foreign body, its removal can be attempted, or the patient may await ophthalmology follow-up in 24 h.
5. Multiple small corneal foreign bodies (e.g., glass or sand) may be removed by irrigating with normal saline or tap water. The instillation of a topical anesthetic facilitates the irrigation process.

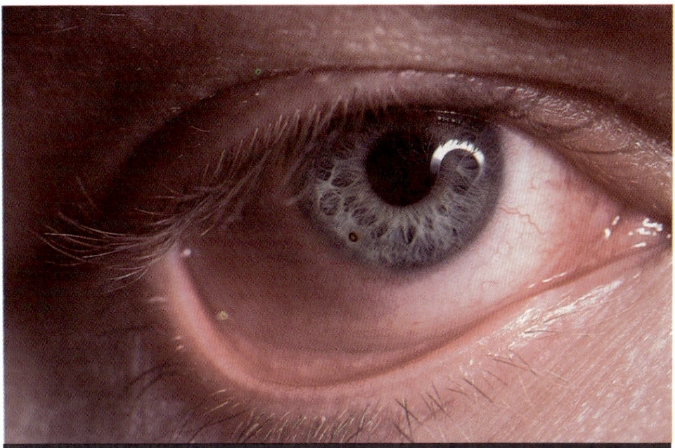

Figure 4.4 "Rust Ring"

A rust ring has formed from a foreign body (likely metallic) in this patient. A burr drill can be used for attempted removal, which if unsuccessful, can be reattempted in 24 h. (Courtesy of Kevin J. Knoop, MD, MS.)

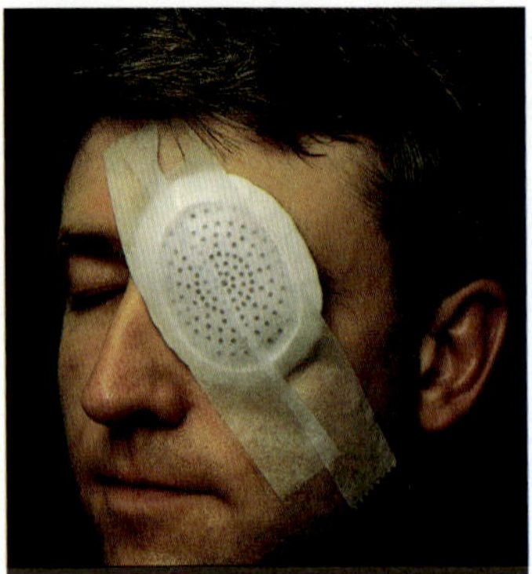

Figure 4.5 Protective Metal (Fox) Shield

A protective shield is used in the setting of a suspected or confirmed perforating injury. A patch may be fashioned from a cup if needed. (Courtesy of Kevin J. Knoop, MD, MS.)

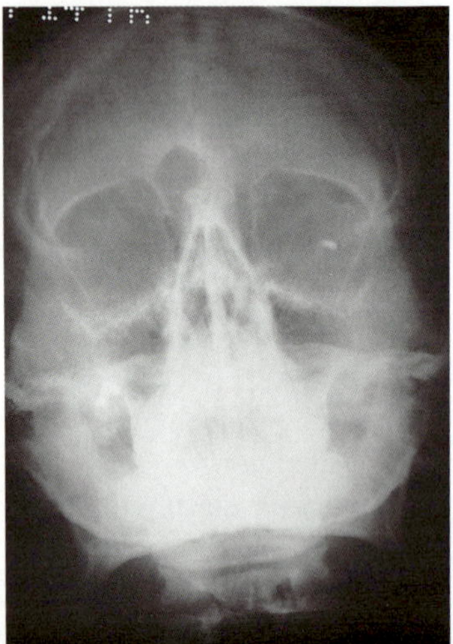

Figure 4.6 Intraocular Foreign Body

A metallic foreign body is seen on a plain radiograph and with comparison with a lateral film indicates the presence of an intraocular foreign body. (Courtesy of Department of Ophthalmology, Naval Medical Center, Portsmouth, VA.)

Associated Clinical Features

Injury to the anterior chamber that disrupts the vasculature supporting the iris or ciliary body results in a hyphema. The blood tends to layer and because of gravity forms a meniscus (Fig. 4.7). Symptoms can include pain, photophobia, and possibly blurred vision secondary to obstructing blood cells. Nausea and vomiting may signal a rise in intraocular pressure (glaucoma) caused by blockage of the trabecular meshwork by blood cells or clot.

Differential Diagnosis

Hypopyon (pus within the anterior chamber), vitreous hemorrhage, iridodialysis, penetrating injury to the globe, and intraocular foreign body should be considered.

ED Treatment and Disposition

Prevention of further hemorrhage is the first goal. The patient should be kept at rest in the supine position with the head elevated slightly. A hard eye shield should be used to prevent further trauma from manipulation. Oral or parenteral pain medication and sedatives are appropriate, but avoid agents with antiplatelet activity (e.g., NSAIDs). Antiemetics should be used if the patient has nausea. Further treatment is at the discretion of specialty consultants, but may include topical and oral steroids, antifibrinolytics such as aminocaproic acid, or surgery. Intraocular pressure should be measured in all patients unless there is a suspicion of penetrating injury to the globe. If elevated, intraocular pressure should be treated with appropriate agents including topical beta blockers, pilocarpine, and if needed, osmotic agents (mannitol, sorbitol) and acetazolamide. The need for admission for small hyphemas is variable, since some centers admit all, whereas others individualize treatment. Ophthalmologic consultation is warranted to determine local practices.

Clinical Pearls

1. The patient should be told specifically not to read or watch television as these activities result in greater than usual ocular activity.
2. Depending on the severity of the initial hyphema, re-bleeding may occur in 10 to 25% of patients, commonly in 2 to 5 days as the original clot retracts and loosens.
3. Blood which is not absorbed from the anterior chamber may infiltrate and stain the cornea leaving a brown discoloration.
4. An "eightball" or total hyphema occurs when blood fills the entire anterior chamber. These require surgical evacuation.
5. Patients with sickle cell and other hemoglobinopathies are at risk for sickling of blood inside the anterior chamber (Fig. 4.8). This can cause a rise in intraocular pressure from physical obstruction of the trabecular meshwork.

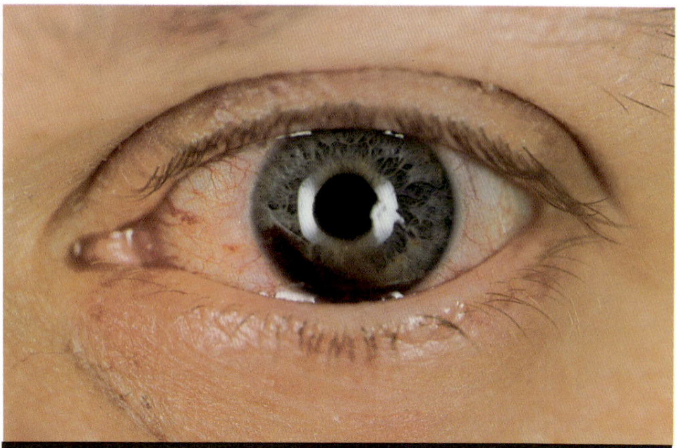

Figure 4.7 Hyphema

This hyphema has almost completely layered while the patient's head was tilted. Note the hazy greenish area at 6 o'clock in contrast to the remainder of the blue iris. This represents blood circulating in the anterior chamber that has not yet layered. (Courtesy of Kevin J. Knoop, MD, MS.)

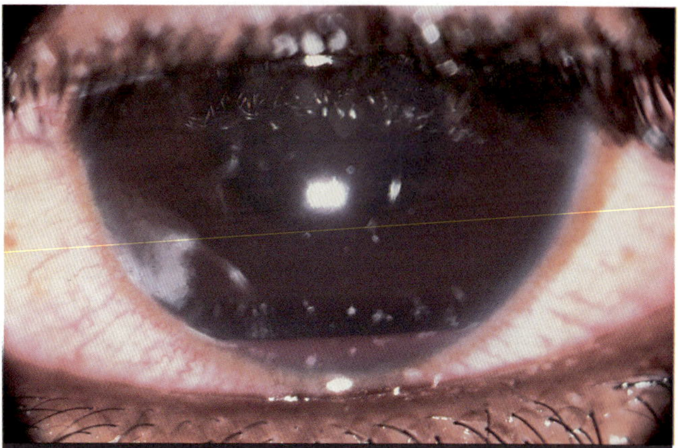

Figure 4.8 Hyphema

A small hyphema (about 5%) in a patient with sickle cell disease that needed to be drained. (Courtesy of Dallas E. Peak, MD.)

Associated Clinical Features

Traumatic iridodialysis is the result of an injury, typically blunt trauma, which pulls the iris away from the ciliary body. The resulting deformity appears as a lens-shaped defect at the outer margin of the iris (Fig. 4.9). Patients may present complaining of a "second pupil." As the iris pulls away from the ciliary body, a small amount of bleeding may result. Look closely for associated traumatic hyphema.

Differential Diagnosis

Traumatic hyphema, penetrating injury to the globe, scleral rupture, intraocular foreign body, and lens dislocation causing billowing of the iris should all be considered.

ED Treatment and Disposition

A remote traumatic iridodialysis requires no specific treatment in the emergency department. Recent history of ocular trauma should prompt a diligent slit-lamp examination for associated hyphema or lens discoloration. If hyphema is present, it should be treated as discussed (see "Hyphema"). Pure cases of iridodialysis may be referred for specialty consultation to exclude other injuries, or if the defect is large enough to result in monocular diplopia, surgical repair may be necessary.

Clinical Pearls

1. The examination should carefully exclude posterior chamber pathology and hyphema.
2. A careful review of the history to exclude penetrating trauma should be made. If the history is unclear, CT scan may be used to exclude the presence of intraocular foreign body.
3. A careful examination includes searching for associated lens dislocation.

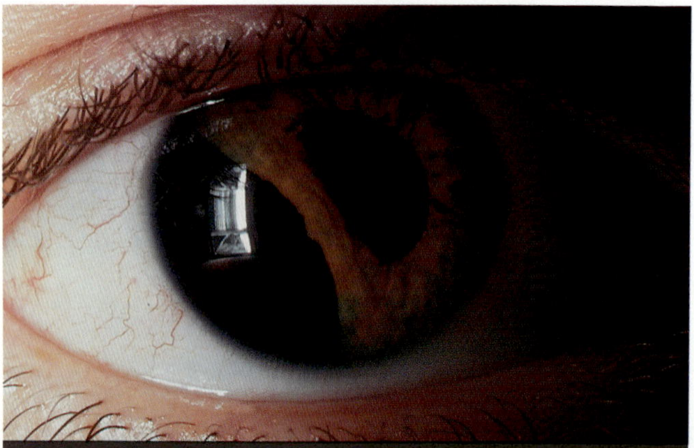

Figure 4.9 Traumatic Iridodialysis

The iris has pulled away from the ciliary body as a result of blunt trauma. (Courtesy of Department of Ophthalmology, Naval Medical Center, Portsmouth, VA.)

Associated Clinical Features

Lens dislocation may result from sudden blow to the globe with resultant stretching of the zonule fibers which hold the lens in place (Fig. 4.10). The patient may experience symptoms of monocular diplopia or gross blurring of images, depending on severity. The edge of the subluxed lens may be visible when the pupil is dilated (Fig. 4.11). If all the zonule fibers tear and the lens is dislocated, it may lodge in the anterior chamber or the vitreous.

Differential Diagnosis

Marfan's syndrome, tertiary syphilis, and homocystinuria may be present and should be considered in patients presenting with lens dislocation.

ED Treatment and Disposition

Almost all require surgery if the lens is totally dislocated; partial subluxations may only require a change in refraction.

Clinical Pearls

1. Patients may experience lens dislocation with seemingly trivial trauma if they have an underlying coloboma of the lens, Marfan's syndrome, homocystinuria, or syphilis.
2. Iridodonesis is a trembling movement of the iris noted after rapid eye movements and is a sign of occult posterior lens dislocation.

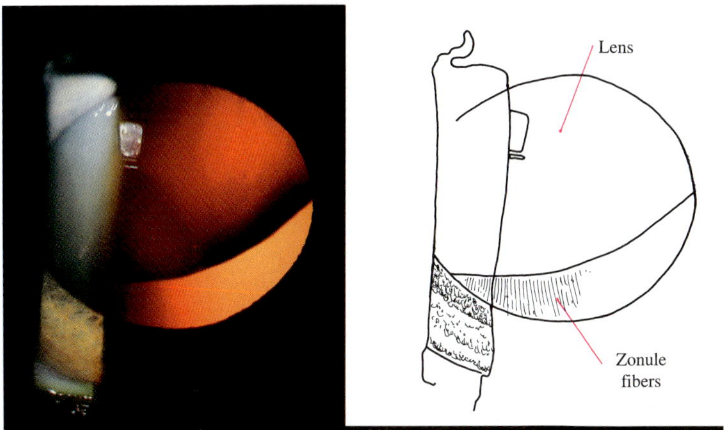

Figure 4.10 Lens Dislocation

Lens dislocation revealed during slit lamp examination. Note the zonule fibers which normally hold the lens in place. (Courtesy of Department of Ophthalmology, Naval Medical Center, Portsmouth, VA.)

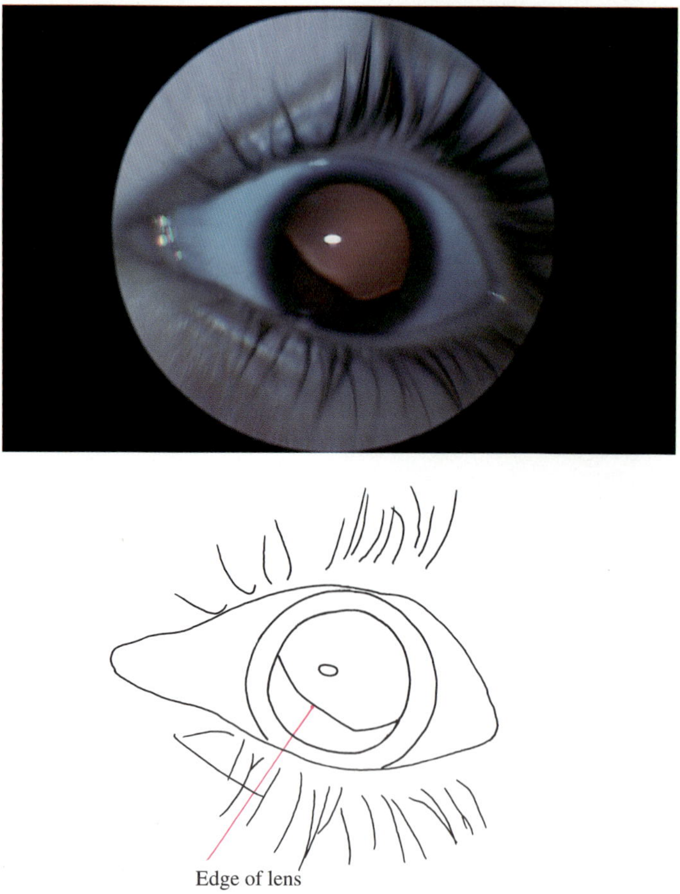

Figure 4.11 Lens Dislocation

The edge of this dislocated lens is visible with the pupil dilated as an altered red reflex. (Courtesy of Department of Ophthalmology, Naval Medical Center, Portsmouth, VA.)

Associated Clinical Features

A subconjunctival hemorrhage or hematoma occurs with often trivial events such as a cough, sneeze, or valsalva. The patient may present with some degree of duress secondary to the appearance of the bloody eye. The blood is usually bright red and appears flat (Fig. 4.12). It is limited to the bulbar conjunctiva and stops abruptly at the limbus. This appearance is important to differentiate from bloody chemosis, which can occur with scleral rupture. Aside from appearance, this condition does not cause the patient any pain or diminution in visual acuity.

Differential Diagnosis

Scleral rupture, nontraumatic bloody chemosis (Fig. 4.13), conjunctivitis, iritis, corneal-scleral laceration, severe hypertension, and coagulopathy may have a similar appearance or presentation.

ED Treatment and Disposition

No treatment is required. The patient should be told to expect the blood to be resorbed in 2 to 3 weeks.

Clinical Pearls

1. Subconjunctival hematoma may be differentiated from bloody chemosis by the flat appearance of the conjunctival membranes.
2. A subconjunctival hematoma involving the extreme lateral globe after blunt trauma is very suspicious for zygomatic arch fracture.
3. Patients with nontraumatic bloody chemosis should be evaluated for an underlying metabolic (coagulopathy) or structural (cavernous sinus thrombosis) disorder.

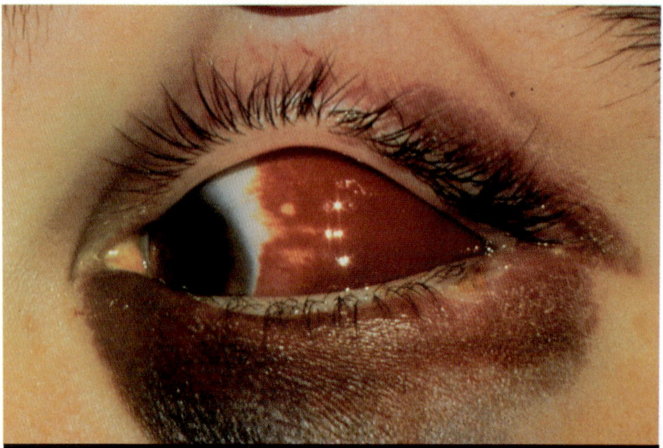

Figure 4.12 Subconjunctival Hemorrhage

Subconjunctival hemorrhage in a patient with blunt trauma. The flat appearance of the hemorrhage indicates its benign nature. (Courtesy of Dallas E. Peak, MD.)

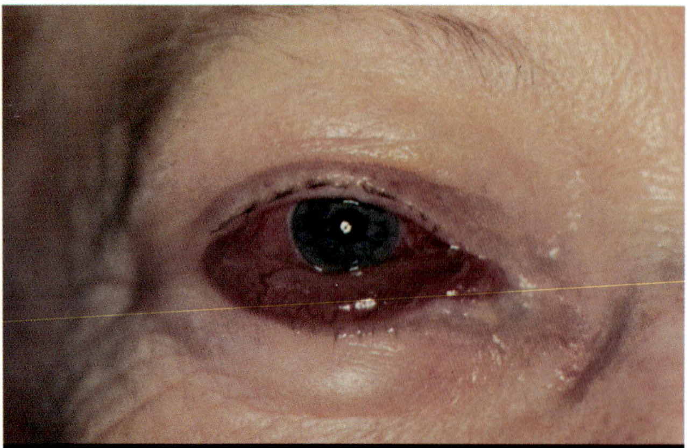

Figure 4.13 Bloody Chemosis

"Bloody chemosis was confused with" "subconjunctival hemorrhage" in this patient with no history of trauma and positive cranial nerve palsies. Cavernous sinus thrombosis was diagnosed. (Courtesy of Eric Einfalt, MD.)

CHAPTER 5

EAR, NOSE, AND THROAT CONDITIONS

Edward C. Jauch
Alexander T. Trott
Kevin J. Knoop

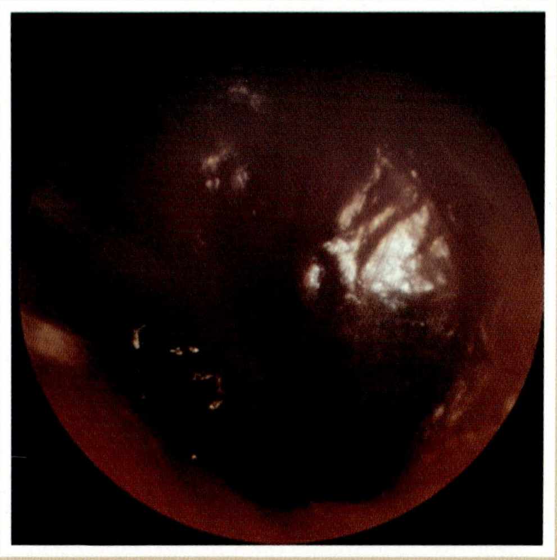

Associated Clinical Features

Children between the ages of 6 months and 2 years are at highest risk of developing otitis media (OM). Males, North American Eskimos, non-breast-fed infants, and children with craniofacial anomalies have the highest incidence of OM. Additionally, children who contract their first episode prior to their first birthday, have a sibling with a history of recurrent OM, are in day care, or have parents who smoke, are at increased risk of recurrent OM.

In its most basic form, OM is defined as an acute inflammation and effusion of the middle ear. Otoscopy of the middle ear should focus on color, position, translucency, and mobility. Compared with the tympanic membrane of a normal ear (Fig. 5.1), acute OM causes the tympanic membrane to appear dull, erythematous or injected, bulging, or less mobile (Figs. 5.2 and 5.3). The light reflex, normal tympanic membrane landmarks, and malleus become obscured.

There are many classifications, and hence presentations, of OM based on symptom duration and clinical presentation. Regardless of classification, the common pathogenesis of OM is eustachian tube dysfunction, allowing retention of secretions (serous otitis) (Figs. 5.4 and 5.5) and seeding of bacteria.

OM is caused by a wide variety of pathogens, including viral, bacterial, and fungal. The most common bacterial isolates are *Streptococcus pneumoniae, Haemophilus influenzae, Moraxella catarrhalis,* and *Streptococcus pyogenes.* Approximately 20% of middle ear effusion aspirations are sterile. The prevalence of β-lactamase–producing strains of *H. influenzae* and *M. catarrhalis* is variable but increasing.

Patient presentation and complaints vary with age. Infants with OM have vague, nonspecific symptoms such as irritability, lethargy, and decreased oral intake. Young children can be irritable, often febrile, and frequently pull at their ears, but they may also be completely asymptomatic. Older children and adults note ear pain, decreased auditory acuity, and occasionally, otorrhea.

Differential Diagnosis

Myringitis, otitis externa, tympanic membrane perforations, and herpes zoster can mimic otitis media. Less common causes of ear pain include temporomandibular joint disorders, odontogenic infections, and sinusitis. Tympanic membrane erythema can be caused by crying children in an otherwise healthy ear.

ED Treatment and Disposition

Although most cases of OM spontaneously resolve, most patients are treated with antibiotics and analgesics. Steroids, decongestants, and antihistamines do not alter the course in OM but may improve upper respiratory tract symptoms. Rarely, myringotomy may be needed for pain relief.

Antibiotic selection is widely variable. Amoxicillin is a suitable first choice for an acute OM. Alternatives for initial therapy include trimethoprim-sulfamethoxazole, erythromycin ethyl succinate with sulfisoxazole, and second-generation cephalosporins. If the patient continues to have symptoms 48 to 72 h after beginning antibiotics, amoxicillin with clavulanate, cefixime, or the newer macrolides may provide broader coverage.

Patients should be instructed to follow up in 10 to 14 days or return if symptoms persist or worsen after 48 h. Patients who have significant hearing loss, failed two complete courses of outpatient antibiotics during a single event, have chronic OM with or without acute exacerbations, or failed prophylactic antibiotics warrant referral to an otolaryngologist for further evaluation and possible tympanostomy tubes (Fig. 5.6).

Clinical Pearls

1. In children, recurrent OM is often due to food allergies.
2. Only 4% of children under 2 years old with OM develop temperatures greater than 104°F. Children with temperatures higher than 104°F or with signs of systemic toxicity should be closely evaluated for other causes of the illness before attributing the fever to OM.

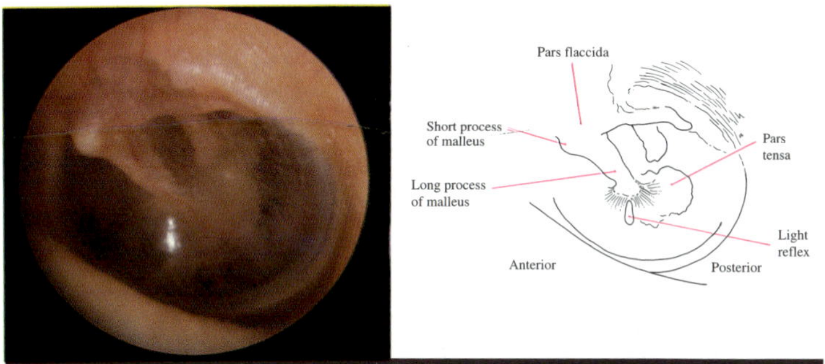

Figure 5.1 Normal Tympanic Membrane

Normal tympanic membrane anatomy and landmarks. (Courtesy of Richard A. Chole, MD, PhD.)

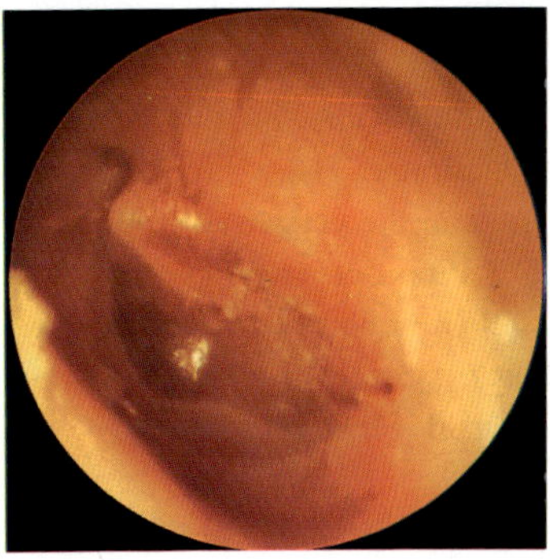

Figure 5.2 Early Acute Otitis Media

A mildly erythematous tympanic membrane is seen with a small purulent effusion in the middle ear. (Courtesy of C. Bruce MacDonald, MD.)

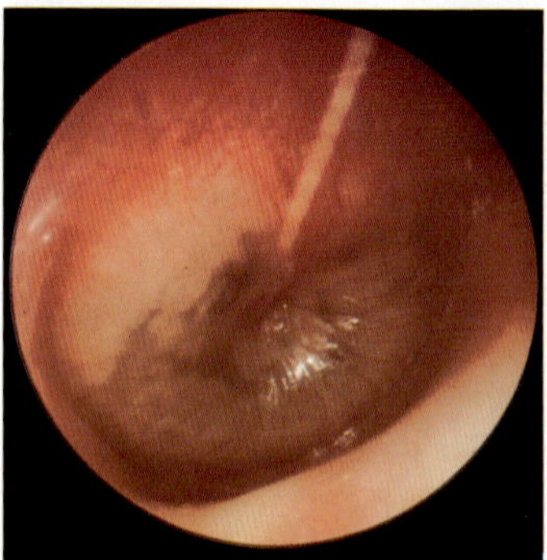

Figure 5.3 Acute Otitis Media

The middle ear is filled with purulent material behind an erythematous, bulging tympanic membrane. (Courtesy of Richard A. Chole, MD, PhD.)

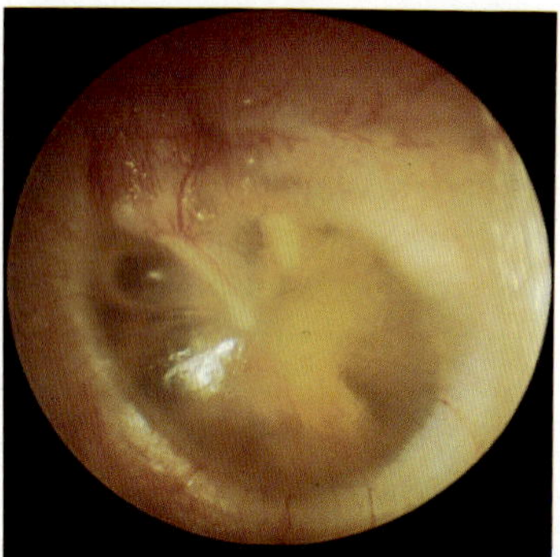

Figure 5.4 Serous Otitis Media with Effusion (OME)

Serous OME is commonly seen after acute otitis media, but is also common without this history. Any process that leads to obstruction of a eustachian tube will cause a middle ear effusion. A clear, amber-colored effusion with a single air-fluid level is seen in the middle ear behind a normal tympanic membrane. (Courtesy of C. Bruce MacDonald, MD.)

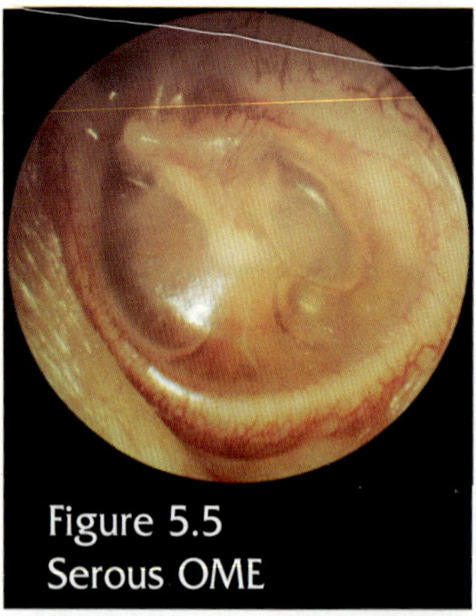

Figure 5.5 Serous OME

A clear, amber-colored effusion with multiple air-fluid levels is seen in the middle ear behind a normal tympanic membrane. (Courtesy of C. Bruce MacDonald, MD.)

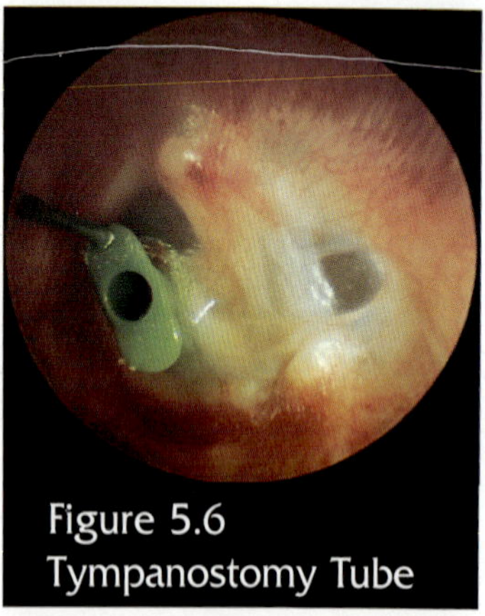

Figure 5.6 Tympanostomy Tube

Typical appearance of a tympanostomy tube in the tympanic membrane. These tubes will migrate to the periphery and eventually drop out. Occassionally, they will be found in the external ear canal. (Courtesy of C. Bruce MacDonald, MD.)

Associated Clinical Features

Bullous myringitis is a direct inflammation and infection of the tympanic membrane (TM) secondary to a viral or bacterial agent. Fluid-filled vesicles or bullae on an infected tympanic membrane are the hallmark of bullous myringitis (Fig. 5.7). Frequently, a concomitant otitis media with effusion is noted. Common bacterial agents are *Mycoplasma pneumoniae, Streptococcus pneumoniae,* and *Haemophilus influenzae.*

The onset of bullous myringitis is preceded by an upper respiratory tract infection and is heralded by sudden onset of ear pain, serosanguinous canal drainage, and frequently some degree of hearing loss. Otoscopy reveals bullae on either the inner or outer surface of the TM, often filled with red bloody fluid. Patients presenting with fever, hearing loss, and purulent drainage are more likely to have other concomitant infections such as otitis media and otitis externa.

Differential Diagnosis

Barotrauma is usually associated with swimming, diving, or airplane travel. Herpes zoster oticus produces facial nerve palsy and facial pain. Otitis externa causes external auditory canal edema and drainage, whereas otitis media distorts the TM but rarely causes bullae.

ED Treatment and Disposition

Differentiation between viral and bacterial etiologies for tympanic membrane bullae is difficult but, fortunately, seldom necessary. Although most episodes spontaneously resolve, many physicians prescribe antibiotics, such as trimethoprim-sulfamethoxazole or a macrolide. Topical or systemic analgesics and oral decongestants may provide symptomatic relief. Referral is not necessary in most cases, unless bullae rupture is required for pain relief.

Clinical Pearl

1. Facial nerve paralysis associated with clear fluid-filled TM vesicles is characteristic of herpes zoster oticus.

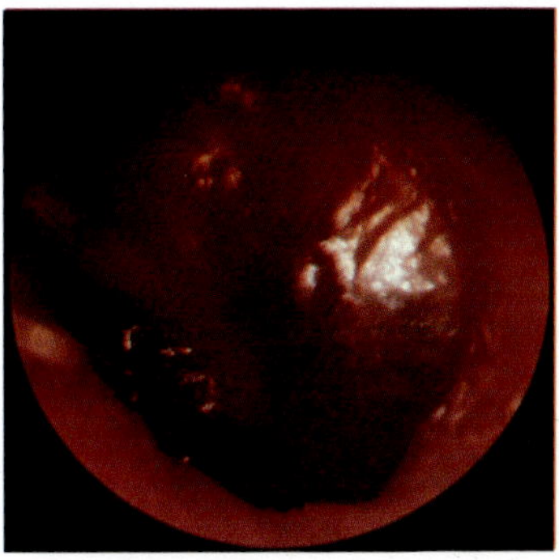

Figure 5.7
Bullous Myringitis

Several bullae, which may be blood- or fluid-filled, are seen distorting the surface of the tympanic membrane. (Courtesy of Richard A. Chole, MD, PhD.)

Associated Clinical Features

Contrary to the origin suggested by their name, cholesteatomas are epidermoid inclusion cysts: collections of desquamating stratified squamous epithelium found in the middle ear or mastoid air cells. Congenital cholesteatomas are most frequently found in children and young adults. Acquired cholesteatomas originate from perforations of the tympanic membrane, usually marginally or in the pars flaccida, allowing migration of external auditory canal stratified squamous epithelium into the middle ear.

Cholesteatomas can be locally destructive of the middle ear ossicles and tympanic membrane and, through the production of collagenases, erode into the temporal bone, inner ear structures, mastoid sinus, or posterior fossa dura. Delays in treatment can lead to permanent conductive hearing loss or infectious complications.

Patients present with progressive hearing loss, foul-smelling ear drainage, and, in advanced stages, pain, headache, dizziness, facial paralysis, fever, or vertigo. Many cholesteatomas have an insidious progression without associated pain or symptoms. Cholesteatomas are seen on otoscopy as either a retraction pocket containing white debris or a yellow crust on the tympanic membrane with or without a perforation (Fig. 5.8). Middle ear cholesteatomas appear as a pearly white or yellow middle ear mass behind the tympanic membrane producing a focal bulge, in contrast to a more diffuse displacement of the tympanic membrane seen in otitis media. Radiographs and CT scans may reveal bony destruction.

Osteomas (sometimes called exostoses) are benign tumors of the external auditory canal (EAC) found in the deep meatus. Osteomas are associated with patients with recurrent cold water exposures, such as swimmers and divers. Osteomas are seen on otoscopy as single or multiple round shiny swellings of the bony external auditory canal (Fig. 5.9). A cerumen impaction or an otitis externa may obscure the examination.

Differential Diagnosis

Wax particles and external auditory canal (EAC) foreign bodies may resemble cholesteatomas on otoscopy. Furuncles are painful to palpation, whereas otitis externa and otitis media have EAC drainage and middle ear effusions, respectively.

ED Treatment and Disposition

Early diagnosis of a cholesteatoma is essential for proper referral. Water avoidance, topical and sometimes systemic antibiotics are important. Small cholesteatomas found in retraction pockets can be excised and a tympanostomy tube placed to equilibrate middle ear pressures. More extensive cholesteatomas may require surgical excision, tympanoplasty, and radical mastoidectomy. Osteomas require no medical or surgical management unless they become symptomatic.

Clinical Pearls

1. Persistent pain associated with headache, facial motor weakness, nystagmus, or vertigo suggests inner ear or intracranial involvement.
2. Polyps found on the tympanic membrane can indicate the presence of a cholesteatoma and require further evaluation to exclude its presence.

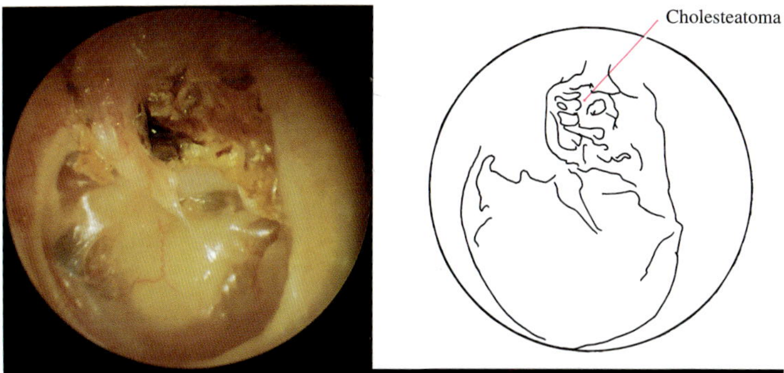

Figure 5.8 Cholesteatoma

A cholesteatoma is seen in this ear. Primary acquired cholesteatomas are thought to arise from gradual invagination of the pars flaccida, usually secondary to trauma. Note the yellow epithelial debris from the cholesteatoma in the area of the pars flaccida. Often there is an effusion and debris, which can distort the anatomy on otoscopy. (Courtesy of C. Bruce MacDonald, MD.)

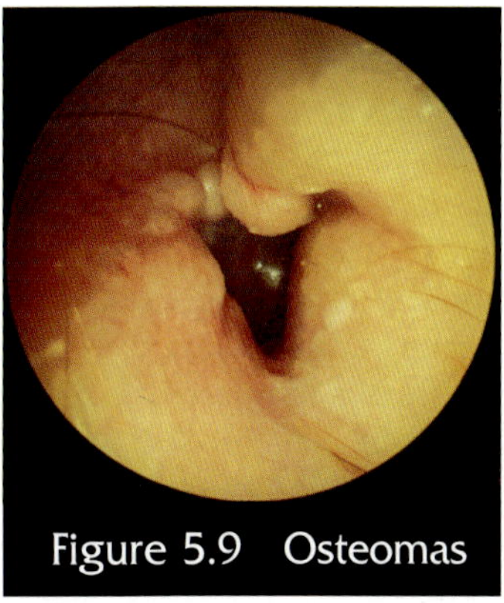

Figure 5.9 Osteomas

Multiple osteomas almost occlude the external auditory canal. The tympanic membrane can be seen in the center, past the osteomas. These are often seen in patients who are cold water swimmers. (Courtesy of C. Bruce MacDonald, MD.)

Associated Clinical Features

Acute tympanic membrane (TM) perforations are often the result of direct penetrating trauma, water or air pressure changes (barotrauma, blast injuries), chronic otitis media, corrosives, thermal injuries (electricity, lightning, heated objects), and iatrogenic causes (foreign body removal, tympanostomy tubes). TM perforations are occasionally complicated by damage to the ossicular chain, producing a more complete conductive hearing loss, temporal bone injuries, and cranial nerve damage.

Patients complain of sudden onset of ear pain, vertigo, tinnitus, and altered hearing after a specific event. Patients with posterior perforations present with a more profound deafness than those with anterior perforation sites. Physical examination of the TM reveals a slit-shaped tear or larger perforation with an irregular border. An acute perforation can have blood on the perforation margin and blood or clot in the canal (Fig. 5.10). The margins are smooth in subacute or chronic perforations (Fig. 5.11).

Differential Diagnosis

Congenital malformations, chronic perforations, residual perforations from tympanostomy tubes, and retraction pockets have more regular borders and no bleeding or TM erythema.

ED Treatment and Disposition

Treatment of acute tympanic membrane perforations is tailored to the mechanism. All easily removable foreign bodies should be extracted. Corrosive exposures require face, eye, and ear decontamination. Antibiotics and irrigation do not improve the rate or completeness of healing unless the injury is associated with otitis media. Systemic antibiotics should be used for perforations associated with otitis media, penetrating injury, and possibly water sport injuries (see "Otitis Media"). Topical steroids impede perforation closure.

Patients are instructed to avoid getting water in the ear while the perforation is healing and to return for symptoms of infection. All TM perforations should be referred to an otolaryngologist for follow-up and possible myringoplasty evaluation. Even though nearly 80% of all TM perforations spontaneously heal, some do not, and complications can develop.

Clinical Pearls

1. Cortisporin eardrops of any formulation have been shown to retard spontaneous healing and should be avoided.
2. Traumatic TM perforation associated with cranial nerve deficits or persistent vertigo requires immediate ENT consultation for possible temporal bone fractures and more extensive injuries.

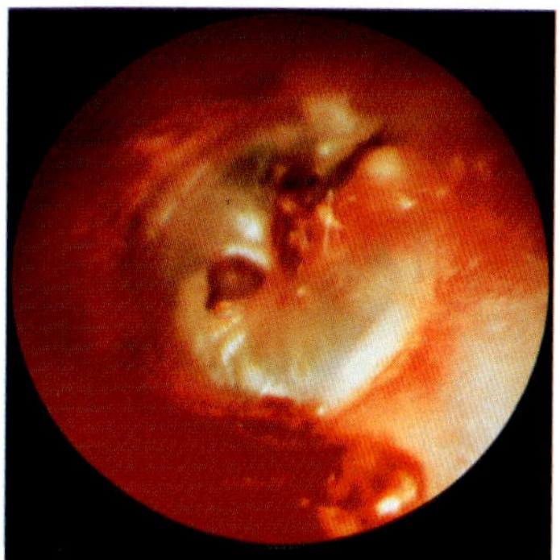

Figure 5.10 Acute Tympanic Membrane Perforation

Acute tympanic membrane perforation with erythema of the canal and tympanic membrane. Note the sharp edges of the perforation. (Courtesy of Robin T. Cotton, MD.)

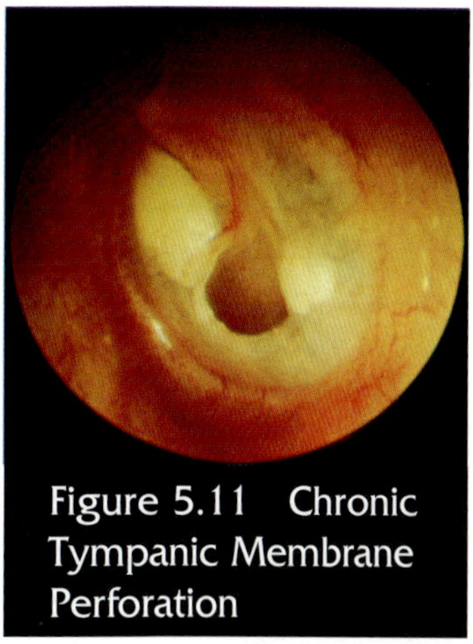

Figure 5.11 Chronic Tympanic Membrane Perforation

Note absence of blood and erythema on the tympanic membrane and the smooth perforation margins. (Courtesy of C. Bruce MacDonald, MD.)

Associated Clinical Features

Otitis externa (OE) or "swimmer's ear" is an inflammation and infection (bacterial or fungal) of the auricle and external auditory canal (EAC). Typical symptoms include otalgia, pruritus, otorrhea, and hearing loss. Physical examination reveals EAC hyperemia and edema (Fig. 5.12), otorrhea, malodorous discharge, occlusion from debris and swelling, pain with auricle manipulation, and periauricular lymphadenopathy.

Several factors predispose the EAC to infection: increased humidity and heat, water immersion, foreign bodies, trauma, hearing aids, and cerumen impaction. Bacterial otitis externa is primarily an infection due to *Pseudomonas* species or *Staphylococcus aureus.* Diabetics are particularly prone to infections by *Pseudomonas, Candida albicans,* and less commonly *Aspergillus niger* (Fig. 5.13).

Differential Diagnosis

Cholesteatomas and foreign bodies can produce a secondary OE. Periauricular cellulitis, herpes zoster oticus (Fig. 5.14), and malignant otitis externa have auricular and facial involvement. EAC dermatitis, eczema, and furuncles rarely produce EAC drainage.

ED Treatment and Disposition

Saline irrigation and suctioning is recommended to thoroughly evaluate the EAC. Topical antibiotic *suspensions* (containing polymyxin, neomycin, and hydrocortisone) with ear wicks are effective. Topical *solutions* are not pH-balanced and thus are irritating and may cause inflammation in the middle ear if a perforation is present. Systemic antibiotics are not indicated unless extension into the periauricular tissues is noted. Patients should avoid swimming and prevent water from entering the ear while bathing. Dry heat aids in resolution, and analgesics provide symptomatic relief. Follow-up should be arranged in 10 days for routine cases.

Clinical Pearls

1. Resistent cases may have an allergic component. These typically present with a dry, scaly EAC and are recurrent and chronic in nature.
2. Drying the EAC after water exposure with a 50:50 mixture of isopropyl alcohol and water, or acetic acid (white vinegar) minimizes recurrence. If the TM is possibly perforated, isopropyl alcohol should be avoided.
3. Often the symptoms are out of proportion to the visible findings, necessitating narcotic analgesia.

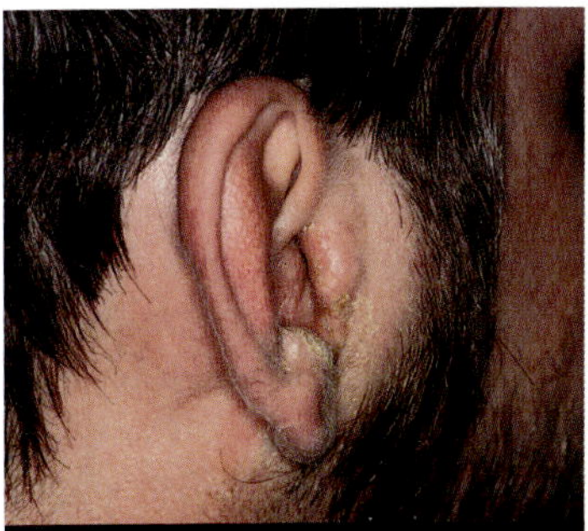

Figure 5.12
Otitis Externa

A discharge is seen coming from the external auditory canal, which is swollen and almost completely occluded. An ear wick placed in the EAC facilitates delivery of topical antibiotic suspension and drainage of debris. (Courtesy of Frank Birinyi, MD.)

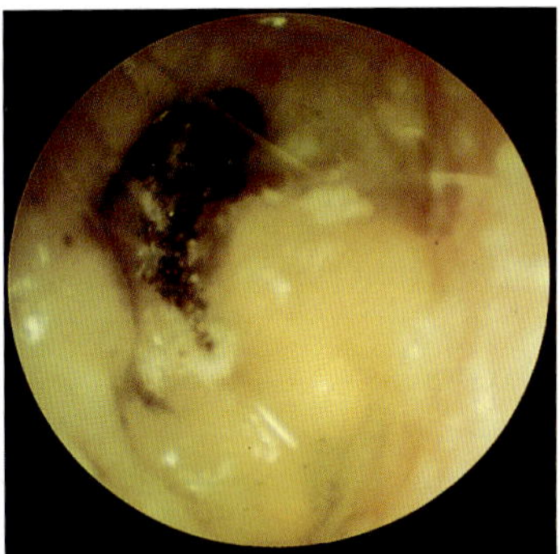

Figure 5.13
Aspergillus Otitis Externa

Chronic otitis externa with copious debris, including black spores from *Aspergillus niger,* cottony fungal elements, and wet debris. This patient had been treated with topical and systemic antibiotics. (Courtesy of C. Bruce MacDonald, MD.)

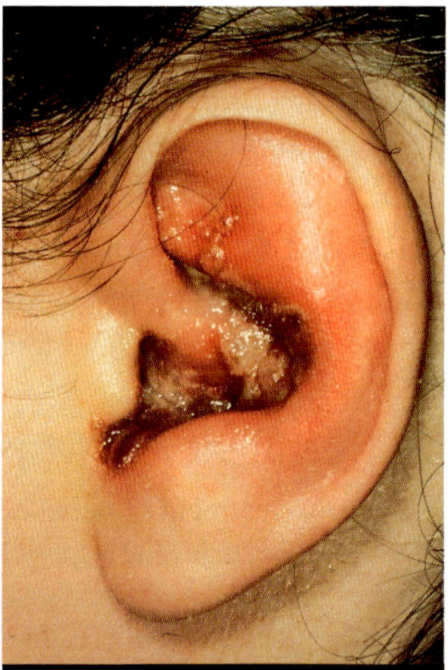

Figure 5.14 Herpes Zoster Oticus

The appearance of erythema and drainage coming from the EAC is seen in this patient with herpes zoster oticus. Otitis externa can have a similar appearance, but does not have vesicles, as seen in this patient. (Courtesy of Robin T. Cotton, MD.)

Associated Clinical Features

Perichondritis is an infection of the auricular cartilage, which can result from trauma hematoma; thermal injuries, frostbite; external auditory canal foreign bodies; chronic otitis media; otitis externa; skin infections; chronic mastoiditis; and surgical procedures. Destruction and necrosis of the auricular cartilage can lead to a flaccid, flat ear.

Infections of skin structures and trauma typically involve streptococci and staphylococci. Ear and mastoid sources frequently involve gram-negative organisms. Untreated perichondritis in the elderly diabetic, and immunocompromised, can lead to malignant external otitis.

Patients present with severe pain and diffuse swelling of the ear. Physical examination reveals an erythematous, swollen, warm, and tender pinna (Fig. 5.15). Advanced cases can present with necrosis of the ear cartilage and spreading cellulitis.

Differential Diagnosis

Cellulitis can mimic perichondritis but has facial involvement. Contact dermatitis can develop from topical ear medications and jewelry.

ED Treatment and Disposition

Immediate treatment of perichondritis is essential to preserve the external ear cartilage. Early perichondritis is treated by irrigation and debridement of any abscess, with administration of broad spectrum antibiotics such as penicillinase-resistant penicillins, amoxicillin-clavulanate, first-generation cephalosporins, or ciprofloxacin. Topical antibiotics are ineffective. A compressive mastoid and auricular dressing is beneficial. Strict follow-up is essential to prevent treatment failure and progression of infection. Advanced perichondritis requires high-dose parenteral antibiotics and early specialist referral for surgical irrigation and debridement.

Clinical Pearl

1. Early diagnosis and treatment is necessary to avoid permanent deformity of the pinna.

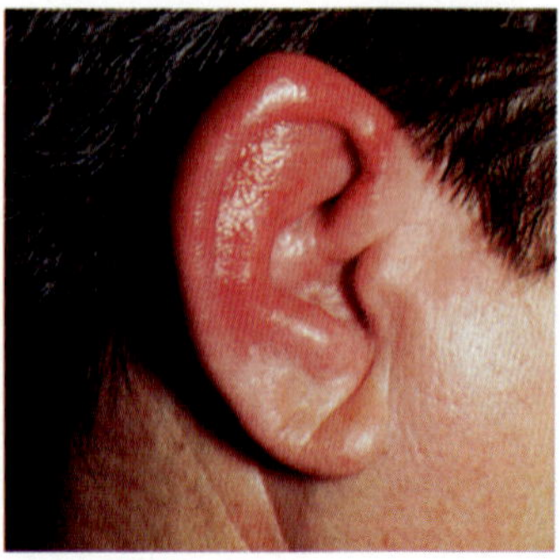

Figure 5.15 Perichondritis

The pinna is swollen and erythematous. No concomitant otitis externa, mastoiditis, or furuncle is noted. (Courtesy of Lawrence B. Stack, MD.)

Associated Clinical Features

The seventh cranial nerve, or facial nerve, provides innervation of the facial muscles via the five branches of the motor root; innervates the submandibular, sublingual, and lacrimal glands, as well as the taste organs on the anterior two-thirds of the tongue; and provides sensation to the pinna of the ear. Seventh-nerve palsies may occur as an isolated finding or as part of a constellation of symptoms. Facial palsies are described as being either central or peripheral. Central seventh-nerve lesions occur before or proximal to the seventh-nerve nucleus in the pons. Lesions that occur distal to the nucleus are classified as peripheral lesions. The hallmark of central lesions is the sparing of the ipsilateral frontalis muscle (Fig. 5.16), since it receives innervation in the nucleus from both ipsilateral and contralateral motor cortices. Peripheral injuries involve the entire side of the face, including the forehead (Fig. 5.17).

The most common etiology of seventh-nerve dysfunction is Bell's palsy, an idiopathic facial nerve dysfunction. Bell's palsy is most likely a viral or postviral syndrome, with 60% of patients having a viral prodrome. Bell's palsy shows no age, sex, or racial predilection. The incidence is higher in pregnant women, diabetics, and in those with a family history of Bell's palsy. It is bilateral in less than 1% of patients.

Patients with Bell's palsy have an acute onset of facial weakness and may note numbness or pain on the ipsilateral face, ear, tongue, and neck, and a decrease or loss of ipsilateral tearing and saliva flow. Hearing in Bell's palsy is preserved.

The prognosis for facial nerve palsies is variable. Facial weakness compared with complete paralysis has a better prognosis for full recovery. Facial palsies due to herpes zoster have a protracted course, and many do not fully resolve. In comparison, 80% of patients with Bell's palsy due to other causes completely recover within 3 months. The recurrence rate of Bell's palsy is 7 to 10%.

Differential Diagnosis

Acoustic neuromas and central nervous system masses have gradual progression of symptoms and cause other neurologic findings. Neurologic disorders, such as Guillain-Barré syndrome, multiple sclerosis, neurosarcoid, and cerebral vascular accidents also cause additional neurologic sequelae. Temporal bone fractures are associated with trauma. The differential diagnosis also includes middle ear infections and parotid tumors.

ED Treatment and Disposition

Initial evaluation is directed by the history. The examination should include a thorough examination of the ear (including sensorineural or conductive hearing loss), the eye (including lacrimation), and the cranial nerves. Motor function of the seventh cranial nerve is evaluated by having the patient raise his or her eyebrows, smile, pucker, and frown. No single laboratory test is diagnostic. A screening head CT is of little value in the absence of additional findings on physical examination.

Most authors empirically recommend steroids for Bell's palsy. A typical regimen is prednisone, 60 mg a day for 10 days, then tapered. If treated within the first 3 weeks, steroids may decrease the sequelae of Bell's palsy. Facial nerve palsies due to Ramsay Hunt syndrome are treated with acyclovir. In all facial nerve palsies, eye lubricants and taping or patching of the eye at night help prevent keratitis and ulceration. Referral to a specialist should be made for follow-up care.

Clinical Pearls

1. Facial nerve paralysis is a symptom, not a diagnosis. The etiology of the paralysis is required before a diagnosis is made.
2. If a provisional diagnosis of Bell's palsy is made and no resolution of symptoms occurs, the diagnosis must be reconsidered. In patients misdiagnosed with Bell's palsy, tumors are the number one missed etiology.
3. Lacrimation is tested by the Schirmer's or litmus test. Asymmetry may indicate a lesion proximal to the geniculate ganglion.

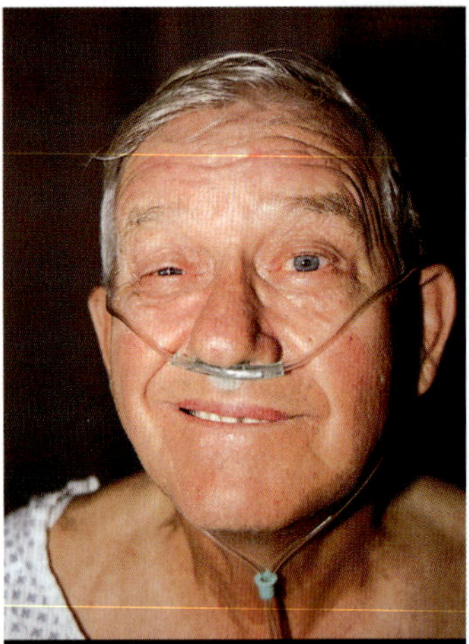

Figure 5.16 Central Seventh-Nerve Palsy

Central facial nerve paralysis with forehead sparing. (Courtesy of Frank Birinyi, MD.)

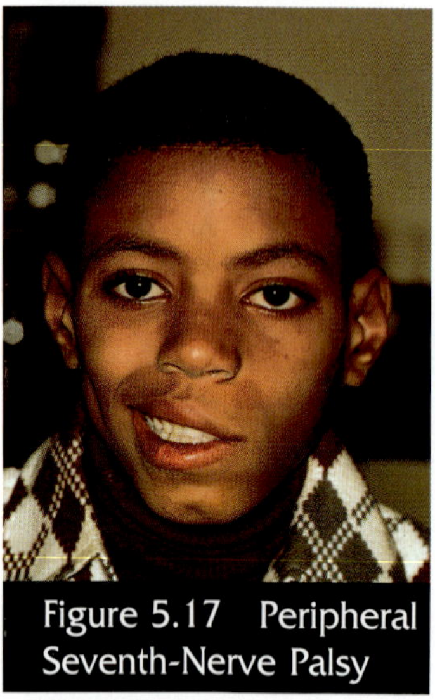

Figure 5.17 Peripheral Seventh-Nerve Palsy

A peripheral nerve paralysis involving the entire ipsilateral face, including the forehead is seen in this patient with Bell's palsy. (Courtesy of Robin T. Cotton, MD.)

Associated Clinical Features

Pharyngitis is an inflammation, and frequently an infection, of the pharynx and its lymphoid tissues, which make up Waldeyer's ring. Most causes of pharyngitis are infectious. Viral infections account for 90% of all cases. Common bacterial agents include group A beta hemolytic streptococci (GABHS, responsible for up to 50% of bacterial cases), other streptococci, *Mycoplasma pneumoniae, Neisseria gonorrhea,* and *Corynebacterium diphtheriae.* In immunocompromised patients and in patients on antibiotics, *Candida* species can cause thrush. Sore throats that last longer than 2 weeks should increase suspicion for either a deep-space neck infection or a neoplastic cause.

Patients with bacterial, and especially GABHS pharyngitis, present with an acute onset of sore throat and fever, and frequently nausea, vomiting, headache, and abdominal cramping. On examination, patients may have a mild to moderate fever, an erythematous posterior pharynx and palatine tonsils, tender cervical lymphadenopathy, and palatal petechiae (Fig. 5.18). Classically, the tonsils have a white or yellow exudate with debris in the crypts; however, many patients may not have exudate on examination. Viral pharyngitis is typically more benign with a gradual onset, lower temperature, and less impressive erythema and swelling of the pharynx. Except for infectious mononucleosis (Fig. 5.19), which can take weeks to resolve, most cases of viral pharyngitis are self-limited with spontaneous resolution in a matter of days. Lingual and adenoid tonsillitis may also be present (Fig. 5.20).

Differential Diagnosis

Deep-space neck infections, diphtheria, epiglottitis, infectious mononucleosis, and Ludwig's angina are other infectious causes of sore throats that should be considered. Allergic rhinitis, angioedema, and pharyngeal neoplasms are noninfectious causes of similar pharyngeal symptoms. Foreign bodies and local pharyngeal trauma produce similar symptoms but usually have an antecedent event.

ED Treatment and Disposition

Treatment is largely symptomatic, except for antibiotics and rehydration. Current first-line antibiotic therapies are intramuscular benzathine penicillin or oral penicillin. Patients allergic to penicillin should receive erythromycin for primary prophylaxis against rheumatic fever. Other suitable antibiotics are macrolides and second-generation cephalosporins. Analgesics, antipyretics, and throat sprays or gargles can provide symptomatic relief.

Clinical Pearls

1. The physical examination should not end at the neck. Auscultation of the chest, palpation of the abdomen, and examination of the skin are also important.
2. Sore throats or chronic pharyngitis that lasts more than 2 weeks must be referred for further evaluation to rule out possible neoplastic or neurologic causes, especially in patients over 50 years old who have a smoking or chewing tobacco history.
3. Recurrent tonsillitis in children merits referral for possible adenoid tonsillectomy.
4. Amoxicillin should be avoided if infectious mononucleosis is a possibility, as a diffuse maculopapular rash will occur in up to 80% of those treated with amoxicillin.
5. Pharyngitis itself may be a prodrome for other pathologic conditions, such as measles, scarlet fever, and influenza.

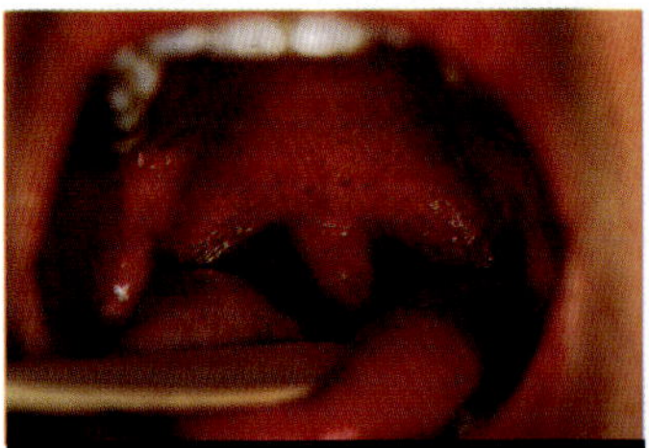

Figure 5.18 Palatal Petechiae

Palatal petechiae and erythema of the tonsillar pillars in a patient with streptococcal pharyngitis. (Courtesy of Kevin J. Knoop, MD, MS.)

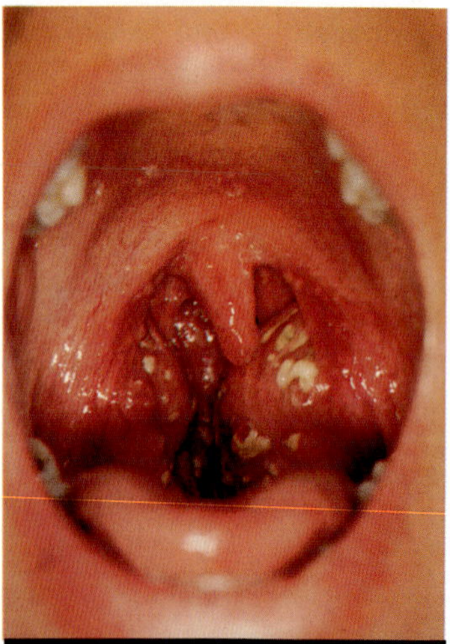

Figure 5.19 Exudative Pharyngitis

Exudative pharyngitis showing erythema and tonsillar exudate in a patient with viral mononucleosis. (Courtesy of George L. Murrell, MD.)

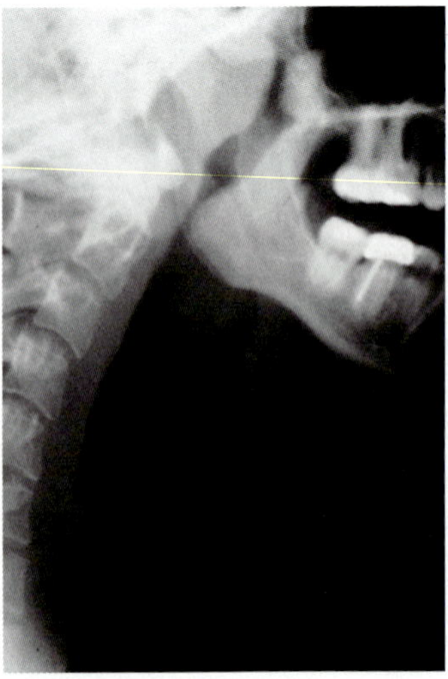

Figure 5.20 Lingual Tonsillitis

A radiograph showing lingual and adenoid tonsillitis. (Courtesy of Edward C. Jauch, MD, MS.)

Associated Clinical Features

Ranulas are mucoceles (mucous retention cysts) that develop in the floor of the mouth, arising from obstructed sublingual or submandibular ducts, or smaller minor salivary glands. At first the cysts are small and barely noticeable, but over time they can expand outward or deeper into the neck (plunging ranula). Large cysts can displace the tongue forward and upward, making the patient uncomfortable. Contrary to sialolithiasis, patients may not always notice an increase in swelling associated with eating. Physical examination reveals a soft, minimally tender translucent cyst with dilated veins running over its surface (Fig. 5.21). Unlike carcinomas, no ulceration is noted, and ranulas are generally softer.

Differential Diagnosis

Torus mandibularis is a hard bony growth off the lingual surface of the mandible. Obstructed major salivary glands are often painful and intermittent. Carcinomas of the mouth are slower growing and firm. Abscesses and local cellulitis also produce sublingual swelling.

ED Treatment and Disposition

Recognition by the physician is essential for proper referral. Definitive treatment is excision or marsupialization, although needle aspiration of the cyst can provide temporary relief. Unless secondarily infected, no antibiotic coverage is required.

Clinical Pearls

1. Most ranulas are painless and are incidental findings on routine examinations.
2. Ranulas often recur, requiring total excision of the offending salivary gland.

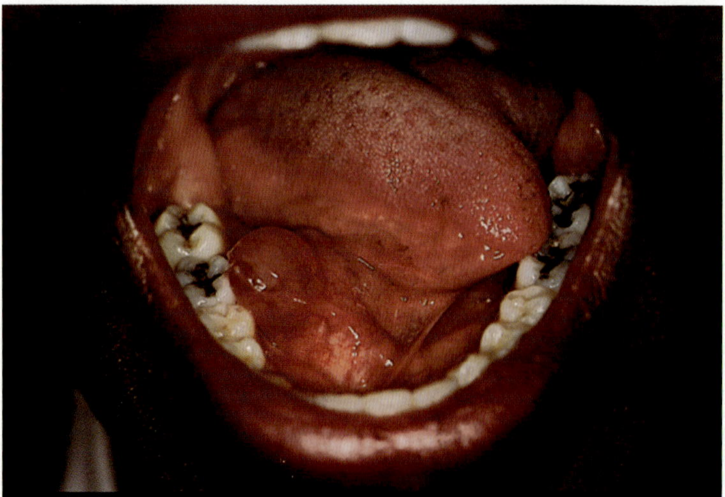

Figure 5.21 Ranula

Sublingual ranula, or mucocele, lateral to Wharton's duct. The patient was asymptomatic except for being aware of the lesion. (Courtesy of Kevin J. Knoop, MD, MS.)

CHAPTER 6

MOUTH

Edwin D. Turner
Edward C. Jauch
Sarah J. Gahm

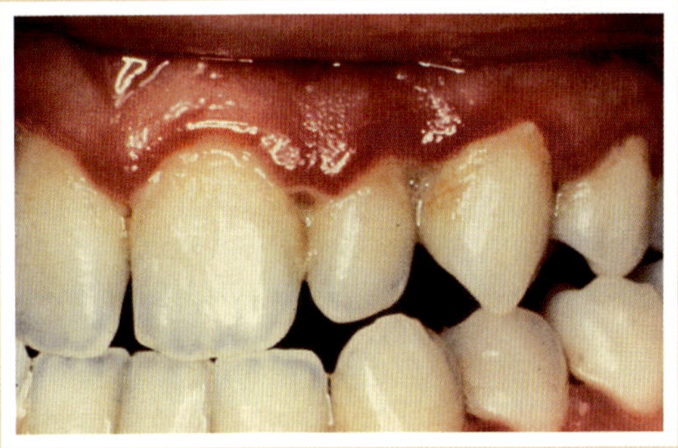

Associated Clinical Features

Tooth subluxation refers to the loosening of a tooth in its alveolar socket. Traumatic oral injury is a common mechanism by which dental subluxation occurs; however, infection and chronic periodontal disease may also produce loosening of teeth. Gingival lacerations and alveolar fractures are commonly associated with dental subluxations. Subluxated, or loosened, teeth are diagnosed by applying gentle pressure to the teeth with a tongue blade or fingertip. Mild displacement may also be noted (Fig. 6.1). Blood along the crevice of the gingiva, where the tooth meets the gingiva, is also a sign of subluxation. Various degrees of tooth mobility may be noted on examination.

Differential Diagnosis

Dental impaction and alveolar ridge fracture should be considered and ruled out clinically and with radiographs.

ED Treatment and Disposition

1. *Primary teeth:* If the subluxated tooth is forced into close proximity to the underlying permanent tooth, extraction by a dentist or oral surgeon is indicated. Otherwise, the patient should be instructed to follow a soft diet for 1 to 2 weeks, allowing the tooth to reimplant.
2. *Permanent teeth:* If the tooth is unstable, it should be temporarily immobilized. This may be accomplished with gauze packing, a figure-eight suture around the tooth and an adjacent tooth, aluminum foil, or a special periodontal dressing (COE-pak). The patient should be referred for dental follow-up.

Clinical Pearls

1. Any evidence of tooth mobility following trauma is a subluxation by definition.
2. Always consider the possibility of an associated underlying alveolar fracture.

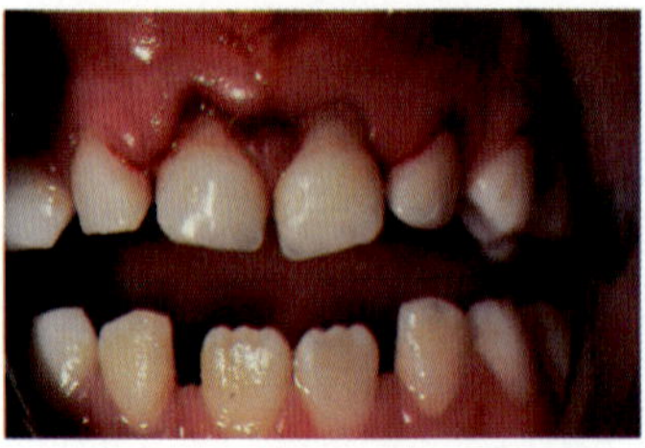

Figure 6.1 Tooth Subluxation

Note the presence of blood along the crevice of the gingival margin of both central incisors—an indication of subluxation following trauma. Mild displacement of the subluxated teeth is noted. (Courtesy of James F. Steiner, DDS.)

Associated Clinical Features

Anatomically, each tooth has a crown and root portion. Externally the crown is covered with white enamel and the root portion with cementum. The cementoenamel junction (cervical line) is where the crown and root meet. The yellow-to-tan dentin is the second innermost layer and composes the bulk of the tooth. The red-to-pink pulp tissue is located in the center of the tooth and furnishes the neurovascular supply to the tooth. The Ellis classification system is used to describe tooth fractures (Fig. 6.2):

Ellis class I: Involves the enamel only (Fig. 6.3).

Ellis class II: Involves the enamel plus exposure of the dentin (Fig. 6.4). The patient may complain of temperature sensitivity.

Ellis class III: Fracture extends into the pulp. A pink or bloody discoloration on the fracture surface is diagnostic of this type of fracture (Fig. 6.5). The patient may have severe pain, but may also have no pain, due to loss of nerve function.

Differential Diagnosis

Subluxation, alveolar fracture, avulsion, or a traumatic impaction are in the differential. Dental fractures may also be occult and occur below the gum line or at the level of root. Radiographic evaluation will aid in differentiating these conditions.

ED Treatment and Disposition

Ellis class I: Pain control should be initiated. Rough tooth edges may be smoothed with an emery board. Immediate dental referral within 24 h is indicated when soft-tissue injury is caused by sharp pieces of the tooth.

Ellis class II: Patients under 12 years of age have less dentin than older patients and are at risk for infection of the pulp. They should have a calcium hydroxide dressing placed, coverage with gauze or aluminum foil, and see a dentist within 24 h. Older patients should be advised to see a dentist within 24 to 48 h.

Ellis class III: This is considered a dental emergency, and immediate dental consultation is indicated. Delay in treatment may result in severe pain and abscess formation.

Clinical Pearls

1. The anterior teeth are most commonly involved because of more direct exposure to trauma.
2. Consider child abuse when dental injuries occur in young children.

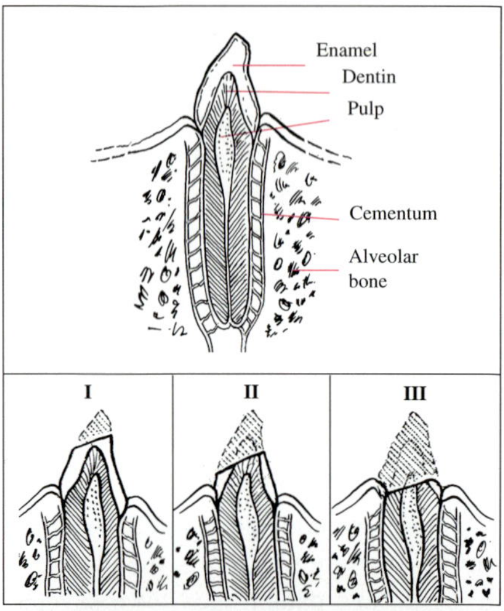

Figure 6.2 Tooth Fractures

Enamel, dentin, and pulp are the anatomic landmarks used in the Ellis classification of tooth fractures.

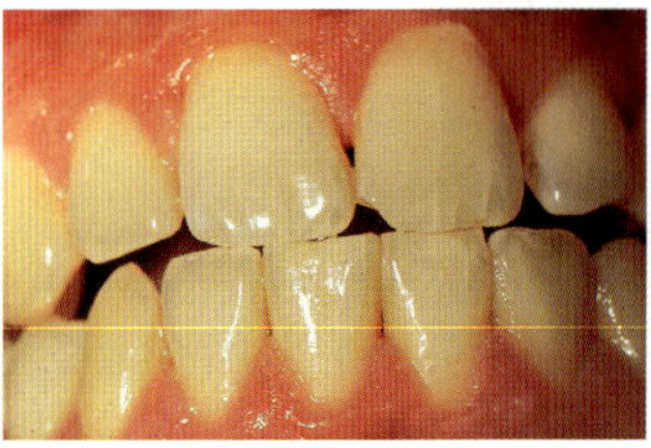

Figure 6.3 Ellis Class I Tooth Fracture

Note the fracture of the left upper central incisor. The sole involvement of the enamel is consistent with an Ellis type I injury. (Courtesy of James F. Steiner, DDS.)

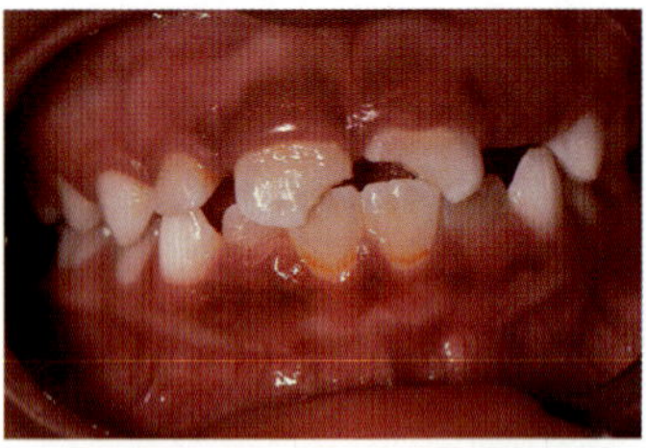

Figure 6.4 Ellis Class II Tooth Fractures

Bilateral maxillary central incisor injuries with exposed enamel and dentin consistent with an Ellis class II fracture. (Courtesy of James F. Steiner, DDS.)

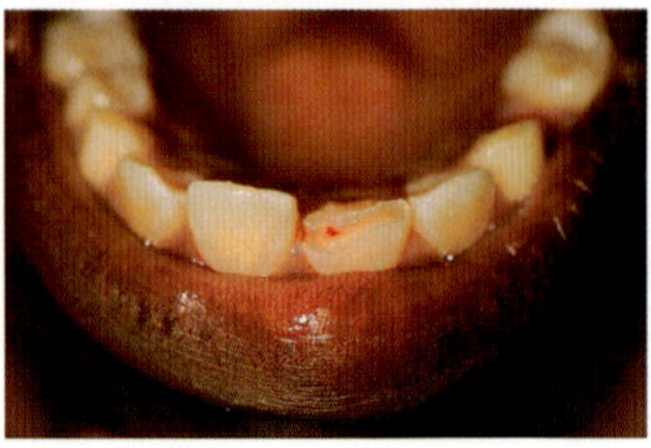

Figure 6.5 Ellis Class III Tooth Fracture

A fracture demonstrating blood at the exposed dental pulp. This sign is pathognomonic for an Ellis class III fracture. (Courtesy of Kevin J. Knoop, MD, MS.)

Associated Clinical Features

Dislocation generally results from direct trauma to the chin while the mouth is open, or more commonly in predisposed individuals after a vigorous yawn. Opening the mouth excessively wide while eating or laughing may also result in dislocation. Acute dislocation occurs when the mandibular condyles displace forward and become locked anterior to the articular eminence. Muscle spasm contributes to prevention of spontaneous relocation. Weakness of the temporal mandibular ligament, an overstretched joint capsule, and a shallow articular eminence are predisposing factors. Patients usually present with an inability to close an open mouth (Fig. 6.6). Other associated symptoms include pain, discomfort, and facial swelling near the temporal mandibular joint (TMJ). Difficulty speaking and swallowing is common. Anterior dislocations are most common; however, posterior dislocation may occur with significant force in association with a basilar skull fracture. Unilateral dislocation results in deviation of the mandible to the unaffected side (Fig. 6.7).

Differential Diagnosis

Temporal mandibular joint hemarthrosis, dystonic reactions, and hysterical dislocation can mimic the true process of TMJ dislocation. Unilateral or bilateral mandible fractures should also be strongly considered, particularly if there is a history of facial trauma.

ED Treatment and Disposition

Acute reduction of pain, muscle spasm, and anxiety is achieved using reassurance, analgesics, and muscle relaxants. Panorex or TMJ x-ray films (pre- and post-reduction) are obtained to exclude a fracture (Fig. 6.8). The patient is typically treated in the sitting position. While facing the patient, the physician grasps the angles of the mandible with both hands. The thumbs are wrapped in gauze for protection and rest on the occlusive surfaces of the molars while downward and backward pressure is applied until the condyle slides back into the articular eminence. Instruct the patient to avoid excessively wide mouth opening while eating and yawning for 3 to 4 weeks. Apply warm compresses to the TMJ areas. A soft diet for 1 week is advised, as is the use of nonsteroidal anti-inflammatory drugs as needed. Dental follow-up should be arranged.

Clinical Pearls

1. Approximately 70% of the general population can subluxate the mandible partially and then spontaneously reduce it.
2. TMJ dysfunction secondary to a neuroleptic or antipsychotic medication–related dystonic reaction is treated with diphenhydramine or benztropine.
3. When trauma is the cause of TMJ dislocation, maintain a high index of suspicion for cervical spine injury.

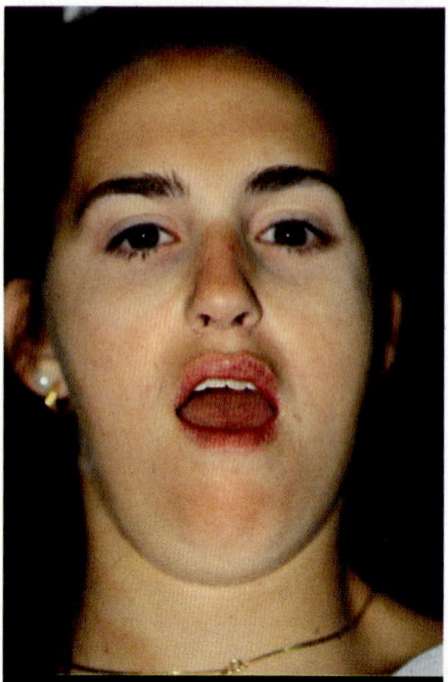

Figure 6.6 TMJ Dislocation (Bilateral)

This patient awoke from sleep with the inability to close her mouth. Note the dry lips and tongue secondary to prolonged exposure. (Courtesy of Warren K. Russell, MD.)

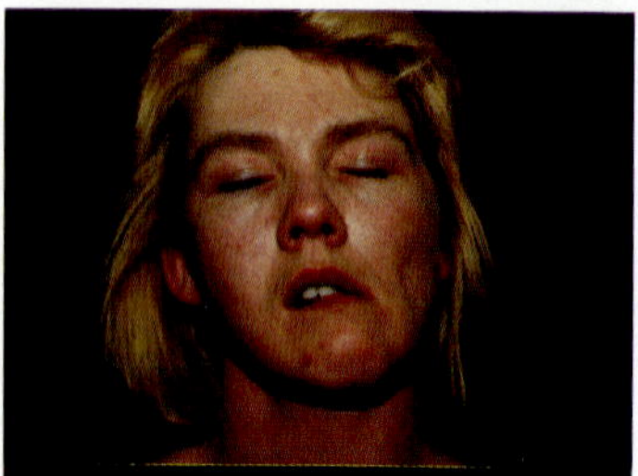

Figure 6.7 TMJ Dislocation (Unilateral)

Note the asymmetric jaw deviation toward the unaffected side. Always consider the possibility of an associated underlying fracture or cervical spine injury. (Courtesy of Kevin J. Knoop, MD, MS.)

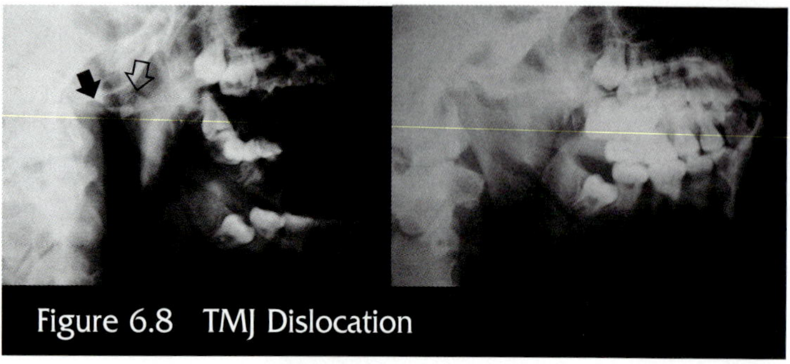

Figure 6.8 TMJ Dislocation

Left. Radiographic demonstration of an anterior TMJ dislocation. The location of the condyle is indicated by the open arrow. The position of the mandibular notch is indicated by the closed arrow. *Right.* Postreduction radiograph showing normal positioning of the condyle in the mandibular notch. (Courtesy of Edwin D. Turner, MD.)

Associated Clinical Features

Gingival abscesses tend to involve the marginal gingiva, and result from entrapment of food and plaque debris in a gingival pocket with subsequent staphylococcal, streptococcal, anaerobic, or mixed bacteria overgrowth leading to abscess formation. Localized swelling, erythema, tenderness, and possible fluctuance in the space between the tooth and the gingiva (the so-called pocket) is the usual location. There may be spontaneous purulent drainage from the gingival margin, or an area of pointing may be seen. In cases of acute gingival abscess formation, pus may be expressed from the gingival margin by gentle digital pressure. When the gingival abscess involves the deeper supporting periodontal structures, it is referred to as a periodontal abscess (Fig. 6.9). These may present as a fluctuant vestibular abscess or with a draining sinus that opens onto the gingival surface.

Differential Diagnosis

Periapical abscesses are deep and not obvious on inspection. They usually present as tenderness to percussion or pain with chewing over the involved tooth, unlike gingival abscesses. A parulis may also simulate a gingival abscess; however, a parulis represents the cutaneous manifestation of a deeper periapical abscess. Unlike a parulis or periapical abscesses, gingival abscesses are not usually associated with dental caries or fillings. Pericoronal abscesses tend to involve the gingiva overlying a partially erupted third molar and should be considered in the differential diagnosis.

ED Treatment and Disposition

The initial management is a small incision with drainage and warm saline irrigation. Removal of entrapped food and debris is performed. Oral antibiotic therapy with penicillin or clindamycin is recommended. Analgesics should be provided along with dental follow-up. The patient's tetanus status should be addressed.

Clinical Pearls

1. Patients with gingival abscesses are usually afebrile.
2. Consider more extensive abscess formation and oral disease processes in the febrile toxic-appearing patient.
3. Patients with chronic deep periodontal abscesses complain of dull gnawing pain as well as a desire to bite down on and grind the tooth.

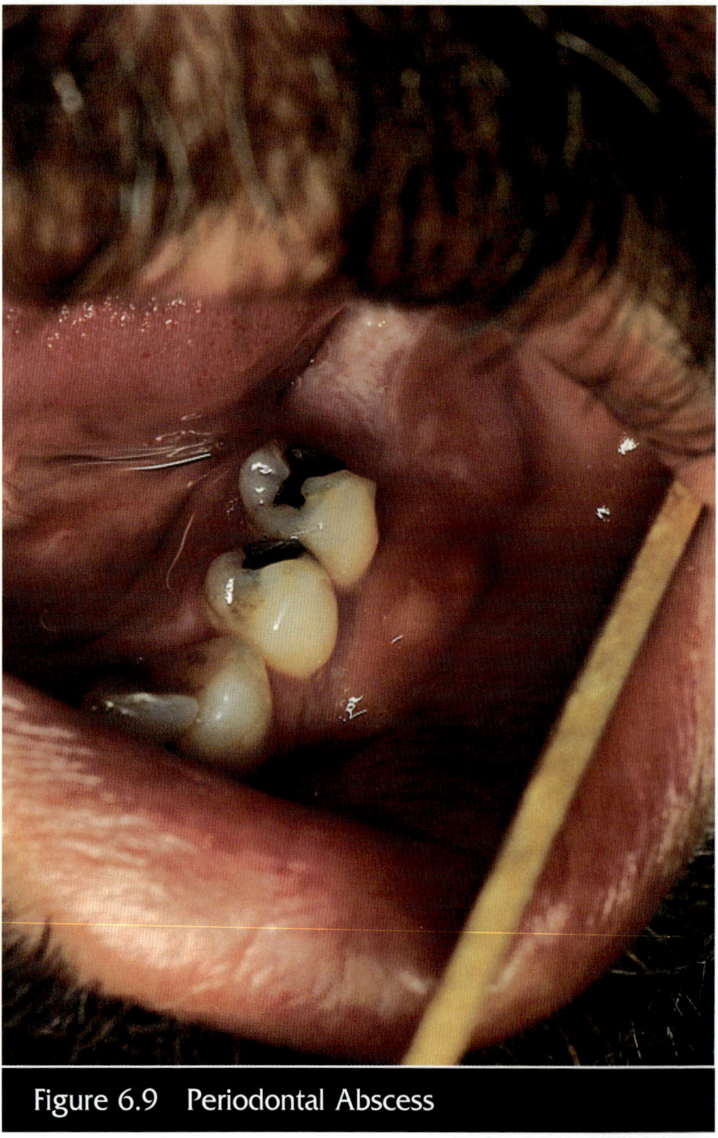

Figure 6.9 Periodontal Abscess

Localized gingival swelling, erythema, and fluctuance are seen in this periodontal abscess with spontaneous purulent drainage. (Courtesy of Kevin J. Knoop, MD, MS.)

Associated Clinical Features

Acute pain, swelling, and mild tooth elevation is characteristic of a periapical abscess. Exquisite sensitivity to percussion or chewing on the involved tooth is a common sign. The involved tooth may have had a root canal treatment, a filling, or a dental carie. Periapical abscesses may enlarge over time and "point" internally on the lingual or buccal mucosal surfaces, or extraorally with swelling and redness of the overlying skin. Occasionally these lesions may tract up to the alveolar periosteum and gingival surface to form a parulis ("gumboil"). Radiographically, these abscesses appear as well circumscribed areas of radiolucency at the dental apex or along the lateral aspect of the root (Fig. 6.10). Early acute periapical abscesses may not demonstrate any radiographic changes. Both deep periodontal and periapical abscesses may have sinuses draining purulent material onto the gingival surface. If the infection is allowed to progress, it can erode through the nearest cortical bone, manifesting itself in a variety of locations (Fig. 6.11).

Differential Diagnosis

Gingival or deep periodontal abscess, buccal space abscess, and unilateral sublingual, parapharyngeal, and submandibular space abscesses should all be considered in the differential diagnosis. All the aforementioned may present with oral pain, tenderness, facial swelling, and possible fever. Panorex films, dental radiographs, or a CT scan may aid in making the diagnosis.

ED Treatment and Disposition

NSAIDs or oral narcotics for pain should be administered as well as oropharyngeal antibiotic therapy. A regional nerve block may be performed with a local anesthetic agent for more immediate temporary relief. Administer tetanus toxoid if indicated. Dental consultation or follow-up in 1 to 2 days is recommended for endodontic evaluation or possible extraction of the involved tooth. Incision and drainage with saline irrigation and prompt referral constitutes the initial treatment of a parulis.

Clinical Pearls

1. More than one tooth may be involved simultaneously.
2. Exquisite tenderness and pain on tooth percussion is a key feature on physical examination and identifies the involved tooth.
3. Periapical abscesses are almost always associated with carious or nonviable teeth.

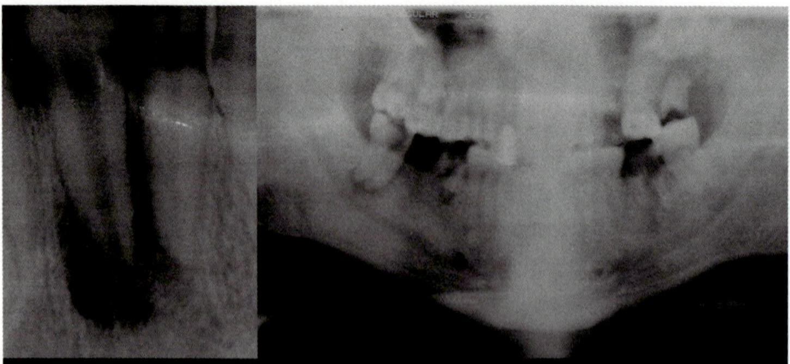

Figure 6.10 Periapical Abscess

Left. Note the well defined radiolucent area at the apex and lateral root of the tooth in this radiograph. (Courtesy of James L. Kretzschmar, DDS, MS.) *Right.* This Panorex film shows several areas consistent with periapical abscesses. (Courtesy of David P. Kretzschmar, DDS, MS.)

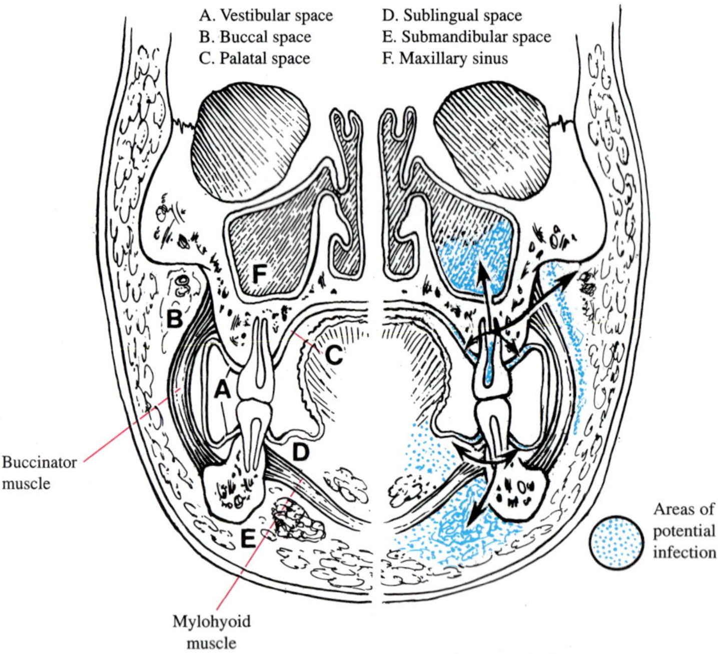

Figure 6.11 Odontogenic Abscesses

As infection progresses from the pulp at the tooth apex, it erodes through the bone and can express itself in a variety of places. This illustration notes several possible locations or spaces. (Adapted with permission from Cummings C, Schuller D (eds): *Otolaryngology Head and Neck Surgery,* 1st ed. Chicago, Mosby-Year Book, 1986.)

Associated Clinical Features

A partially erupted or impacted third molar (wisdom tooth) is the most common site of pericoronitis and pericoronal abscesses. The accumulation of food and debris between the overlying gingival flap and crown of the tooth sets up the foci for pericoronitis and subsequent abscess formation. The gingival flap becomes irritated and inflamed. The area is also repeatedly traumatized by the opposing molar tooth and may interfere with complete jaw closure as swelling and tenderness increases. The inflamed gingival process may eventually become infected and form a fluctuant abscess (Fig. 6.12). Foul taste, inability to close the jaw, and fever may occur. Swelling of the cheek and angle of the jaw as well as localized lymphadenopathy are also characteristic. More advanced disease may spread posteriorly to the base of the tongue and oropharyngeal area. Potential spread into the deep cervical spaces is also an important concern with extensive processes.

Differential Diagnosis

Ludwig's angina, peritonsillar abscess, gingival abscess, buccal space abscess, and a severe periapical abscess may all present similar to a pericoronal abscess. Ludwig's angina and peritonsillar abscesses are in fact potential sequelae of acute pericoronitis and pericoronal abscesses.

ED Treatment and Disposition

Superficial incision and drainage with warm saline irrigation may be performed initially in the emergency department. Adequate analgesia and antibiotic coverage should be provided. Consultation or referral to an oral and maxillofacial surgeon for follow-up is indicated for possible extraction of the involved teeth.

Clinical Pearls

1. Pericoronitis and abscess formation rarely occur in the pediatric population and tend to be late adolescent and adult processes.
2. The mandibular third molar is the most commonly involved tooth.
3. Airway compromise is a potential complication with posterior extension of a pericoronal abscess.

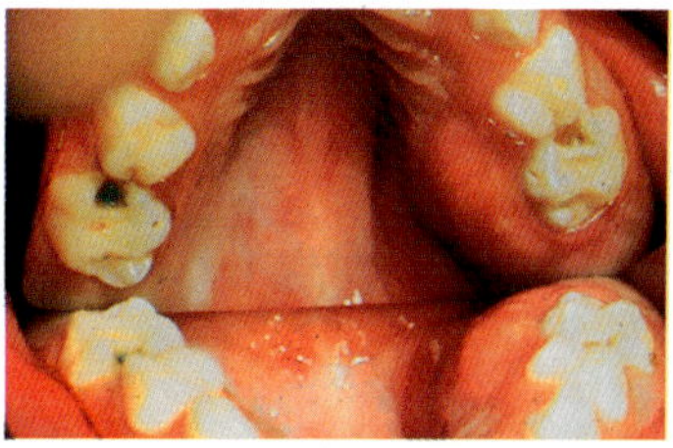

Figure 6.12 Pericoronal Abscess

Note the inflamed fluctuant gingival tissue approximating the incompletely erupted third molar. (Courtesy of James F. Steiner, DDS.)

Associated Clinical Features

The buccal space lies anatomically between the buccinator muscle and the overlying superficial fascia and skin. The maxillary second and third molar teeth are the usual source of infection contributing to buccal space abscesses. Infection from the involved teeth erodes through the maxillary alveolar bone superiorly into the buccal space (Fig. 6.13). Rarely, the third mandibular molar may be the source. In this instance, the infection erodes through the mandibular alveolar bone inferiorly into the buccal space. These patients present with unilateral facial swelling, redness, and tenderness to the cheek (Fig. 6.14). Trismus is generally not present.

Differential Diagnosis

Canine space abscess, parapharyngeal abscess, facial cellulitis, Ludwig's angina, and masticator space abscess formation are all conditions that may resemble buccal space abscesses. Inspection of all the maxillary and third mandibular molar teeth is essential to help make the diagnosis. A CT scan can aid in localizing the space involved.

ED Treatment and Disposition

Parenteral antibiotic therapy with penicillin or a third-generation cephalosporin is recommended. Antibiotic coverage for anaerobic organisms may also be added to the treatment regimen. NSAIDs or mild oral narcotic analgesics should be provided as indicated. Dental or oral surgical consultation is necessary for intramural abscess drainage and endodontic therapy versus extraction of the involved molar teeth.

Clinical Pearls

1. Ovoid cheek swelling with sparing of the nasolabial fold helps to identify buccal space abscesses and differentiates it from canine space abscesses.
2. Odontogenic infections of the second or third maxillary molars is the most common source for buccal space abscesses.

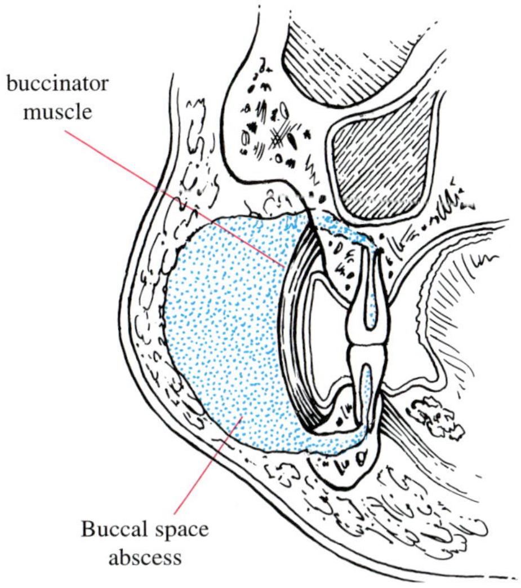

Figure 6.13 Buccal Space Anatomy

The buccal space lies between the buccinator muscle and the overlying skin and superficial fascia. This potential space may become involved by maxillary or mandibular molars. (Adapted with permission from Cummings C, Schuller D (eds): *Otolaryngology Head and Neck Surgery,* 2d ed. Chicago, Mosby-Year Book, 1993.)

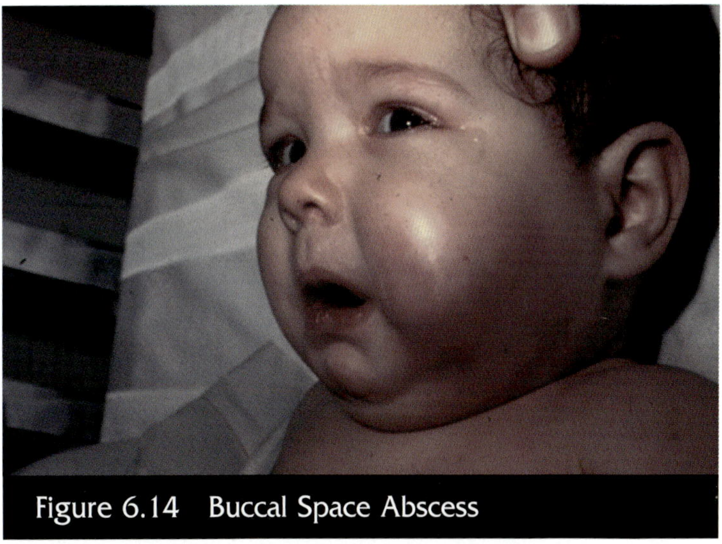

Figure 6.14 Buccal Space Abscess

Note the ovoid cheek swelling with sparing of the nasolabial fold. This finding along with accompanying redness and tenderness helps to identify buccal space abscess formation. (Courtesy of Michael J. Nowicki, MD.)

Associated Clinical Features

The canine space lies between the anterior surface of the maxilla and levator labii superioris muscle of the face. The origin of these abscesses can be from upper anterior teeth and bicuspids, although it is almost exclusively from the maxillary canine tooth. Erosion of maxillary tooth infection through the alveolar bone into the canine space leads to abscess formation, although cutaneous infections from the upper lip and nose are a rare source. Unilateral facial redness, pain, and swelling lateral to the nose with obliteration of the nasolabial fold is characteristic (Fig. 6.15). Severe upper lip and lower eyelid swelling may cause eye closure and drooling at the corner of the mouth.

Differential Diagnosis

Buccal space infection, facial cellulitis, and maxillary sinusitis may present with various clinical features similar to canine space abscesses. Examination of the anterior maxillary teeth may provide very helpful clues to the origin and diagnosis of canine space abscesses. CT scan and sinus x-rays may aid in defining these lesions.

ED Treatment and Disposition

Parenteral antibiotic therapy is to include anaerobic coverage indicated for treatment. Dental or oral surgical consultation for intramural incision and drainage represents the most definitive treatment for canine space abscesses. Extraction or endodontic treatment of the involved anterior maxillary teeth is usually necessary.

Clinical Pearls

1. The maxillary canine (cuspid) teeth are the most common source for canine space abscesses.
2. Although these patients may drool when significant upper lip swelling is present, they typically do not have trismus, dysphagia, or odynophagia.

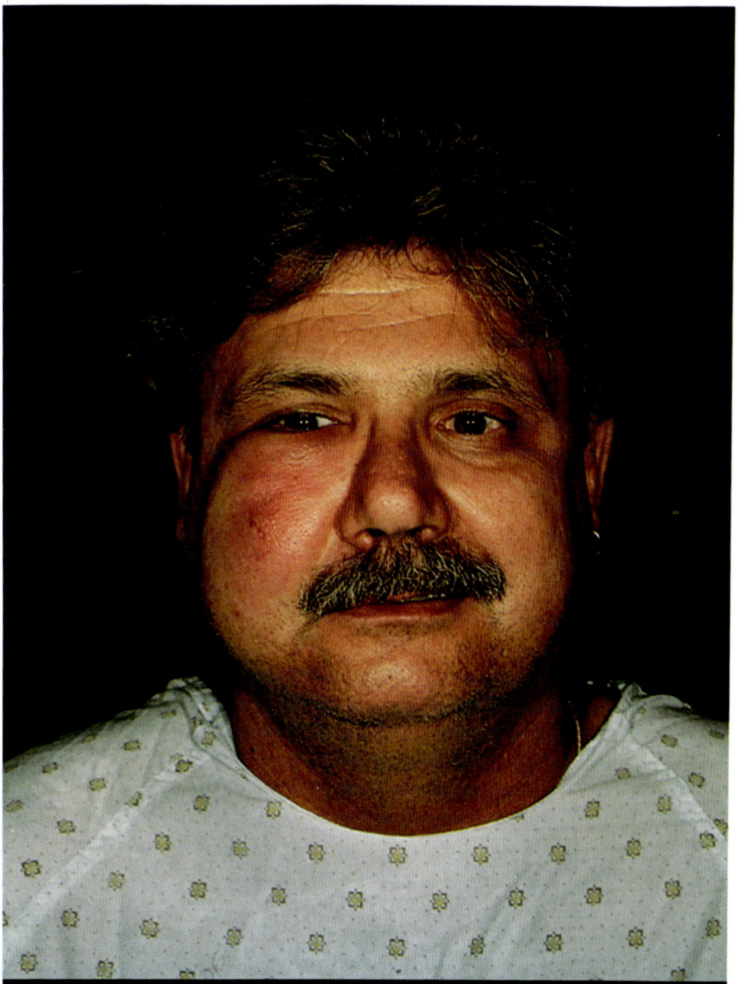

Figure 6.15 Canine Space Abscess

Unilateral facial swelling lateral to the nose with associated redness and the typical loss of the nasolabial fold is shown. The maxillary canine tooth is usually the source of this process. (Courtesy of Frank Birinyi, MD.)

Associated Clinical Features

Painful, severely edematous interdental papillae is characteristic of acute necrotizing ulcerative gingivitis (ANUG). Other associated features include the presence of ulcers with an overlying grayish pseudomembrane and "punched out" appearance (Fig. 6.16). The inflamed gingival tissue is very friable, necrotic, and represents an acute destructive disease process of the periodontium. Fever, malaise, and regional lymphadenopathy are commonly associated signs. Patients may also complain of foul breath and a strong metallic taste. Poor hygiene, emotional stress, smoking, and immunocompromised states all may contribute to predisposition for ANUG. Anaerobic *Fusobacterium* and spirochetes are the predominant bacterial organisms involved. The anterior incisor and posterior molar gingival regions are the most commonly affected oral tissue.

Differential Diagnosis

Acute herpetic gingivostomatitis, aphthous stomatitis, desquamative gingivitis, gonococcal and streptococcal gingivostomatitis, and chronic periodontal disease all represent oral diseases which may mimic ANUG. Differentiating these oral conditions from one another is based primarily on history and a thorough oropharyngeal examination.

ED Treatment and Disposition

Initial management includes warm saline irrigation. Systemic analgesics and topical anesthetics such as viscous lidocaine may facilitate oral hygiene measures. Antibiotic treatment is initiated immediately with oropharyngial coverage. Dilute 1.5 to 2% hydrogen peroxide oral rinses are also helpful. Follow-up with a dentist or periodontist in 1 to 2 days is recommended. Patients with more advanced disease may require admission and oral surgical consultation.

Clinical Pearls

1. Dramatic relief of symptoms within 24 h of initiating antibiotics supportive treatment is characteristic.
2. Periodontal abscesses and underlying alveolar bone destruction are common complications of ANUG and dental follow-up.
3. There is no evidence that ANUG is a communicable disease.
4. Gingivitis is a nontender inflammatory disorder.

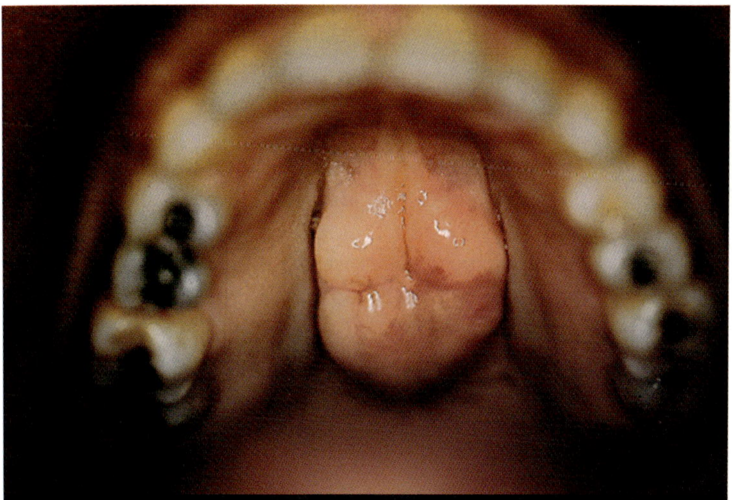

Figure 6.16 Acute Necrotizing Ulcerative Gingivitis

Note the inflamed, friable, and necrotic gingival tissue. An overlying grayish pseudomembrane or punched-out ulcerations of the interdental papillae are pathognomonic. (Courtesy of David P. Kretzschmar, DDS, MS.)

Associated Clinical Features

White, flaky, curdlike plaques covering the tongue and buccal mucosa with an erythematous base is typical of thrush (Fig. 6.17). These lesions tend to be painless; however, painful inflammatory erosions or ulcers may be noted, particularly in adults. Decreased oral intake secondary to pain is common. Colonization of surface epithelium by *Candida* may be opportunistic as a result of an altered oral milieu. Predisposing factors include antibiotic use, corticosteroids, radiation to the head and neck, extremes of ages, patients with immunologic deficiencies, and chronic irritation (e.g., denture use and xerostomia).

Differential Diagnosis

Hairy leukoplakia, lingual lichen planus, flecks of milk or food debris, and liquid antacid adhering to the tongue may be confused with candidiasis. Hairy leukoplakia cannot be brushed off with a tongue depressor. This helps differentiate this process from thrush or residue from ingested materials. Microscopic examination of the removed specimen for the presence of hyphae in potassium hydroxide mount will aid in the identification of *Candida*.

ED Treatment and Disposition

Nystatin oral tablets, nystatin suspension, or clotrimazole oral troches are usually adequate therapy. Topical analgesic cocktails may also provide comfort for patients (e.g., Maalox™, diphenhydramine, viscous lidocaine oral rinse).

Clinical Pearls

1. Thrush is most common in premature infants and immunosuppressed patients.
2. In young adults thrush may be the first sign of AIDS; a history of HIV risk factors should be elicited.

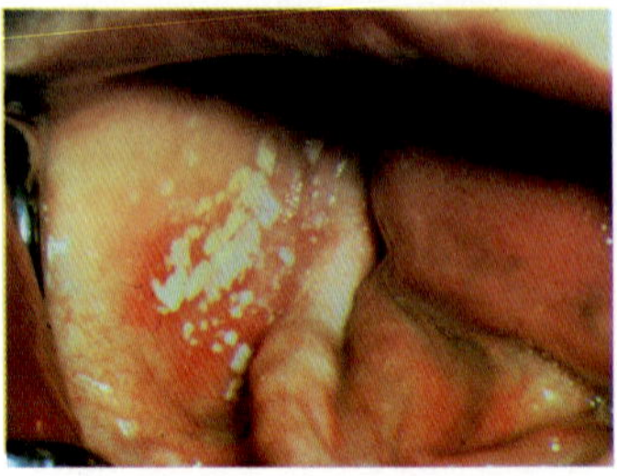

Figure 6.17 Oral Candidiasis (Thrush)

Whitish plaques are seen here on the buccal mucosa. These plaques are easily removed with a tongue blade, differentiating them from lichen planus or leukoplakia. (Courtesy of James F. Steiner, DDS.)

Associated Clinical Features

Kaposi's sarcoma is the most common AIDS-related malignancy. For unknown reasons, it is more common in homosexual men with HIV than in other HIV-positive groups. The most common intraoral site for Kaposi's sarcoma is the palate (Fig. 6.18). It may, however, be found anywhere in the mouth or in different locations of the body. It appears as vascularlike, flat, bluish-red patches with irregular borders. Kaposi's sarcoma alone is generally not associated with a significant morbidity or mortality.

Differential Diagnosis

Ecchymosis, hemangioma, purpura, lymphoma, and oral nevus formation all represent oral conditions which may mimic Kaposi's sarcoma.

ED Treatment and Disposition

Referral for HIV testing, counseling, and biopsy of the lesion is the recommended management. Radiation and chemotherapy are generally reserved for cosmetically disfiguring, extensive, and very painful lesions.

Clinical Pearls

1. Kaposi's sarcoma is the most common cutaneous manifestation of AIDS.
2. Kaposi's sarcoma is the second most common overall manifestation of AIDS, *Pneumocystis carinii* being the first.

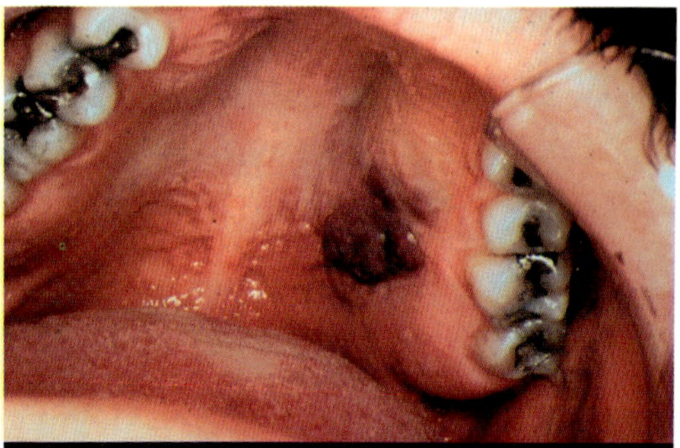

Figure 6.18 Oral Kaposi's Sarcoma

Note the typical bluish-red coloration and the irregular borders commonly found with these lesions. The palate is the most common intraoral location for Kaposi's sarcoma. (Courtesy of James F. Steiner, DDS.)

Associated Clinical Features

Oral herpes simplex may present acutely as a primary gingivostomatitis, or as a recurrence. Painful vesicular eruptions on the oral mucosa, tongue, palate, vermilion borders, and gingiva are highly characteristic (Fig. 6.19). A 2- to 3-day prodromal period of malaise, fever, and cervical adenopathy is common. The vesicular lesions rupture to form a tender ulcer with yellow crusting and an erythematous margin. Pain may be severe enough to cause drooling and odynophagia, which can discourage eating and drinking, particularly in children. The disease tends to run its course in a 7- to 10-day period with resolution of the lesions without scarring. Recurrent herpes labialis may present with an aura of burning, itching, or tingling prior to vesicle formation. Oral trauma, sunburn, stress, and any variety of febrile illnesses can precipitate this condition.

Differential Diagnosis

Oral erythema multiforme or Stevens-Johnson syndrome, aphthous lesions, oral pemphigus, and hand-foot-mouth (HFM) syndrome are in the differential diagnosis. It should be noted that aphthous ulcers tend to occur on movable oral mucosa and rarely on immovable mucosa (i.e., hard palate and gingiva). The vermilion border is a characteristic location for herpes labialis as opposed to aphthous lesions. Posterior oropharyngeal ulcerations with associated hand and foot lesions help to define HFM syndrome. Painful hemorrhagic oral ulcers in association with anorectal and conjunctival lesions aid in identifying erythema multiforme or Stevens-Johnson syndrome. Oral pemphigus is commonly found in elderly patients. Cutaneous skin bullae and several weeks of vague constitutional symptoms are also characteristic of pemphigus. A thorough history is invaluable in differentiating the aforementioned disorders.

ED Treatment and Disposition

Supportive care with rehydration and pain control are the mainstays of therapy. Temporary pain relief may be achieved with topical analgesics. Viscous lidocaine, 2%, may be used as an oral rinse, 5 mL every 3 to 4 h. Oral acyclovir, 200 mg capsules five times per day, may be useful in adults with primary infections. Topical acyclovir ointment may also be of use by preventing viral spreading and acting as a lubricant to prevent lip cracking and bleeding. Secondary infection of herpetic lesions should be treated with oral penicillin or erythromycin.

Clinical Pearls

1. Oral herpetic lesions tend to occur commonly on the vermilion border, gingiva, and hard palate.
2. Fatal viremia and systemic involvement may occur in infants and children with herpetic gingivostomatitis.
3. Primary acute oral herpetic infection occurs most commonly in children and young adults.
4. Corticosteroid use is contraindicated in herpetic gingivostomatitis because of potential worsening of the condition.

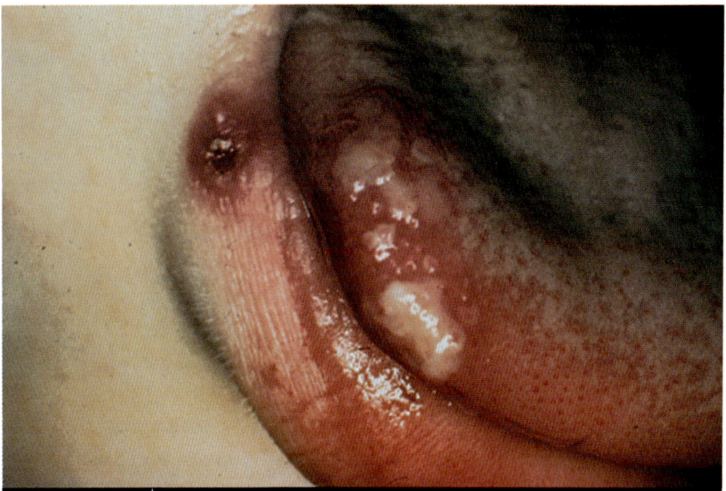

Figure 6.19 Herpes Simplex Virus (HSV) Stomatitis

Note the vermilion border and lingual lesions that are common in this condition. A prodromal period of fever, malaise, and cervical adenopathy may herald the onset of these painful ulcerations. (Courtesy of James F. Steiner, DDS.)

Associated Clinical Features

Aphthous ulcers are painful mucosal lesions varying in size from 1 to 15 mm. A prodromal burning sensation in the affected area may be noted 2 to 48 h before an ulcer is noted. The initial lesion is a small, white papule, which ulcerates and enlarges over the subsequent 48 to 72 h (Fig. 6.20). The lesions are typically round or ovoid with a raised yellow border and surrounding erythema. Multiple aphthous ulcers may occur on the lips, tongue, buccal mucosa, floor of the mouth, or soft palate (Fig. 6.21). Spontaneous healing of lesions occurs in 7 to 10 days without scarring. The exact etiology of aphthous lesions is unknown. Deficiencies of vitamin B_{12}, folic acid, and iron and viruses have all been implicated. Stress, local trauma, and immunocompromised states have all been cited as possible precipitating factors.

Differential Diagnosis

Primary or recurrent herpetic oral lesions may present with a near identical prodrome and similar appearance to aphthous ulcerations. Herpetic lesions, unlike aphthous ones, tend to occur on the gingiva, hard palate, and vermilion border. Oral erythema multiforme may also present similar to aphthous stomatitis; however, like oral herpes, it may tend to present with multiple vesicles in the early stages. Stevens-Johnson syndrome represents a severe form of erythema multiforme characterized by hemorrhagic anogenital and conjunctival lesions as well as oral lesions. Herpangina results from coxsackie and echo viruses with oral ulcerations typically involving the posterior pharynx. Oral pemphigus should also be considered in the differential. Behçet's syndrome can present with recurrent oral lesions, but also demonstrates genital ulcers and uveitis.

ED Treatment and Disposition

Supportive care, rehydration, and pain control constitutes the focus of therapy. A topical anesthetic agent such as 2% viscous lidocaine as an oral rinse every 3 to 4 h is palliative. Protective dental paste (Orabase) may be applied every 6 h to prevent irritation of lesions. Triamcinolone acetonide in an emollient dental paste applied three to four times daily may also reduce pain and promote healing of the lesions.

Clinical Pearls

1. Aphthous ulcers may be associated with Crohn's disease.
2. Women are more commonly affected by aphthous lesions than men.
3. The first aphthous episode occurs most commonly in the second decade of life.
4. Aphthous lesions almost never occur on the gums or hard palate.

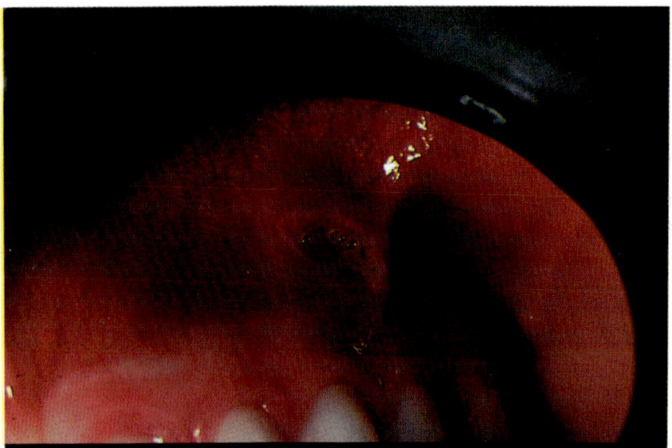

Figure 6.20 Aphthous Ulcer (Single Lesion)

Raised yellow borders with surrounding erythema are typical of aphthous ulcers. (Courtesy of James F. Steiner, DDS.)

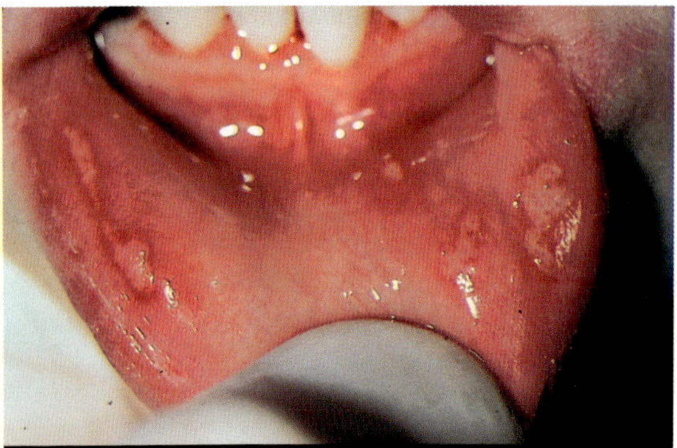

Figure 6.21 Aphthous Ulcerations

Note the multiple ulcers of various sizes located on the lip and gingival mucosa. These lesions rarely occur on the immobile oral mucosa of the gingiva or hard palate. (Courtesy of James F. Steiner, DDS.)

Associated Clinical Features

Reddened, hypertrophied lingual papillae, called strawberry tongue, is associated primarily with scarlet fever, which is caused by group A streptococcus. The tongue initially appears white with the erythematous papillae sticking through. After several days, the white coating is lost and the tongue appears bright red (Fig. 6.22). Other signs of group A streptococcal infection include fever, an exudative pharyngitis, a scarlatiniform rash, and the presence of Pastia's lines (petechial linear rash in the skin folds).

Differential Diagnosis

Kawasaki syndrome may also present with an injected pharynx and a erythematous strawberrylike tongue. It is essential to make the distinction between streptococcal infection and Kawasaki syndrome, since the latter is associated with a high incidence of coronary artery aneurysm if left untreated. Also consider toxic shock syndrome (TSS), in which one-half to three-fourths of patients tend to have pharyngitis with a strawberry-red tongue. Patients with TSS also have skin rashes as with scarlet fever; however, the rash in TSS is macular and "sunburnlike." Erythema multiforme can also be associated with fever, pharyngeal erythema, and lingual lesions; however, it has a more distinct pathognomonic cutaneous rash called target, or iris, lesions.

ED Treatment and Disposition

Penicillin or erythromycin is the drug of choice for group A streptococci. Pharyngeal cultures are useful for confirming the diagnosis. Antistreptolysin O (ASO) titers can be used for confirmation in the convalescent stage if the diagnosis is in question.

Clinical Pearls

1. A course, palpable, sandpaperlike rash of the skin is highly characteristic of scarlet fever.
2. Strawberry tongue initially appears white in color, with prominent red papillae bulging through the white exudate. After several days, the tongue becomes completely beefy red.

Associated Clinical Features

Koplik's spots are oral lesions pathognomonic for measles. They appear 1 to 2 days before the generalized measles rash. The spots are bright red with a tiny bluish-white center. They are most often seen on the buccal mucosa opposite the posterior teeth. By the second or third day, the spots coalesce. The patient generally complains of prodromal symptoms such as fever, conjunctivitis, cough, and malaise for 1 to 2 days before the Koplik's spots appear.

Differential Diagnosis

Before the onset of rash, the syndrome may be mistaken for any number of viral syndromes. Aphthous lesions, herpes simplex virus, and lesions from herpangina should be considered. Forschheimer's spots are nonspecific pinpoint petechiae found on the soft palate of some patients with rubella (German measles). Koplik's spots, however, are nonpetechial, nonulcerated lesions and are nontender.

ED Treatment and Disposition

Measles is a highly contagious infection transmitted by respiratory droplets. Almost all unprotected household contacts are either infected or at considerable risk for infection. Supportive care including rest, antipyretics, and fluids is usually adequate. For more definitive treatment recommendations see Chapter 14.

Clinical Pearls

1. Measles is now an unusual infection because of routine vaccination.
2. Koplik's spots may occur on any mucosal surface in the oral cavity except the tongue.
3. The oral mucosa opposite the first and second molars is the most common location for these lesions.
4. Koplik's spots are nontender and do not cause odynophagia.

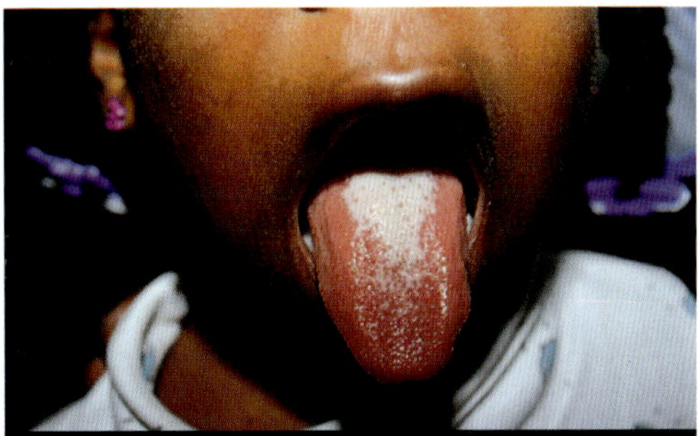

Figure 6.22 Strawberry Tongue

Note the white exudate with bulging red papillae. The white coating is eventually lost after several days, and the tongue then appears bright red. (Courtesy of Michael Nowicki, MD.)

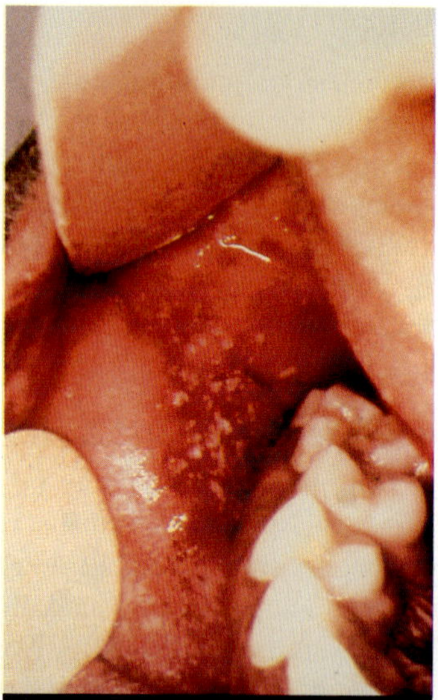

Figure 6.23
Koplik's Spots

The presence of bright red buccal mucosal spots with a whitish center near the molars is most consistent with Koplik's spots. (Courtesy of Michael J. Nowicki, MD.)

Associated Clinical Features

Tori are benign nodular overgrowths of the cortical bone. Although their physical appearance can be somewhat alarming to those unfamiliar with this entity, there is generally no need for concern. These bony protuberances occur in the midline of the palate where the maxilla fuses (Fig. 6.24). Tori may also be located on the mandible, typically on the lingual aspect of the molar teeth. Tori are covered by a thin epithelium, which is easily traumatized and ulcerated. These ulcerations tend to heal very slowly because of the poor vascularization of the tori. Torus palatinus, in particular, is slow growing and may occur at any age; however, it is most commonly noted prior to age 30 in adults. Torus palatinus affects females twice as frequently as males.

Differential Diagnosis

There are a variety of oral conditions that may be confused with mandibular or palatal tori. Gingival fibromatosis, fibroma formation secondary to irritation, granulomas, abscesses, and oral neurofibromatosis located on the palate may all be similar in appearance to torus palatinus. Nodular bony enlargement in the oral cavity may also result from fibrous dysplasia, osteomas, and Paget's disease. Biopsies, oral radiographs, and CT scans may aid in differentiating these conditions.

ED Treatment and Disposition

Tori are a normal structural variant and do not represent any inflammatory or neoplastic process. Therefore, they are of no clinical significance and require no treatment unless associated with a complication. Tori may enlarge enough to interfere with eating or speaking and impair proper fitting of dental prosthesis. For some patients the mere presence of torus palatinus may be bothersome and undesirable. Oral and maxillofacial consultation is indicated when complications call for surgical excision of the lesion. Reassurance is otherwise all that is indicated. However, elective removal can be undertaken for the overly anxious patient who is preoccupied with or annoyed by their presence.

Clinical Pearls

1. Torus palatinus almost always occurs in the midline of the hard palate.
2. Both torus palatinus and torus mandibularis are nontender and otherwise asymptomatic.

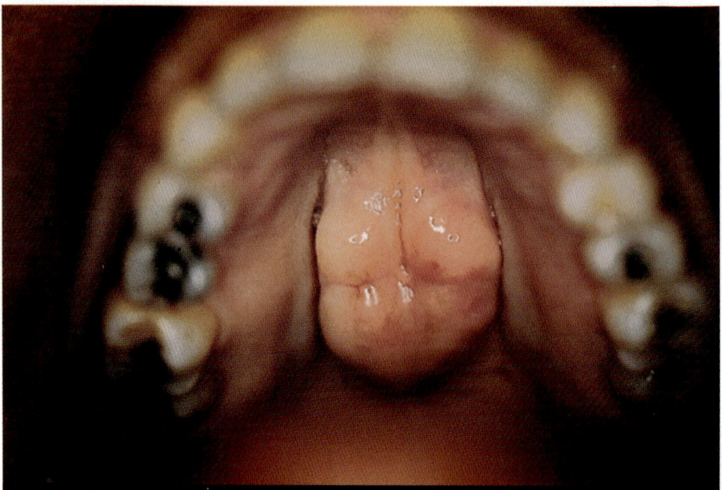

Figure 6.24 Torus Palatinus

Note the nodular appearance and characteristic central palatal location. Abrasions and ulcerations can occur on the thin overlying epithelium secondary to trauma by food and oral objects. (Courtesy of Kevin J. Knoop, MD, MS.)

CHAPTER 7

CHEST AND ABDOMEN

Stephen Corbett
Lawrence B. Stack
Kevin J. Knoop

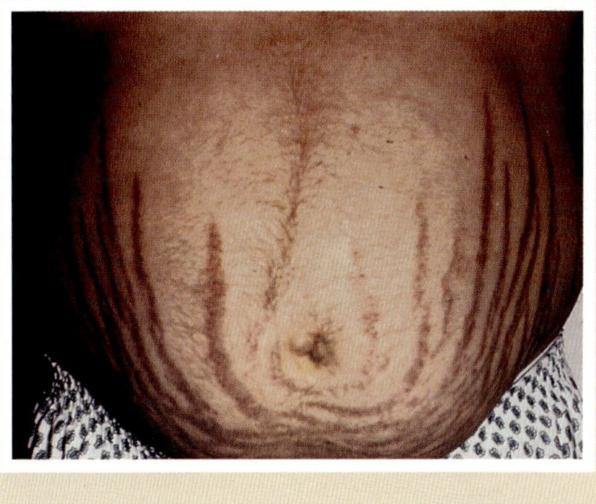

Associated Clinical Features

Increased respiratory effort may be manifest by increased respiratory rate, increased chest wall excursion, and retractions of the less rigid structures of the thorax. Retractions of the sternum (Fig. 7.1), suprasternal notch (Fig. 7.2), and intercostal retractions reflect increased respiratory effort. This may be due to obstructive disease such as asthma, or tracheal obstruction, pneumonia, or restrictive disease. The presence of stridor, wheezing, or rhonchi will help distinguish the cause.

Differential Diagnosis

Asthma, chronic obstructive pulmonary disease (COPD), emphysema, epiglottitis, croup, foreign body aspiration, esophageal foreign body, bacterial tracheitis, posterior pharyngeal abscess, and anaphylaxis are all conditions that must be considered in a patient with retractions.

ED Treatment and Disposition

An aggressive search for the cause of the retractions is required to direct therapy. Rapid evaluation of the airway for patency, and breathing for oxygenation should be done immediately on presentation. High-flow oxygen by face mask is appropriate for patients in respiratory distress. Preparations for securing an airway should be underway for those patients in severe distress or respiratory failure. Routine measures for the mildly symptomatic patient depend on the cause of the retractions. For asthma or COPD exacerbations, nebulized β_2 agonists and steroid therapy may be appropriate. Patients with croup may require nebulized normal saline and possibly epinephrine or dexamethasone as initial therapy. Foreign body aspiration requires consultation for confirmation of the suspected diagnosis and removal.

Clinical Pearls

1. Retractions are best observed with the patient at rest and their chest exposed.
2. Retractions from obstructive airway disease can be intercostal and supraclavicular, and are usually accompanied by nasal flaring, increased expiratory phase, and increased respiratory rate.

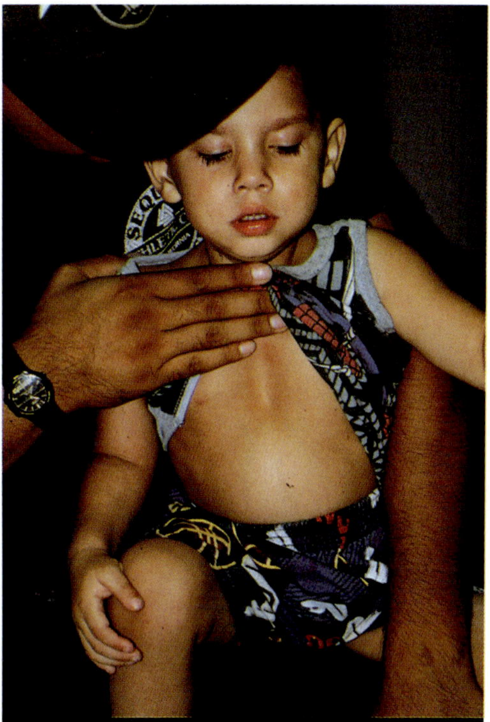

Figure 7.1 Sternal Retractions

Sternal retractions in a patient with croup. (Courtesy of Stephen Corbett, MD.)

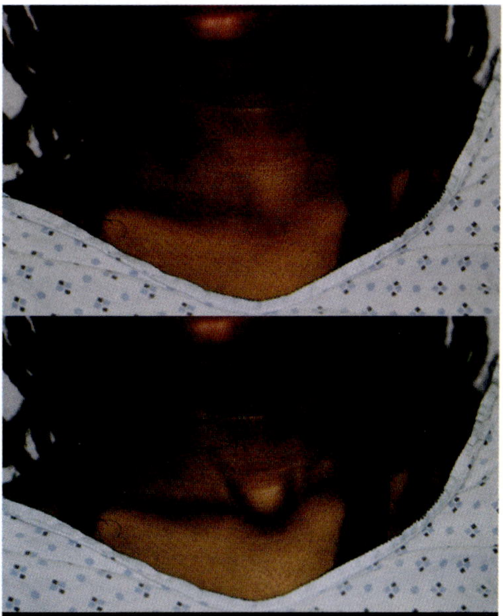

Figure 7.2 Suprasternal Retractions

Suprasternal retractions in an adolescent with severe asthma. (Courtesy of Kevin J. Knoop, MD, MS.)

Associated Clinical Features

A hernia is a tissue protrusion through an abnormal body cavity opening. Most abdominal wall hernias occur at the groin and umbilicus. Incarceration is defined as the inability to reduce the protruding tissue to its normal position. Strangulation occurs when the blood supply of the hernia's contents is obstructed and tissue necrosis ensues. An *incisional* hernia (Fig. 7.3) may be manifest clinically by a mass or palpable defect adjacent to a surgical incision and can be reproduced by having the patient perform Valsalva's maneuver. Obesity and wound infection, which interfere with wound healing, predispose to the formation of incisional hernias. The defect of an *indirect* inguinal hernia (Fig. 7.4) is the internal (abdominal) inguinal ring, and may be manifest in either sex by a bulge over the midpoint of the inguinal ligament that increases in size with Valsalva's maneuver. A fingertip placed into the external ring through the inguinal canal may palpate the defect. A *direct* hernia (Fig. 7.5) may be manifest by a bulge midway adjacent to the pubic tubercle and may be felt by the pad of the finger placed in the inguinal canal. The defect is in the posterior wall of the inguinal canal. Direct inguinal hernias are usually painless and occur in males.

Nausea and vomiting may be present if incarceration with bowel obstruction occurs. Strangulation can lead to fever, peritonitis, and sepsis.

Differential Diagnosis

Tumor, aneurysm, lymphadenopathy, bowel obstruction, ascites, lipoma, femoral hernia, hydrocele, testicular torsion, and epididymitis may have similar presentations.

ED Treatment and Disposition

When patients present without clinical evidence of strangulation (fever, leukocytosis, systemic signs of toxicity), reduction should be attempted. In the presence of these signs, prompt surgical consultation is warranted for surgical reduction. Reduction in the ED is facilitated with systemic analgesia (as most patients present with significant pain), placing the patient in the supine position, and applying a cold pack to the hernia. Routine consultation for operative repair is indicated in asymptomatic patients with reducible hernias.

Clinical Pearls

1. Acutely strangulated or incarcerated hernias require immediate surgical evaluation.
2. Direct inguinal hernias are usually painless.
3. Evaluation and treatment of concomitant exacerbating conditions (cough, constipation, vomiting) prevents recurrences.

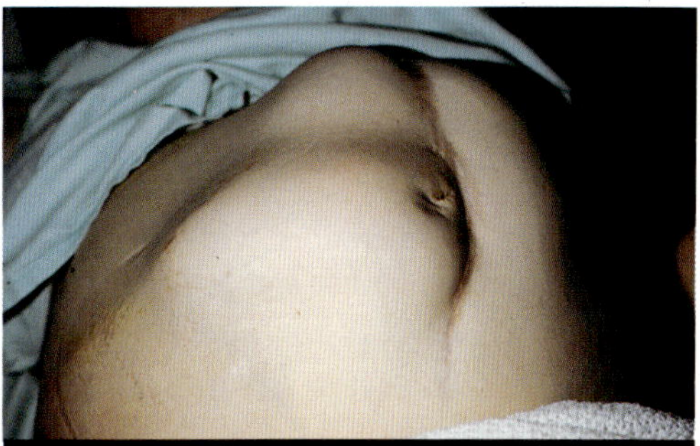

Figure 7.3 Incisional Hernia

An incisional hernia in an obese female. (Courtesy of Stephen Corbett, MD.)

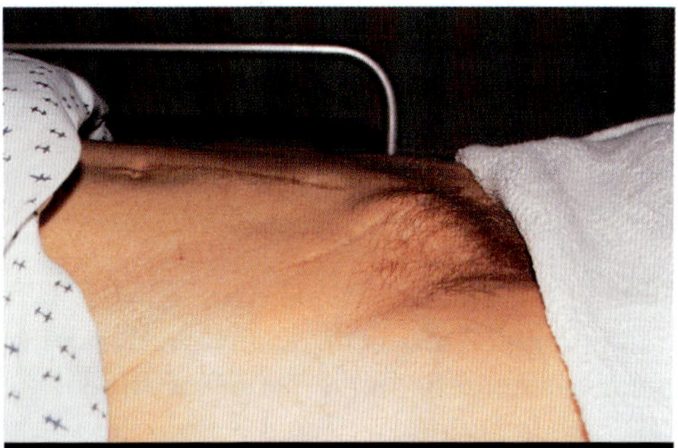

Figure 7.4 Indirect Inguinal Hernia

A recurrent indirect inguinal hernia in a female patient. (Courtesy of Frank Birinyi, MD.)

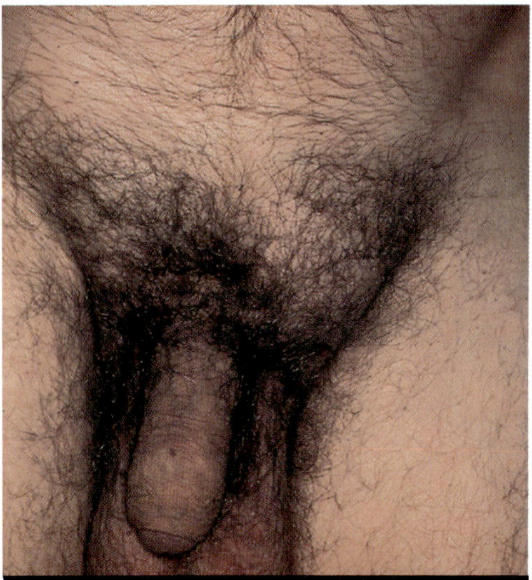

Figure 7.5 Direct Inguinal Hernia

A direct inguinal hernia. Note the bulge adjacent to the left pubic tubercle. (Courtesy of Daniel L. Savitt, MD.)

Associated Clinical Features

The umbilicus is a common site of abdominal hernias. Predisposing conditions in adults most commonly include ascites and prior abdominal surgery. The size of the defect determines the symptomatology and incidence of incarceration, with smaller defects resulting in more pronounced symptoms and an increased incidence of incarceration. Pain is located in the area of the fascial defect. Contents of the hernia may be palpable and tender. Symptoms of obstruction (nausea, vomiting, and abdominal distention) may be present. If the hernia becomes strangulated (Fig. 7.6), erythema of the overlying skin with fever and hypotension may occur.

Differential Diagnosis

An omphalocele, gastroschisis, or urachal duct may present as an umbilical mass.

ED Treatment and Disposition

Reduction is attempted in the stable patient without clinical evidence of strangulation. Treatment of any predisposing conditions (i.e., abdominal paracentesis in the patient with tense ascites) may cause spontaneous reduction and avoid progression of the hernia to strangulation. Routine consultation for elective repair is indicated in asymptomatic patients with reducible hernias.

Clinical Pearls

1. Umbilical hernias in children usually resolve without treatment.
2. Umbilical hernias in adults usually become worse and require elective repair.

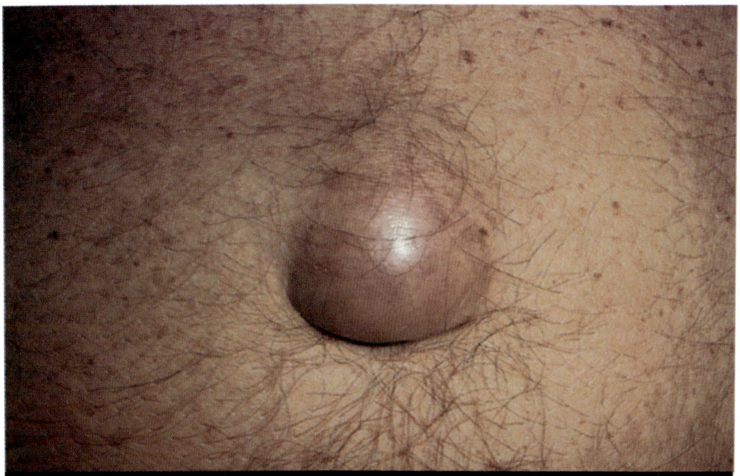

Figure 7.6 Strangulated Umbilical Hernia

The overlying skin of a strangulated umbilical hernia is erythematous and tender. (Courtesy of Lawrence B. Stack, MD.)

Associated Clinical Features

Abdominal striae are linear, depressed pink or bluish scarlike lesions (Fig. 7.7) that may later become silver or white. They are caused by weakening of the elastic cutaneous tissues from chronic stretching. They most commonly occur on the abdomen, but are also seen on the buttocks, breasts, and thighs. Striae are commonly seen in obesity, pregnancy, Cushing's syndrome, and chronic topical corticosteroid treatment. In Cushing's syndrome, a state of adrenal hypercorticism, the skin becomes fragile and easily breaks from normal stretching.

Differential Diagnosis

Obesity, pregnancy, Cushing's syndrome, and chronic topical corticosteroid treatment should be considered.

ED Treatment and Disposition

This finding seldom presents as a condition requiring acute treatment; thus, attention is directed to determining and treating the underlying cause.

Clinical Pearls

1. Recent striae (pink or blue) with moon facies, hypertension, renal calculi, osteoporosis, and psychiatric disorders are suggestive of Cushing's syndrome.
2. The striae caused by pregnancy typically fade with time, unlike those associate with Cushings syndrome.

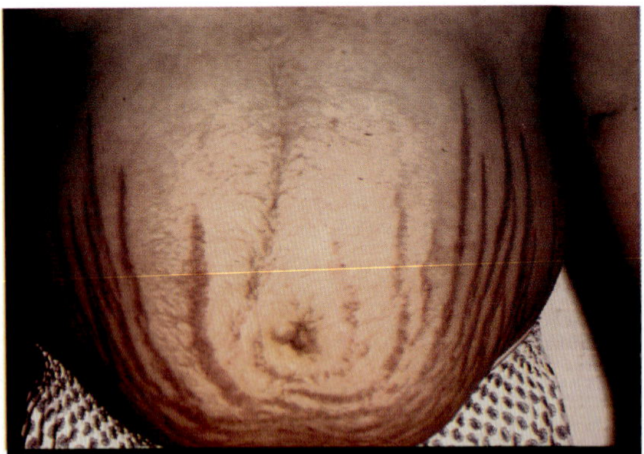

Figure 7.7 Abdominal Striae

These striae are from a patient with recent weight gain, moon facies, and altered mental status. The patient was diagnosed with Cushing's syndrome. (Courtesy of Geisinger Medical Center, Dept. of Emergency Medicine, Danville, Pennsylvania.)

CHAPTER 8

UROLOGIC CONDITIONS

Jeffrey D. Bondesson

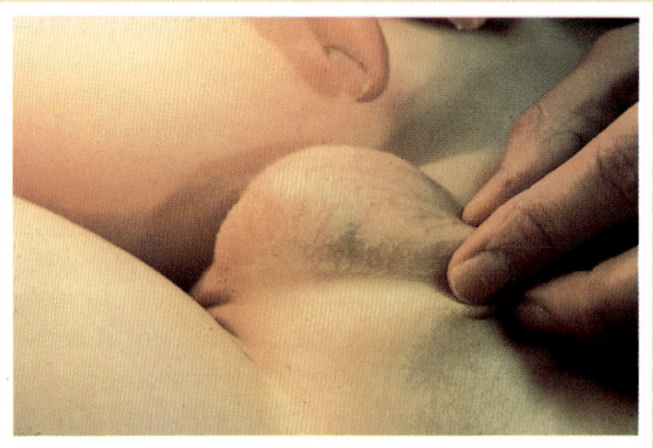

Associated Clinical Features

These patients are most often young men (average age 16 to 17.5 years) who present complaining of the sudden onset of pain in one testicle. The pain is then followed by swelling of the affected testicle, reddening of the overlying scrotal skin, lower abdominal pain, nausea, and vomiting. An examination reveals a swollen, tender, retracted testicle (Fig. 8.1) that often lies in the horizontal plane (bell clapper deformity) (Fig. 8.2). The spermatic cord is frequently swollen on the affected side. Delayed presentations may present with the entire hemiscrotum swollen, tender, and firm (Fig. 8.3). The urine is usually clear with a normal urinalysis. In one-third of cases there is a peripheral leukocytosis.

Differential Diagnosis

Alternative diagnoses that should be considered include acute epididymitis, torsion of the testicular appendix (Fig. 8.4), trauma, acute orchitis (mumps), hydrocele, spermatocele, varicocele, hernia, and tumor. A good history and physical examination helps narrow the diagnosis.

ED Treatment and Disposition

Urologic consultation should be obtained immediately and preparation made to go to the operating room without delay. Doppler ultrasound or technetium scanning may be helpful if they will not delay surgery. In the interim, detorsion may be attempted if the patient is seen within a few hours of onset: the affected testicle should initially be opened like a book, that is, the right testicle turned counterclockwise when viewed from below, and the left testicle turned clockwise when viewed from below. Pain relief should be immediate. Decreased pain should prompt additional turns (as many as three) to complete detorsion; increased pain should prompt detorsion in the opposite direction. Ancillary studies should not delay operative intervention, since testicular infarction will occur within 6 to 12 h after torsion.

Clinical Pearls

1. The cremasteric reflex is almost always absent in testicular torsion.
2. Patients may report similar, less severe episodes that spontaneously resolved in the recent past.
3. Half of all torsions occur during sleep.
4. Abdominal or inguinal pain is sometimes present without pain to the scrotum.
5. The age of presentation has a bimodal pattern, since torsion is also more prevalent during infancy.

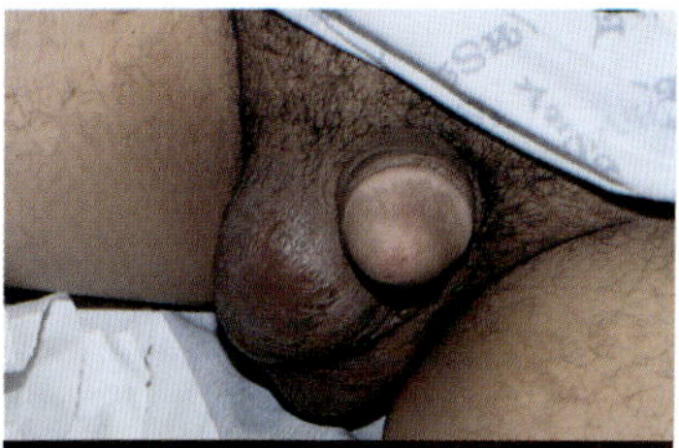

Figure 8.1 Testicular Torsion

Swollen, tender hemiscrotum, with erythema of scrotal skin and retracted testicle. (Courtesy of Stephen Corbett, MD.)

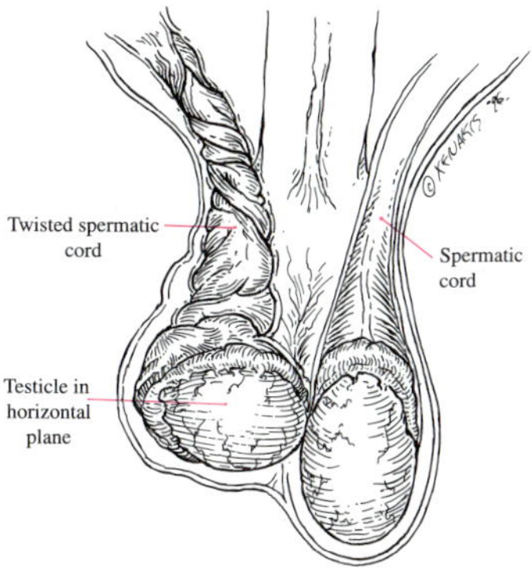

Figure 8.2 Bell Clapper Deformity

A bell clapper deformity in testicular tortion results from the twisting of the spermatic cord and causes the testis to be elevated with a horizontal lie. The lack of fixation of the tunica vaginalis to the posterior scrotum predisposes the freely movable testis to rotation and subsequent torsion. An elevated testis with a horizontal lie may be seen in asymptomatic patients at risk for torsion.

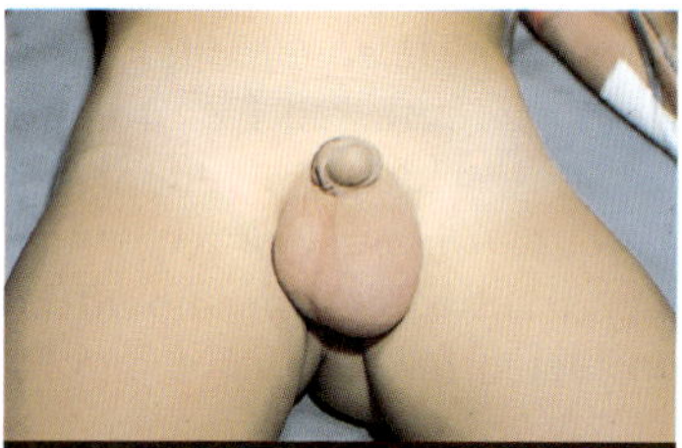

Figure 8.3 Testicular Torsion

Swollen, tender scrotal mass. (Courtesy of Patrick McKenna, MD.)

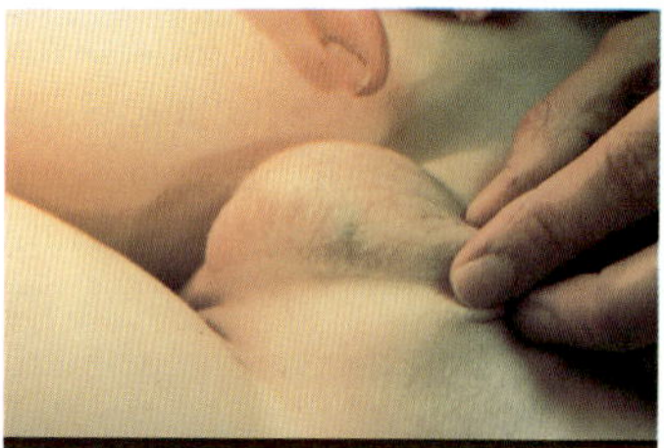

Figure 8.4 Blue Dot Sign

A blue dot sign is caused by torsion of the testicular appendix. It is best seen with the skin held taut over the testicular appendix. (Courtesy of Javier A. Gonzalez del Rey, MD.)

Associated Clinical Features

Acute epididymitis causes pain in the scrotum on the affected side, with referred pain to the groin, inguinal canal, or lower abdominal quadrant. The onset of pain is gradual, occurring over hours. When the patient presents early in the course, a tender, indurated, edematous epididymis can be palpated separately from the nontender testis. Late presentations will have generalized scrotal swelling and pain, making examination and differentiation more difficult (Fig. 8.5). The urinalysis will reveal pyuria or bacteriuria half of the time, and the peripheral white blood cell count is frequently elevated. Patients can present with fever and signs of sepsis.

Differential Diagnosis

Torsion of the testis, torsion of the testicular appendix, orchitis, trauma, tumor, or hernia may present in a similar fashion. Nuclear isotope scanning or ultrasound may be helpful by demonstrating increased testicular and epididymal blood flow.

ED Treatment and Disposition

Treatment is usually outpatient (NSAIDs, scrotal support), and based on the most likely causative organism. Younger men (under 35 years) tend to have the sexually transmitted organisms of *Chlamydia trachomatis* and *Neisseria gonorrhoeae* as the most frequent offenders, whereas older men tend to have infections caused by bacteria commonly associated with urinary tract infections, that is, *Escherichia coli, Enterococcus* species and *Pseudomonas aeruginosa.* Adolescents and children should be referred for urologic evaluation to rule out congenital anomalies, which are common in nongonococcal infections in this age group. A history of recent urinary tract instrumentation or urinary tract infection should be sought. Febrile patients should be considered for admission and IV antibiotics.

Clinical Pearls

1. Elevation of the affected hemiscrotum may provide relief of symptoms (Prehn's sign).
2. Older men should be evaluated for urinary retention, as this is a frequent cause of epididymitis.
3. Testicular tumors are most frequently misdiagnosed as epididymitis.
4. The absence of pyuria or bacteriuria does not exclude the diagnosis.

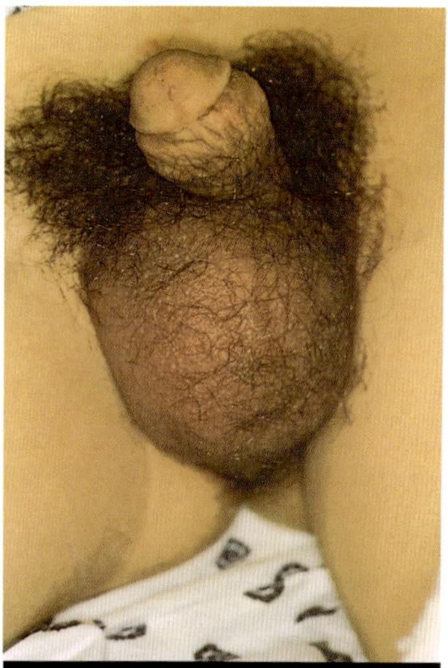

Figure 8.5 Acute Epididymitis

Swelling of the right hemiscrotum shown here is nonspecific. Tenderness was localized to the epididymis in this patient. (Courtesy of Adam R. Saperston, MD, MS.)

Associated Clinical Features

Most hydroceles occur in older patients and develop gradually without any significant symptoms. They are generally a soft, pear-shaped, fluid-filled cystic mass anterior to the testicle and epididymis that will transilluminate (Fig. 8.6). However, they can be tense and firm and transilluminate poorly if the tunica vaginalis is thickened. Almost all hydroceles in children are communicating, resulting from the same mechanism that causes inguinal hernia. A persistent narrow processus vaginalis acts like a one-way valve, thus permitting the accumulation of dependent peritoneal fluid in the scrotum. Acute symptomatic hydroceles are more rare, and can occur in association with epididymitis, trauma, or tumor.

Differential Diagnosis

Painless masses that must be differentiated from hydrocele include spermatocele, varicocele, inguinal hernia, and tumor. Painful masses to be differentiated include traumatic hematocele, epididymitis, orchitis, and torsion.

ED Treatment and Disposition

In an acute hydrocele, treatment must be directed at discovering a possible underlying cause. A positive urinalysis may point toward an infectious etiology. Transillumination helps demonstrate whether the mass is cystic or solid. Ultrasound can be very helpful in imaging the scrotal contents and delineating mass composition. Acute hydroceles should not be considered benign and require referral to a urologist to rule out tumor or infection. Chronic accumulations are referred to a urologist on a more routine basis for elective drainage.

Clinical Pearls

1. Ten percent of testicular tumors have a reactive hydrocele as the presenting complaint.
2. An inguinal hernia with a loop of bowel in it will transilluminate.
3. Hydroceles are almost never symptomatic.
4. Acute reactive hydroceles may be caused by infection, trauma, or torsion.

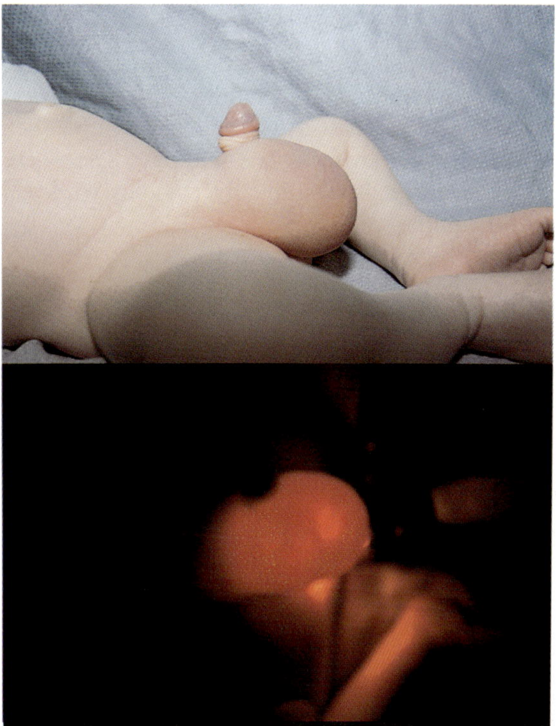

Figure 8.6 Hydrocele

Painless swelling in the scrotum of a young boy (top). Transillumination of the swelling (bottom) identifies the hydrocele. (Courtesy of Michael J. Nowicki, MD.)

Associated Clinical Features

In testicular tumor, a painless, firm testicular mass (Fig. 8.7) is palpated, with the patient often complaining of a "heaviness" of his testicle. If the patient presents early, the mass will be distinct from the testis, whereas later presentations will have generalized testicular or scrotal swelling. It occasionally presents with pain due to infarction of the tumor.

Differential Diagnosis

Epididymitis is the most frequent misdiagnosis, which unfortunately may delay surgical intervention. When the tumor presents with infarction pain, differentiation from epididymitis or torsion can be difficult. In some cases, ultrasound can help differentiate these entities.

ED Treatment and Disposition

Patients should be promptly referred to a urologist for surgical exploration.

Clinical Pearls

1. Acute hydroceles and hematoceles should prompt the physician to consider a tumor as the cause.
2. Pain from tumor infarction is usually not as severe as pain due to torsion or epididymitis.
3. Findings of an unexplained supraclavicular lymph node, abdominal mass, or chronic nonproductive cough resistant to conventional therapy should prompt a testicular examination for tumor.

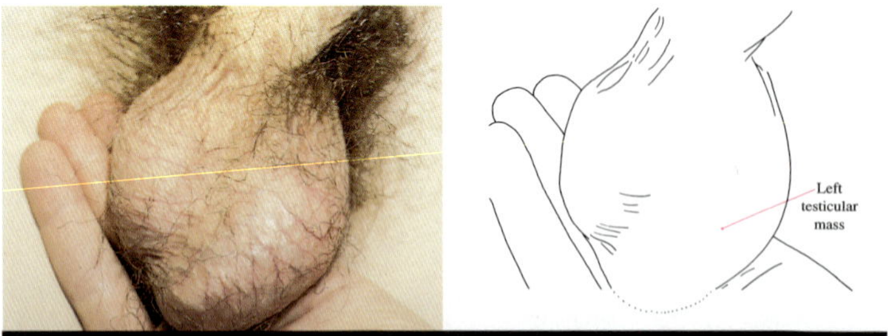

Figure 8.7 Testicular Tumor

This painless left testicular mass is highly suspicious for tumor, as was the case in this patient. (Courtesy of Patrick McKenna, MD.)

Associated Clinical Features

Paraphimosis is the entrapment of a retracted foreskin behind the coronal sulcus that cannot be reduced (Fig. 8.8). Pain, swelling, and erythema are common. If severe, the constriction causes edema and venous engorgement of the glans (Fig. 8.9) that can lead to arterial compromise with subsequent tissue necrosis.

Differential Diagnosis

In contrast to paraphimosis, phimosis is the inability to retract the foreskin, usually a chronic condition. Other diagnoses to consider include superficial balanitis, hair tourniquet, contact dermatitis, and urticaria.

ED Treatment and Disposition

Squeezing the glans firmly for 5 min to reduce the swelling can lead to successful reduction of the foreskin. Local infiltration of anesthesia with vertical incision of the constricting band should be performed by a urologist if manual reduction fails.

Clinical Pearls

1. In the presence of arterial compromise, the emergency physician should incise the constricting band if a urologist is not immediately available.
2. The patient should be referred to a urologist for circumcision if successfully reduced.
3. Phimosis is "physiologic" in young males (generally less than 5 to 6 years old).
4. Phimosis, if "reduced" (retracted proximally over the glans), can cause a paraphimosis—a true emergency.

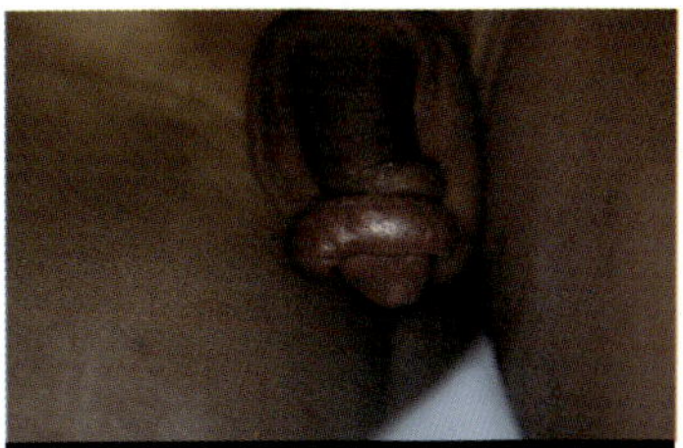

Figure 8.8 Paraphimosis

Moderate edema of the retracted foreskin, which is entrapped behind the coronal sulcus. (Courtesy of Anthony J. Musielewicz, MD.)

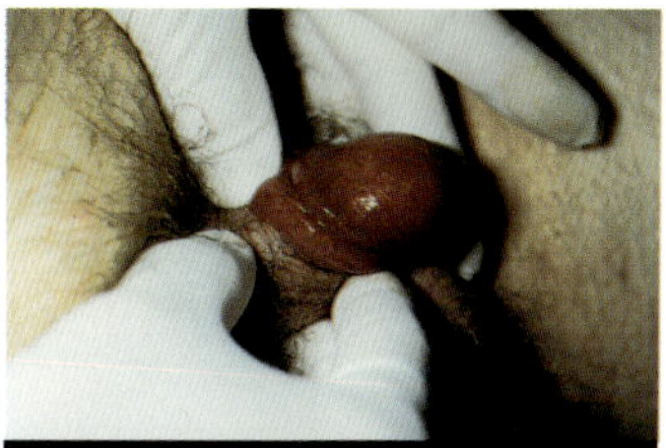

Figure 8.9 Paraphimosis

Mild swelling with erythema of the entrapped foreskin and engorgement of the glans. (Courtesy of Alan B. Storrow, MD.)

Associated Clinical Features

In straddle injury, the patient has pain, swelling, contusion, and hematoma of the perineum or scrotum following direct blunt trauma (Fig. 8.10 and 8.11). This injury is commonly caused by falls onto bicycle frame cross-tubes, playground equipment, or a toilet seat. Swelling can be severe enough to interfere with urination. Scrotal contents can also be contused or crushed with this injury.

Differential Diagnosis

Fournier's gangrene, cellulitis, and urticaria are similar in appearance, but without the history of trauma. Sexual or physical abuse should be considered.

ED Treatment and Disposition

Treatment is supportive and includes cold packs, elevation, rest, and analgesics. If unable to void, the patient may require catheterization.

Clinical Pearls

1. Laceration of the perineum can be obscured by swelling if a careful examination is not performed.
2. Pelvis radiographs should be obtained in all perineal injuries.
3. Males and females are at high risk for urethral injuries with this type of injury.
4. Straddle injury is differentiated from abuse with a good history that matches the injury from a reliable caregiver.

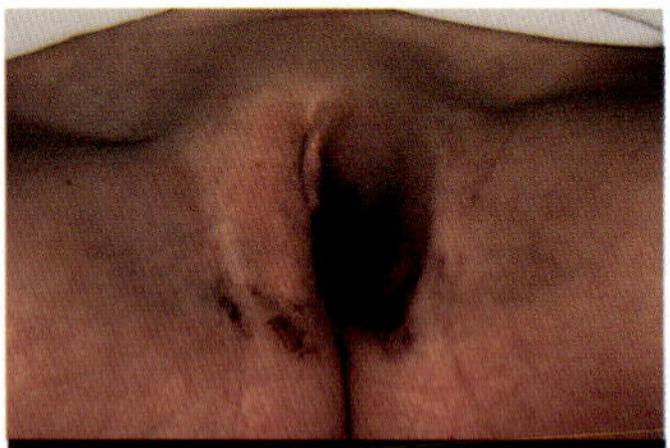

Figure 8.10 Straddle Injury

Ecchymosis, swelling, and contusion of the perineum in a 3-year-old female who tripped and fell on a large plastic toy. (Courtesy of James Mensching, MD.)

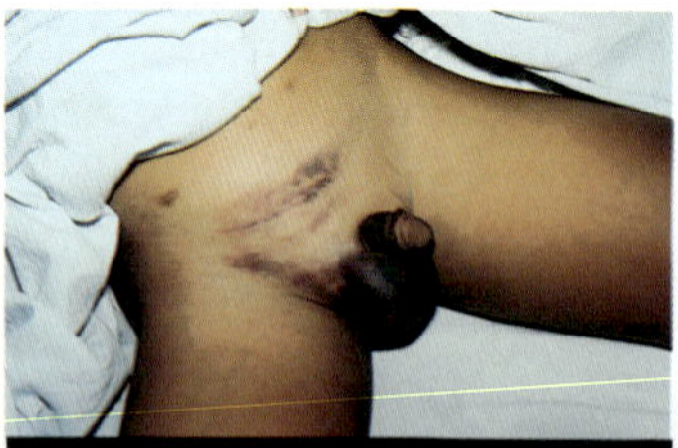

Figure 8.11 Straddle Injury

Contusion of the scrotum and lower abdomen in a young boy consistent with a straddle injury. (Courtesy of David W. Munter, MD.)

Associated Clinical Features

Balanoposthitis is an infection and inflammation of the glans penis that also involves the overlying foreskin (prepuce) (Fig. 8.12). *Balanitis* is isolated to the glans, whereas *posthitis* involves only the prepuce. Pain, erythema, and edema of the affected parts of the penis are typically present. Patients may refrain from urination secondary to dysuria, or the edema may induce meatal occlusion, leading to urinary retention or obstruction. Common etiologies include overgrowth of normal bacterial flora secondary to poor hygiene (pediatric), sexually transmitted diseases (adolescents and adults), and candidal infections (elderly or immunocompromised) (Fig. 8.13).

Differential Diagnosis

The diagnosis is usually straightforward; however, the underlying etiology often must also be addressed. Examples are sexually transmitted diseases in healthy adults and diseases associated with immunocompromise (e.g. diabetes mellitus, AIDS, alcoholism). Phimosis occurs when chronic infection due to poor hygiene causes fibrosis and contracture of the preputial opening. Other diagnoses to consider include contact dermatitis, fixed drug eruptions, lichen sclerosus et atrophicus, and squamous cell carcinoma.

ED Treatment and Disposition

Treatment is directed at the suspected etiology. Warm soaks and topical antibiotics (bacitracin) are the mainstay of therapy for infectious etiologies owing to poor hygiene. Parents should be counseled about proper cleansing and handling of the prepuce. Oral or intravenous antibiotics may be indicated if there is an accompanying cellulitis. If urinary obstruction is present, catheterization may be attempted using a small catheter. If catheterization is unsuccessful, urologic consultation for emergent surgical correction of the prepuce is required. Candidal infections are treated with meticulous hygiene and topical antifungal agents. Routine urologic referral is indicated for suspected lichen sclerosus et atrophicus and squamous cell carcinoma.

Clinical Pearls

1. The inability to retract the foreskin completely is normal in young males up to age 4 or 5. Attempting to do so could cause a paraphimosis, a true emergency.
2. Placing the child in a bathtub with warm water will help alleviate difficulty with micturition, assuming no obstruction is present.
3. Candidal balanitis or balanoposthitis may be associated with an undiagnosed immunocompromised state.
4. Suspected sexually transmitted diseases require treatment for the partners as well.

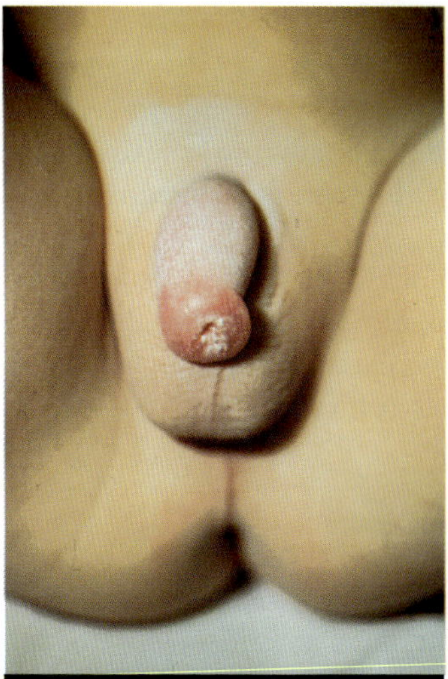

Figure 8.12 Balanoposthitis

Note the erythema, localized edema, and significantly constricted preputial orifice of the distal penis. (Courtesy of Lawrence B. Stack, MD.)

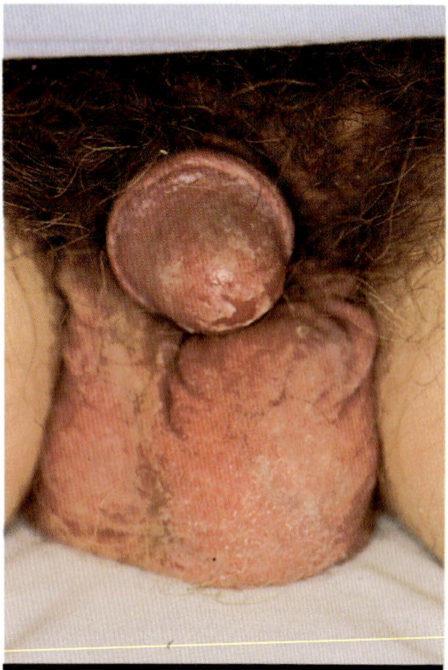

Figure 8.13 Balanitis

Candidal balanitis in an elderly patient with no other complaints. New onset diabetes was diagnosed. (Courtesy of Kevin J. Knoop, MD, MS.)

CHAPTER 9

SEXUALLY TRANSMITTED DISEASES AND ANORECTAL CONDITIONS

Diane M. Birnbaumer
Lynn K. Flowers

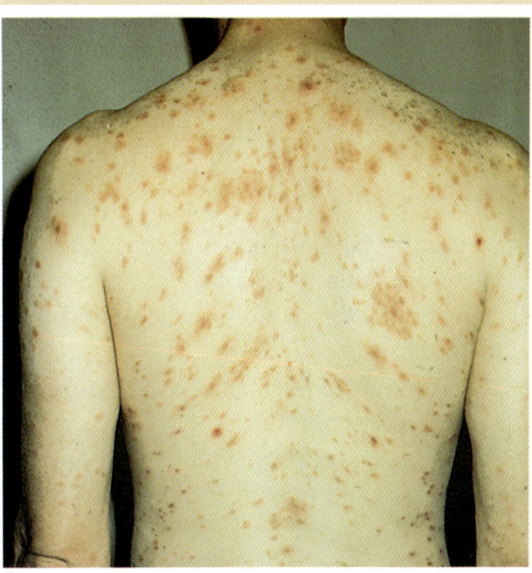

Associated Clinical Features

Lesions of primary syphilis generally appear after an incubation period of 2 to 6 weeks, but may appear up to 3 months after exposure. The patient usually presents with a solitary, round to oval, painless genital ulcer (Figs. 9.1 and 9.2). However, the ulcer may be slightly painful, and several lesions are sometimes seen. The base of the genital ulcer is dry in males, moist in females; purulent fluid in the base is uncommon. The borders of the ulcer are often indurated. Patients may develop ulcers at any site of inoculation on the body. Bilateral, nontender, nonfluctuant adenopathy is common. Lesions resolve spontaneously in 3 to 12 weeks without treatment as the infection progresses to the secondary stage. Patients with primary syphilis are at risk for concurrent infection with other sexually transmitted diseases.

Differential Diagnosis

Behçet's disease, fixed drug eruption, recurrent genital herpes, chancroid, squamous cell carcinoma, and lesions caused by trauma can have a similar appearance.

ED Treatment and Disposition

Treat with benzathine penicillin G, 2.4 million units IM once. Penicillin-allergic patients should be given doxycycline, 100 mg PO bid for 2 weeks. Other alternatives include tetracycline, 500 mg PO qid for 2 weeks; erythromycin base, 500 mg PO qid for 2 weeks; or ceftriaxone, 250 mg IM once daily for 10 days. An RPR or VDRL should be checked. Partners within the last 90 days should be treated presumptively; partners over the last 90 days should be treated on the basis of their serologic testing results. This is a reportable disease, and appropriate paperwork should be filed.

Clinical Pearls

1. Lesions are usually painless and solitary, but may be slightly painful and two or three lesions may also be seen.
2. Consider dark-field examination of the lesion to rapidly confirm the diagnosis.
3. Chancres of primary syphilis can occur anywhere on the body at the site of inoculation.
4. Evaluate patients with primary syphilis for concurrent sexually transmitted diseases and treat accordingly.

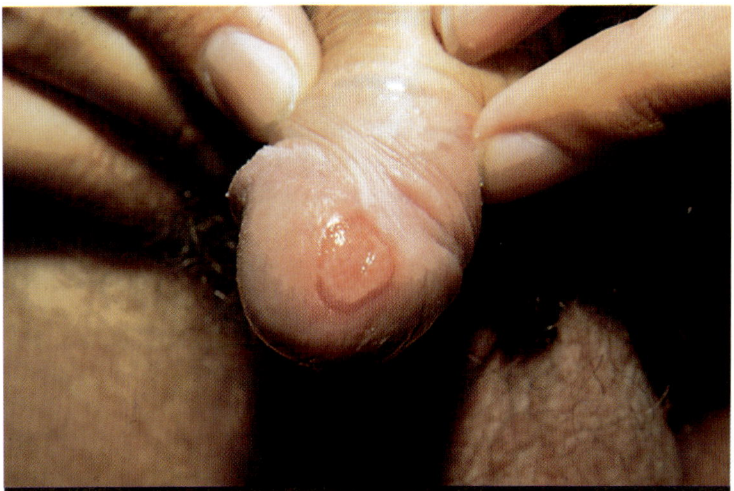

Figure 9.1 Primary Chancre—Male

This dry-based, painless ulcer with indurated borders is typical for a primary chancre in a male patient. (Courtesy of A. Wisdom: *Sexually Transmitted Diseases.* London, Mosby-Wolfe, 1992.)

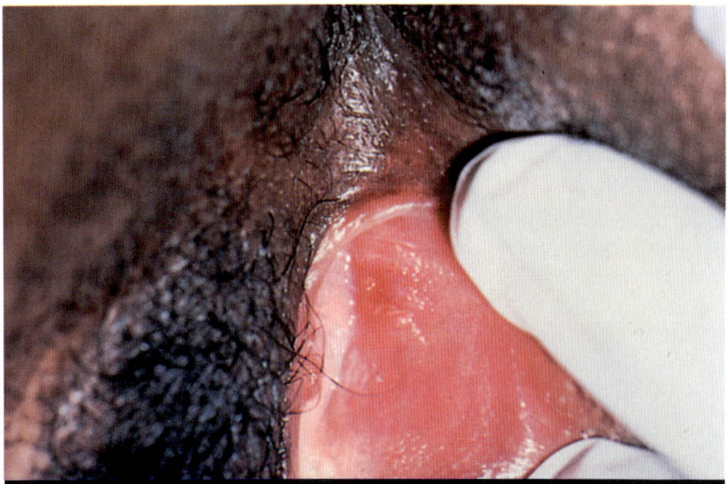

Figure 9.2 Primary Chancre—Female

A solitary, painless genital chancre with a clean base in a patient with primary syphilis. (Courtesy of the Dept. of Dermatology, Naval Medical Center, Portsmouth.)

Associated Clinical Features

The rash of secondary syphilis often occurs 2 to 10 weeks after resolution of the primary lesions. It begins as a nonpruritic macular rash that evolves into a papulosquamous rash involving primarily the trunk, palms, and soles (Figs. 9.3, 9.4, 9.5). The rash is often annular in shape. Diffuse, painless lymphadenopathy is also seen at this stage. Mucous patches represent mucous membrane involvement of the tongue and buccal mucosa (Fig. 9.6). Condyloma lata (Fig. 9.7) can be seen during this stage, as can patchy alopecia. The manifestations of this stage resolve without treatment in several months.

Differential Diagnosis

The differential diagnosis depends on the site involved:

Rash: Pityriasis rosea, psoriasis, lichen planus, Reiter's, viral syndrome, allergic rash

Mucous patches: Apthous ulcerations, thrush

Condyloma lata: Condyloma accuminata, squamous cell carcinoma, granuloma inguinale

ED Treatment and Disposition

Benzathine penicillin G, 2.4 million units IM once; penicillin allergic patients should receive doxycycline, 100 mg PO bid for 2 weeks. RPR or VDRL should be sent and titers followed to determine adequate response to therapy. Suspected and confirmed cases of syphilis must be reported.

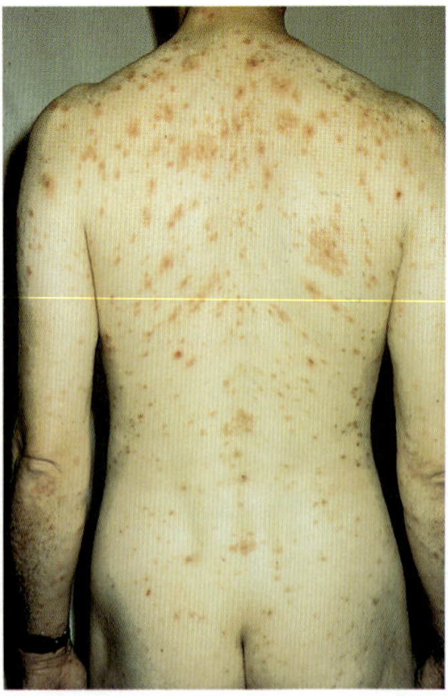

Figure 9.3 Secondary Syphilis—Trunk

Rash on trunk in secondary syphilis. (Courtesy of A. Wisdom: *Sexually Transmitted Diseases.* London, Mosby-Wolfe, 1992.)

Clinical Pearls

1. Lesions of secondary syphilis are very infectious. It is prudent to always wear gloves when examining a patient with a rash that may be due to secondary syphilis.
2. Consider using dark-field examination of scrapings of the rash, mucous patches, and condyloma lata to make a rapid diagnosis.
3. Patients should be warned about the potential development of the Jarish-Herxheimer reaction after they are treated. This syndrome, characterized by fever, headache, malaise, and myalgias, occurs within 24 h of treatment and is caused by massive release of pyrogens by the dying spirochetes.

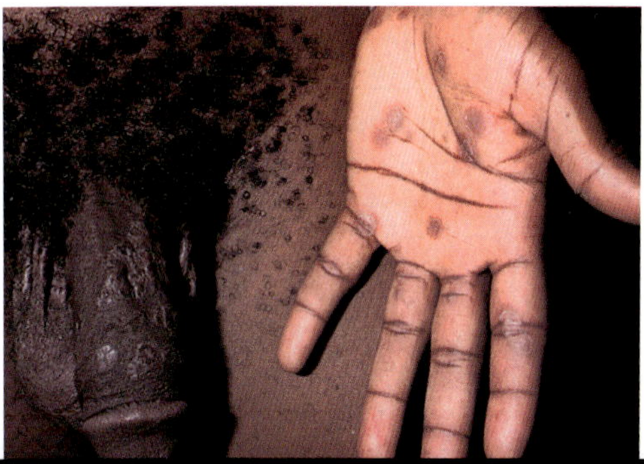

Figure 9.4 Secondary Syphilis—Palms

Papulosquamous rash of secondary syphilis. Note the annular appearance of the palmar rash. (Courtesy of H. Hunter Handsfield: *Atlas of Sexually Transmitted Diseases.* New York, McGraw-Hill, 1992.)

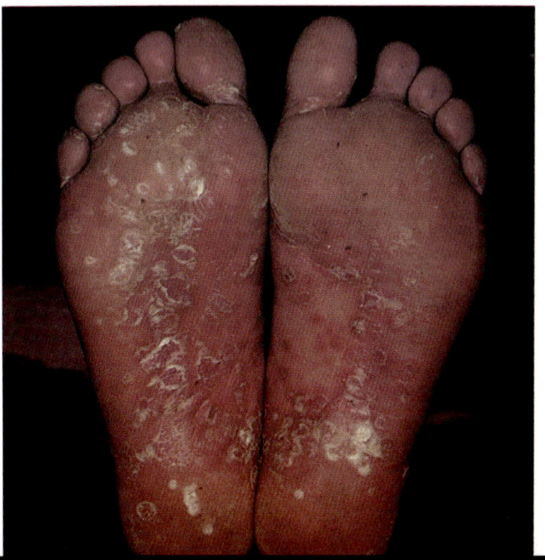

Figure 9.5 Secondary Syphilis—Soles

Hyperkeratotic plantar rash in a patient with secondary syphilis. (Courtesy of H. Hunter Handsfield: *Atlas of Sexually Transmitted Diseases.* New York, McGraw-Hill, 1992.)

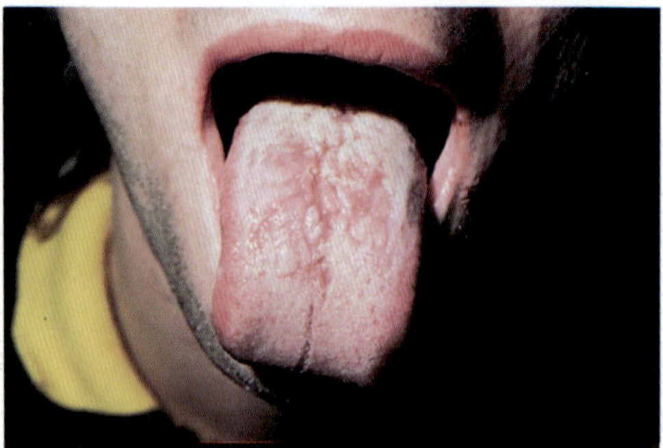

Figure 9.6 Mucous Patches

Oral involvement in secondary syphilis manifested by mucous patches. These lesions are very infectious, and dark-field examination is often positive for spirochetes. (Courtesy of Morse, Moreland, Thompson: *Atlas of Sexually Transmitted Diseases.* London, Mosby-Wolfe, 1990.)

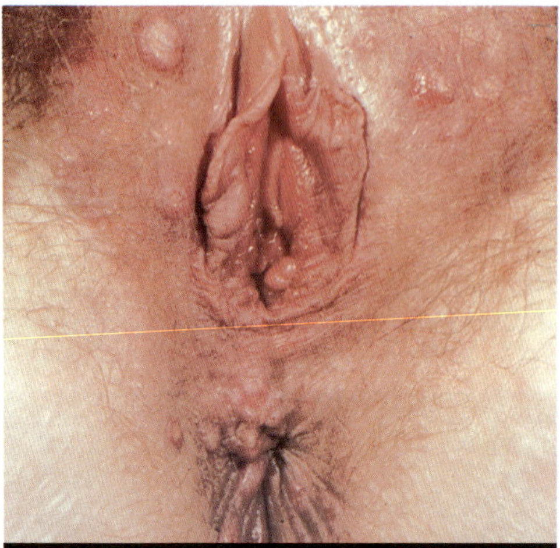

Figure 9.7 Condyloma Lata

Typical appearance of the verrucous, heaped-up lesions of condyloma lata, a manifestation of secondary syphilis. (Courtesy of H. Hunter Handsfield: *Atlas of Sexually Transmitted Diseases.* New York, McGraw-Hill, 1992.)

Associated Clinical Features

Gonorrhea often manifests after a short incubation period of 2 to 5 days. In men, urethritis is characterized by purulent, usually copious urethral discharge (Fig. 9.8) with dysuria; however, up to 10% of men are asymptomatic. Women may also develop urethritis (Fig. 9.9) and complain of dysuria. Cervicitis is often asymptomatic. If symptomatic, women may complain of increased vaginal discharge or vaginal spotting, particularly after intercourse. On speculum examination, the cervix is friable with a mucopurulent endocervical exudate (Fig. 9.10). Patients with gonococcal conjunctivitis have chemosis and copious, purulent exudate (Fig. 9.11); untreated, these patients can develop endophthalmitis and globe perforation. Untreated gonorrhea may disseminate, and more commonly does so in women. Disseminated gonococcal infection (DGI) presents with a monoarticular or oligorticular septic arthritis usually involving the knees, ankles, elbows, or wrists. Skin lesions are necrotic pustules on an erythematous base, may ulcerate, and are more commonly found on the distal extremities (Fig. 9.12).

Differential Diagnosis

The differential diagnosis depends on the site involved:

Urethritis and cervicitis: Chlamydia, mycoplasma, ureaplasma

Conjunctivitis: Bacterial conjunctivitis, chemical conjunctivitis

Arthritis: Septic arthritis, rheumatic fever, hepatitis B prodrome, immune complex disease, Reiter's syndrome, systemic lupus erythematosus

Skin lesions: Folliculitis, subacute bacterial endocarditis (septic emboli)

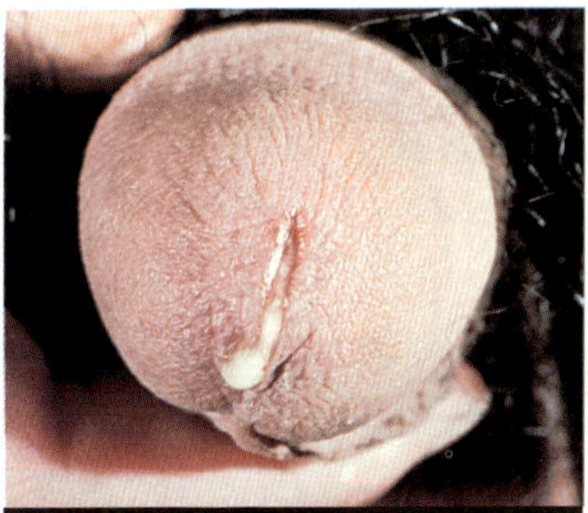

Figure 9.8
Male Urethritis

Purulent, copious urethral discharge in a patient with gonococcal urethritis. (Courtesy of H. Hunter Handsfield: *Atlas of Sexually Transmitted Diseases.* New York, McGraw-Hill, 1992.)

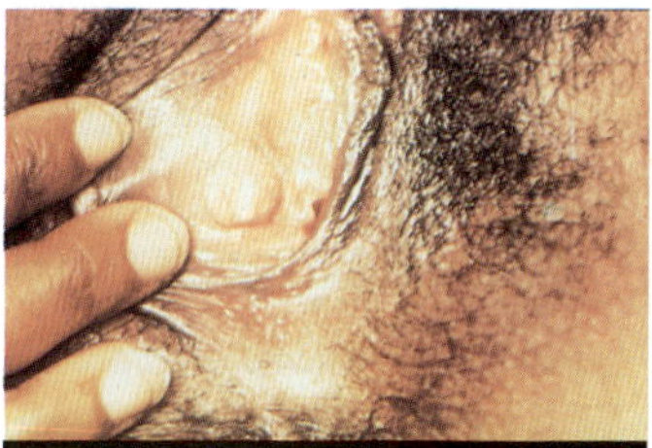

Figure 9.9
Female Urethritis

Gonococcal urethritis in a female patient; note the purulent urethral discharge. (Courtesy of Morse, Moreland, Thompson: *Atlas of Sexually Transmitted Diseases.* London, Mosby-Wolfe, 1990.)

ED Treatment and Disposition

Treatment is dependent on the site of infection:

Urethritis and cervicitis: Ceftriaxone, 125 mg IM once; cefixime, 400 mg PO once; ciprofloxacin, 500 mg PO once; ofloxacin, 400 mg PO once

Conjunctivitis: Ceftriaxone 1 g IM once; eye irrigation

Disseminated gonococcal infection: Ceftriaxone, 1 g IV or IM daily for 7 to 10 days; may treat with 1 to 2 days of IM ceftriaxone and then change to cefixime, 400 mg PO bid, or ciprofloxacin, 500 mg PO bid, to complete a 7- to 10-day course. Sexual partners should be notified and treated. Gonorrhea is a reportable disease.

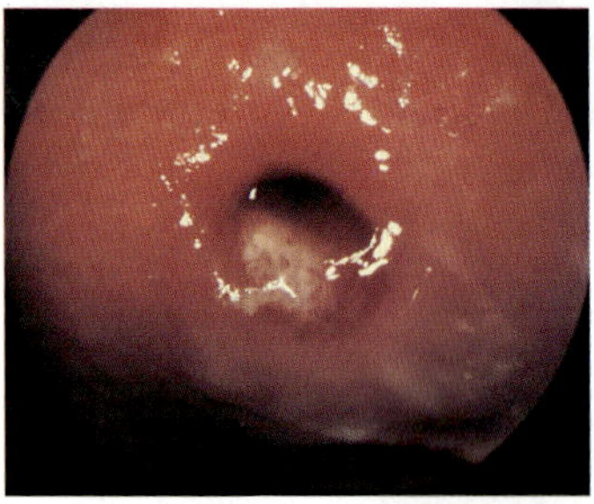

Figure 9.10 Cervicitis

Endocervical purulent exudate in an asymptomatic patient with gonococcal cervicitis. The cervix is very friable. (Courtesy of King K. Holmes, MD from H. Hunter Handsfield: *Atlas of Sexually Transmitted Diseases.* New York, McGraw-Hill, 1992.)

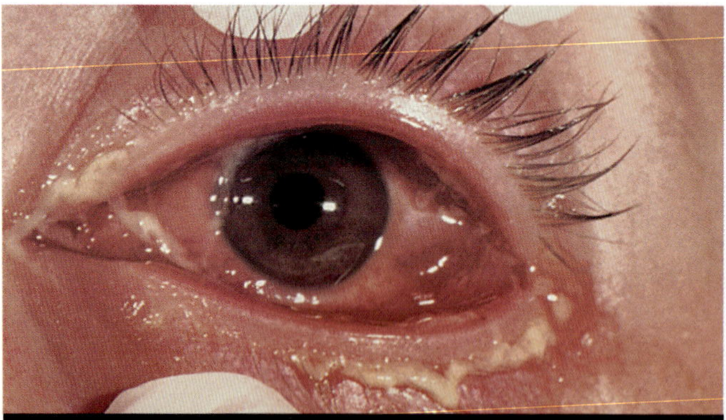

Figure 9.11 Conjunctivitis

Chemotic conjunctiva and copious purulent exudate in a patient with gonococcal conjunctivitis. (Courtesy of H. Hunter Handsfield: *Atlas of Sexually Transmitted Diseases.* New York, McGraw-Hill, 1992.)

Clinical Pearls

1. Patients with gonorrhea need to be treated for concurrent infection with *Chlamydia.* Coinfection with these organisms is seen in 30% of men with urethritis and 50% of women with cervicitis.
2. Gonococcal arthritis is the most common cause of monoarticular arthritis in young, sexually active patients.
3. Suspect gonococcal conjunctivitis in patients with copious eye discharge and chemosis.
4. Enlarged, fluctuant, tender Bartholin's abscess of the labia, usually but not always a result of gonorrhea.
5. Cultures are the gold standard for confirming the diagnosis of gonorrhea. Selective media should be used when specimens are obtained from the cervix, pharynx, urethra, or rectum. Nonselective medium (blood agar) should be used when culturing joint fluid, blood, or cerebrospinal fluid.

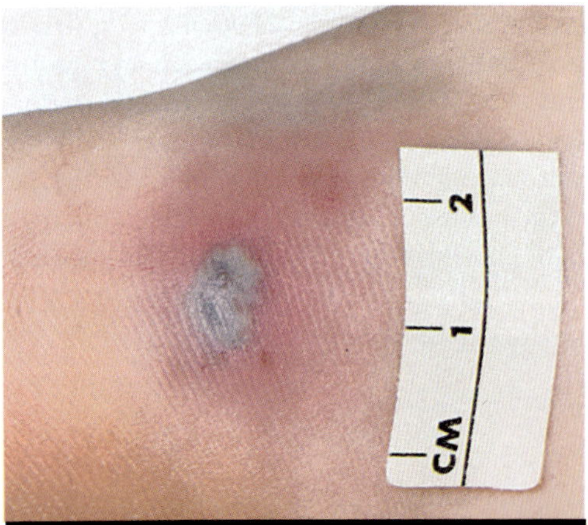

Figure 9.12 Skin Lesions

Small pustules with hemorrhage suggestive of the skin lesions of disseminated gonococcal infection. (Courtesy of H. Hunter Handsfield: *Atlas of Sexually Transmitted Diseases.* New York, McGraw-Hill, 1992.)

Associated Clinical Features

Herpes genitalis presents in several ways: symptomatic primary infection, first-episode nonprimary infection, and recurrent infection. Symptomatic primary infection occurs when the patient develops symptoms when first acquiring the virus. Some patients may be asymptomatic when primarily infected with the virus, however, and present at a later time with their first symptomatic episode of nonprimary genital herpes. Patients with either symptomatic primary infection or first-episode nonprimary infection may develop recurrences.

Symptomatic primary genital herpes is characterized by multiple vesicles that quickly ulcerate into shallow, painful ulcers (Figs. 9.14, 9.15). The ulcers may coalesce. The lesions are accompanied by a viral syndrome with low-grade fever and myalgias. Up to 10% of patients may develop aseptic meningitis. Women may develop sacral autonomic dysfunction and require urinary catheterization because of urinary retention. The lesions last up to 3 weeks and heal without scarring.

First-episode nonprimary genital herpes and recurrent genital herpes are less dramatic (Fig. 9.16). Patients with first-episode nonprimary genital herpes do not have systemic symptoms, have solitary to several painful lesions, and resolve their symptoms in 1 to 2 weeks. Recurrences of genital herpes are often heralded by a warning prodrome of tingling or numbness in the perineal area. Vesicles and their subsequent ulcers are often solitary. Duration of symptoms is often several days and usually less than a week.

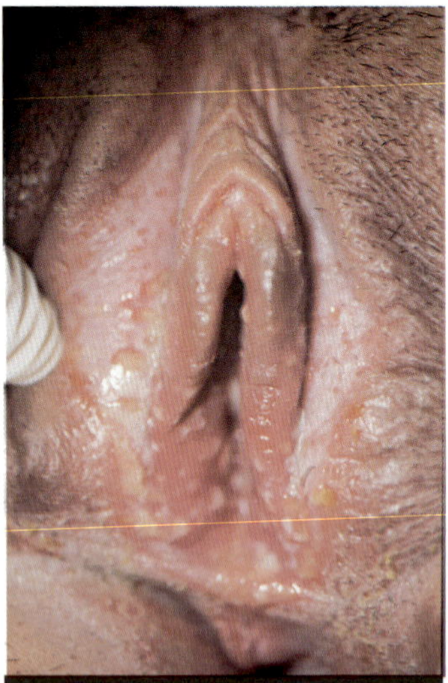

Figure 9.14 Primary Lesions—Female

Multiple, coalescing superficial ulcerations of primary genital herpes. (Courtesy of Lawrence B. Stack, MD.)

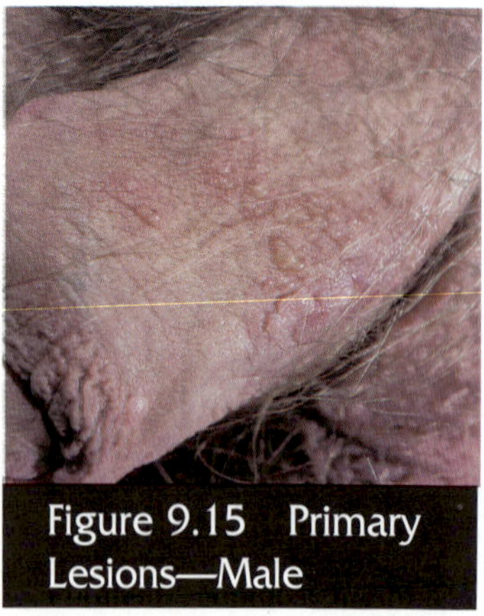

Figure 9.15 Primary Lesions—Male

Multiple genital vesicles of primary genital herpes. (Courtesy of H. Hunter Handsfield: *Atlas of Sexually Transmitted Diseases.* New York, McGraw-Hill, 1992.)

Differential Diagnosis

Pustular psoriasis, chancroid, erythema multiforme, fixed drug eruption, Behçet's disease, Stevens-Johnson syndrome, pyoderma gangrenosum, syphilis, and pyodermic infection may have a similar appearance.

ED Treatment and Disposition

Primary genital herpes: Acyclovir, 200 mg PO five times daily for 7 to 10 days or until symptoms resolve; 400 mg PO tid may be substituted for patient convenience.
Recurrent genital herpes: Acyclovir, 200 mg PO five times daily; 400 mg PO tid for 5 to 7 days; or Famciclovir, 125 mg PO BID for 5 days.

Clinical Pearls

1. Women with genital herpes must be counseled to inform their obstetrician of this history of herpes when they become pregnant.
2. Genital herpes is the most common cause of ulcerating genital lesions.
3. Patients may initially present with full-blown primary genital herpes symptoms or may have their first clinical presentation as a recurrence of an asymptomatically acquired infection (Fig. 9.17).

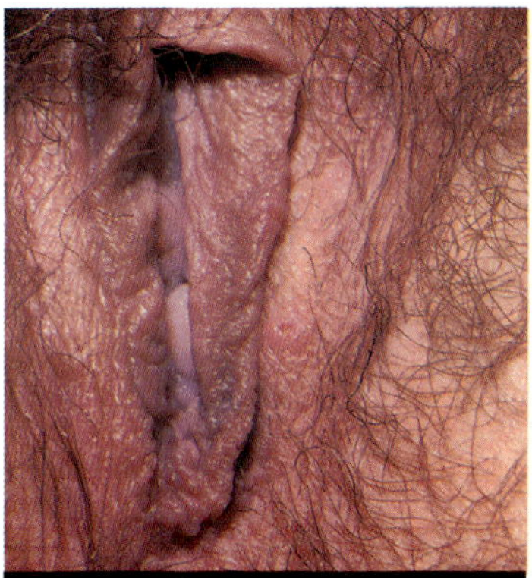

Figure 9.16 Recurrent Lesions—Female

Solitary, minimally painful lesion of recurrent genital herpes. (Courtesy of H. Hunter Handsfield: *Atlas of Sexually Transmitted Diseases.* New York, McGraw-Hill, 1992.)

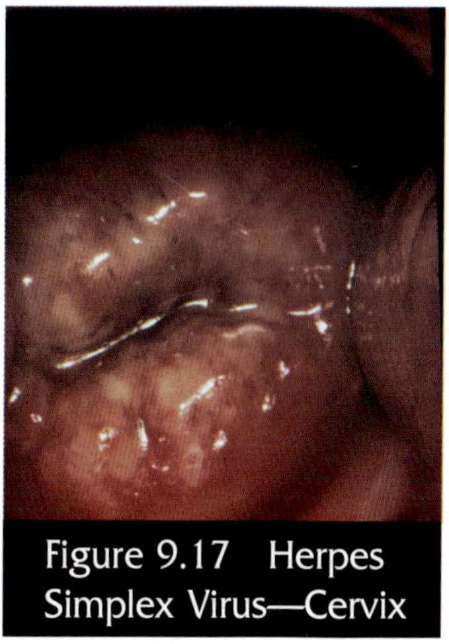

Figure 9.17 Herpes Simplex Virus—Cervix

Erosive ulcerations of the cervix in a patient with genital herpes infection. This patient may be completely asymptomatic and may transmit the disease. (Courtesy of A. Wisdom: *Sexually Transmitted Diseases.* London, Mosby-Wolfe, 1992.)

Associated Clinical Features

Pediculosis can be caused by either the body louse or the crab louse. Body lice (Fig. 17.13) are not sexually transmitted and tend to cluster around the waist, shoulders, axillae, neck, and head. Extremely itchy, patients may present with excoriations and intense pruritus. The lice are very small and may not be easily seen. The larval form of the louse, the nit, may be mistaken for dandruff in the hair. Unlike dandruff, however, the nits are extremely adherent to the hair shaft and cannot be brushed out of the hair. The adult lice and their eggs are often found in the seams of clothing.

Pubic infestation is caused by *Phthirus pubis,* the crab louse (Fig. 9.18, 17.12). Patients may present with intense itching in the pubic area; however, as many as half of patients with this infestation may be asymptomatic. Patients may notice the lice or may note tiny rust-colored spots on their underwear, which represent bleeding from the sites of louse bites. Nits may be found at the base of pubic hairs and hatch in 5 to 10 days.

Differential Diagnosis

Tinea, contact dermatitis, scabies, and heat rash may have a similar appearance.

ED Treatment and Disposition

Lindane shampoo (Kevell™) should be lathered into the pubic, perineal, and perianal hair, or lindane lotion applied in the affected areas and left on for 10 min and rinsed off. Synergized pyrethrins (RID™), or synthetic pyrethrins (NIX™, Elmite™), may also be used. Since lindane may be toxic, pyrethrins are preferred in pregnant women and children. Treatment should be repeated in 1 week to treat any nits that may have hatched. Clothing worn or linen used in the preceding 24 h should be washed. Mechanical removal of nits attached to hairs should be attempted. Petrolatum jelly or any bland ophthalmic ointment can be applied to the eyelashes twice daily for a week to treat infestation of the eyelashes (Fig. 9.19). Sexual contacts should be examined.

Clinical Pearls

1. Nits are easier to find on examination than are mature lice; the average number of lice in an infestation is only 10.
2. Patients with pediculosis pubis should be considered at risk for other sexually transmitted diseases and examined.
3. Lindane shampoo or lotion should not be used in infants under 1 year of age or in pregnant women.

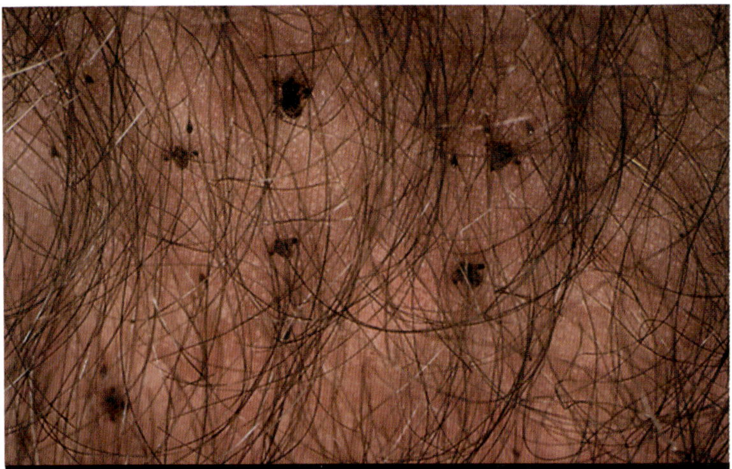

Figure 9.18 Pediculosis Pubis—on Hairs

Phthirus pubis, or the crab louse, in the pubic hair of a patient complaining of itching. Note also the nits attached to the hairs. (Courtesy of Morse, Moreland, Thompson: *Atlas of Sexually Transmitted Diseases.* London, Mosby-Wolfe, 1990.)

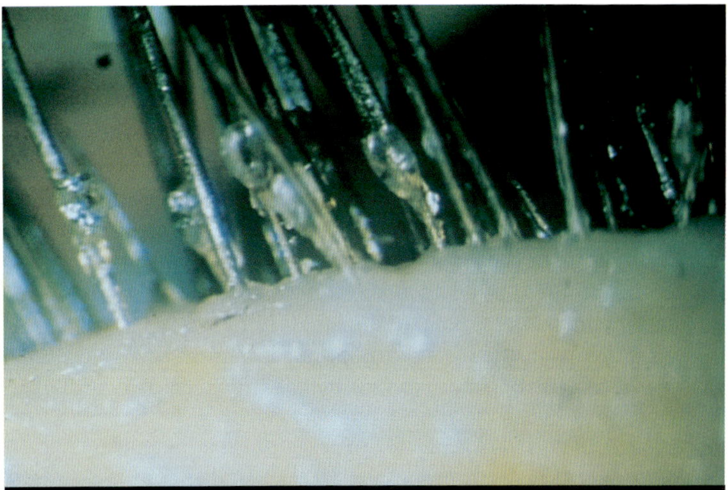

Figure 9.19 Pediculosis Pubis—on Eyelashes

Phthirus pubis lice noted in the eyelashes. (Courtesy of Spalton, Hitchings, Hunter: *Atlas of Clinical Ophthalmology,* 2d ed. London, Mosby-Year Book Europe, 1994.)

Associated Clinical Features

Caused by human papilloma virus (HPV), these flesh-colored lesions may be flat, sessile, or pedunculated (Figs. 9.20, 9.21). They often have a cauliflowerlike appearance and are usually asymptomatic, but may be seen or felt by patients or their sexual partners. They range in size from 1 to 4 mm to masses that may be several centimeters large (giant warts, Figs. 9.22 to 9.23).

Differential Diagnosis

Condyloma lata due to secondary syphilis is the primary alternative diagnosis (Fig. 9.7). Bowen's disease, molluscum contagiosum, and carcinoma may have a similar appearance.

ED Treatment and Disposition

Local caustic agents (e.g., podophyllin) are used to treat the lesions; multiple treatment is often needed, and recurrence is common. Other therapies include cryotherapy, electrocautery, and trichloracetic acid. Laser therapy or surgery may be needed in cases of giant warts.

Clinical Pearls

1. Evidence suggests that HPV is linked with increased risk of cervical cancer.
2. Women with genital warts need to have a Pap smear to rule out coexisting carcinoma in situ.
3. Large lesions should be biopsied to rule out cancer.
4. Patients should be advised that it may take several to many visits to completely eradicate the condyloma.
5. In cases where the diagnosis is not obvious, rule out condyloma lata (secondary syphilis) by sending serologic studies.

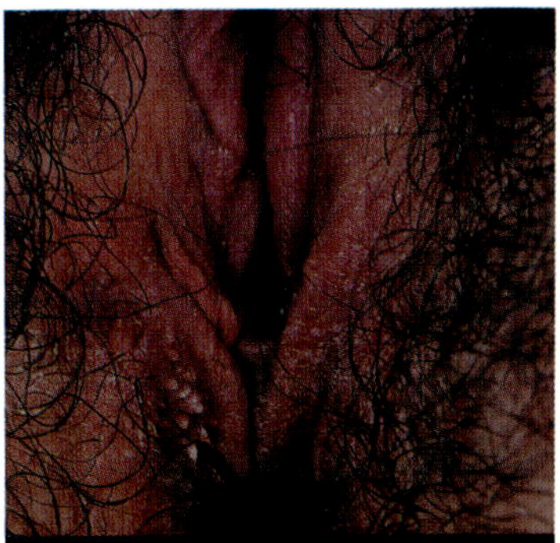

Figure 9.20 Genital Warts—Female

Verrucous lesions of the posterior fourchette in a patient with condyloma acuminata. (Used with permission from H. Hunter Handsfield: *Atlas of Sexually Transmitted Diseases.* New York, McGraw-Hill, 1992.)

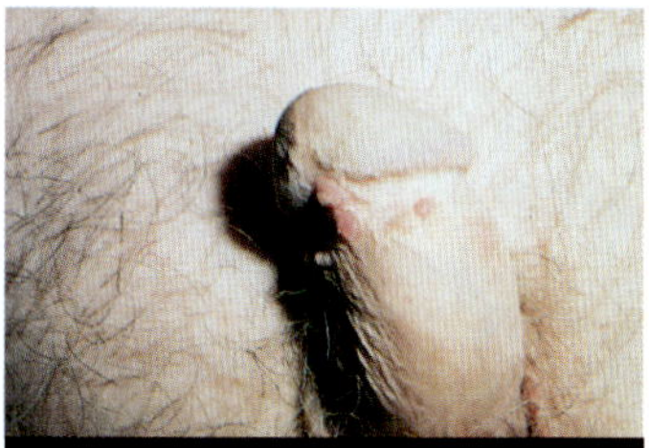

Figure 9.21 Genital Warts—Male

Typical appearance of condyloma acuminata of the glans penis. (Courtesy of Morse, Moreland, Thompson: *Atlas of Sexually Transmitted Diseases.* London, Mosby-Wolfe, 1990.)

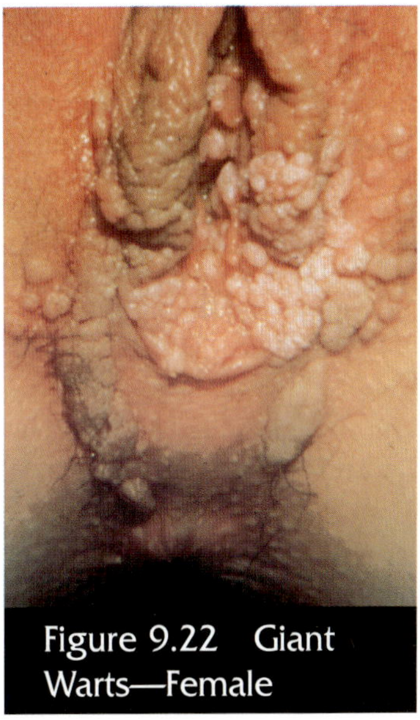

Figure 9.22 Giant Warts—Female

Giant warts of a female patient with extensive condyloma acuminata. (Courtesy of Morse, Moreland, Thompson: *Atlas of Sexually Transmitted Diseases.* London, Mosby-Wolfe, 1990.)

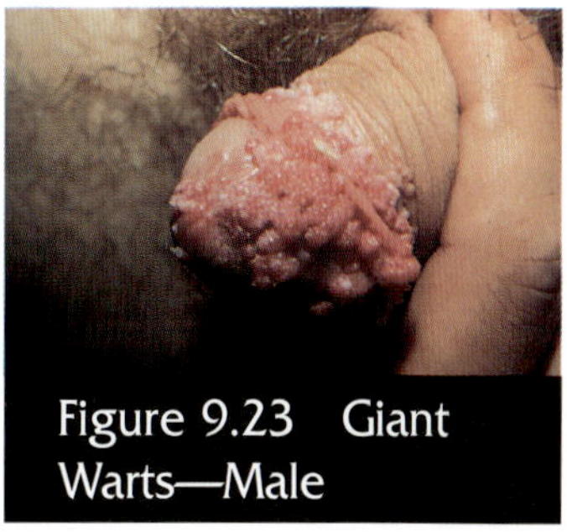

Figure 9.23 Giant Warts—Male

Giant warts in a male patient with extensive condyloma acuminata. (Courtesy of A. Wisdom: *Sexually Transmitted Diseases.* London, Mosby-Wolfe, 1992.)

Associated Clinical Features

An anal fissure is a longitudinal tear in the skin of the anal canal and usually extends from the dentate line to the anal verge. Fissures are thought to be caused by the passage of hard or large stools with constipation, but may also be seen with diarrhea. The fissures are typically a few millimeters wide and occur in the posterior midline (Fig. 9.24), but can occur elsewhere. An anal fissure that is off the midline may have a secondary cause such as inflammatory bowel disease or sexually transmitted infection. Although often seen in infants, this condition is found mostly in young and middle-aged adults. Patients present with the complaint of intense sharp, burning pain during and after bowel movements. They may also note bright red blood at the time or shortly after the passage of stool. Gentle examination with separation of the buttocks usually provides good visualization (Fig. 9.24). Anoscopy should be performed, if possible.

Differential Diagnosis

The diagnosis of inflammatory bowel disease, ulcerative colitis or Crohn's disease should be considered, particularly if the fissure is atypical. Anal fissures may be the result of a sexually transmitted disease such as *Chlamydia,* gonorrhea, herpes, and syphilis. Tuberculosis, anal neoplasms, and sickle cell disease can also present as an anal fissure. An anal abscess and thrombosed hemorrhoids may cause similar symptoms, but can usually be ruled out on physical examination.

ED Treatment and Disposition

Acute treatment of anal fissures consists of anal hygiene, bulk fiber diet supplements to soften stools, warm sitz baths, and topical anesthetics. Oral pain medication and muscle relaxants such as diazepam may be required in certain patients.

Clinical Pearls

1. Pain and involuntary sphincter spasm may preclude a routine digital or anoscopic examination and require an examination under anesthesia.
2. A proctoscopic examination should be done at some point to rule out secondary causes.
3. Most anal fissures heal spontaneously, but refractory cases may require surgical repair.

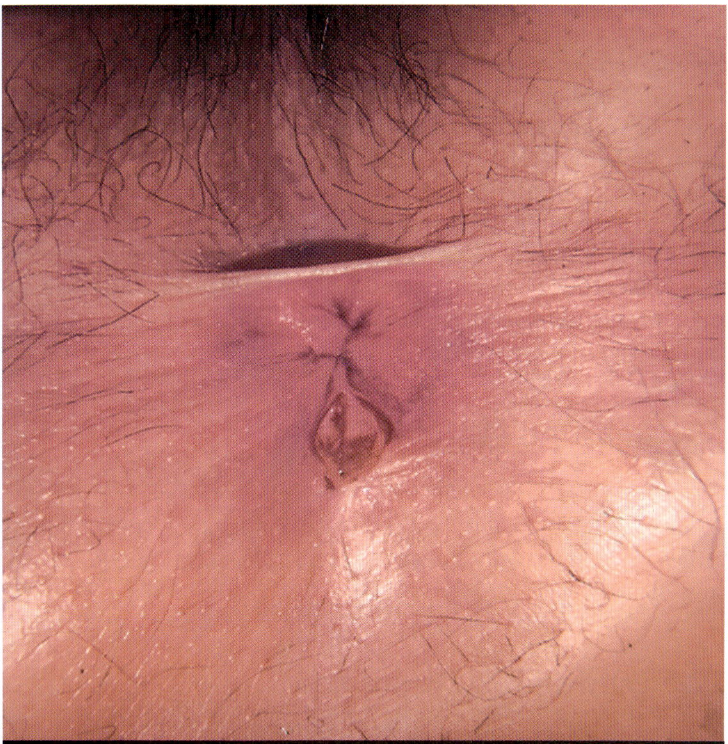

Figure 9.24 Anal Fissure

A typical anal fissure located in the posterior midline. (Courtesy of Paul J. Kovalcik, MD.)

Associated Clinical Features

External hemorrhoids result from the dilatation of the venules of the inferior hemorrhoidal plexus below the dentate line. They have a covering of skin, or anoderm, versus internal hemorrhoids that have a mucosal covering. Hemorrhoids commonly present with an episode of rectal bleeding of bright red blood after defecation. This results from the passage of the fecal mass over the thin-walled venules, causing abrasions and bleeding. Symptoms from external hemorrhoids include complaints of swelling and burning rectal pain. Numerous associated factors exist, such as constipation, family history, pregnancy, portal hypertension, or increased intraabdominal pressure. Hemorrhoids are commonly found at three anatomic locations: right anterior, right posterior, and left lateral positions (Fig. 9.25). A thrombosed external hemorrhoid contains intravascular clots and causes exquisite pain the first 48 h.

Internal hemorrhoids (Fig. 9.26) present with painless rectal bleeding or possibly the sensation of prolapse. They are graded according to the degree of prolapse where the first degree is identifiable at the dentate line and the fourth degree shows irreducible prolapse through the anus. Internal hemorrhoids are not typically painful, whereas external hemorrhoids do cause pain.

Differential Diagnosis

Other diagnoses to consider include infection, perianal or perirectal abscess, inflammatory bowel disease, malignancy, local trauma, herpes or other sexually transmitted infection, rectal polyp, or rectal prolapse.

ED Treatment and Disposition

In the case of severe bleeding, fluid resuscitation would need to be instituted and the bleeding vessel located, clamped, and ligated. The treatment for less severe cases warrants more conservative therapy, including increased dietary fiber, increased fluid intake, hot sitz baths, bedrest, and nonnarcotic pain medication. Advanced cases may require surgical consultation and treatment. ED treatment of thrombosed external hemorrhoids includes an elliptical excision and extrusion of the clot under local anesthesia.

Clinical Pearls

1. Many patients with any anorectal problem complain of hemorrhoids. Therefore, careful examination and consideration of the differential diagnosis should be undertaken with each patient.
2. Having the patient strain during the examination may reveal bleeding or prolapse that may otherwise go unnoticed.
3. Hemorrhoids are a rare cause of anorectal pruritus.

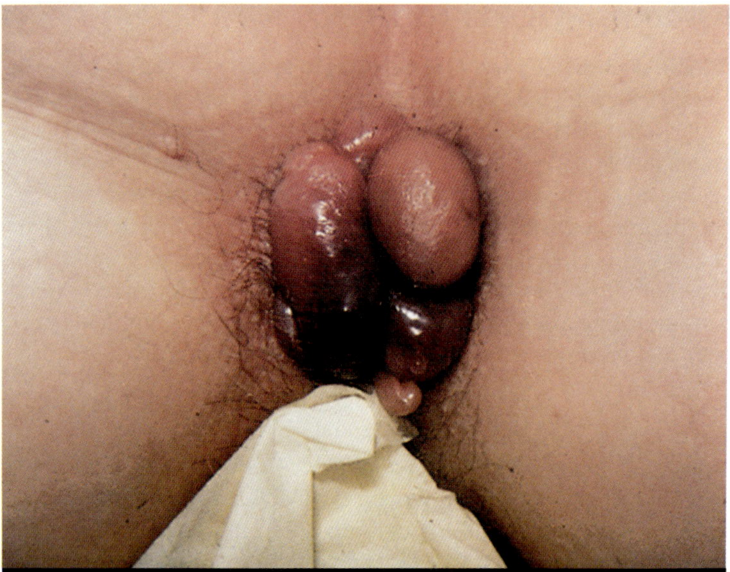

Figure 9.25 External Hemorrhoids

Multiple engorged external hemorrhoids are seen in all quadrants. (Courtesy of the American Society of Colon and Rectal Surgeons.)

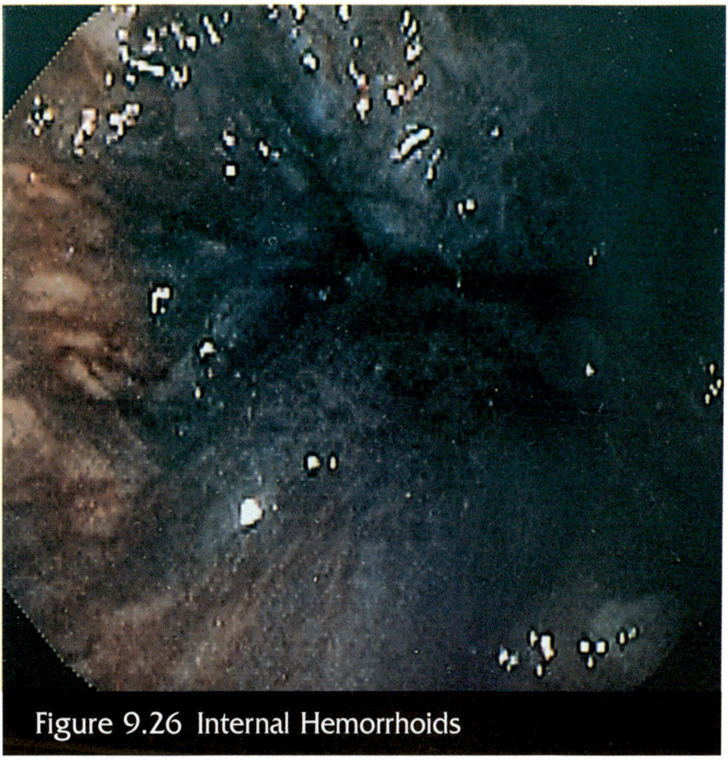

Figure 9.26 Internal Hemorrhoids

Internal hemorrhoids are seen in this endoscopic view of the rectum. (Courtesy of Virender K. Sharman, MD.)

Associated Clinical Features

Pilonidal abscesses are typically seen at or just superior to the gluteal fold (Fig. 9.27) and are more common in teenage and young adult males. Patients complain of localized pain, swelling, and drainage, but usually do not have systemic symptoms. The abscess begins with the formation of a small opening in the skin that develops into a cystic structure involving surrounding hairs. This opening is occluded by hair or keratin, creating a closed space that does not allow drainage. The acute abscess contains mixed organisms including *Staphylococcus aureus* and *Streptococcus,* but anaerobes and gram-negative organisms may also be present.

Differential Diagnosis

Evidence of cellulitis in the sacrococcygeal area may result from a simple abscess or furuncle. However, other causes should be considered such as anal fistulae, hidradenitis, inflammatory bowel disease, or tuberculosis.

ED Disposition and Treatment

An acutely fluctuant abscess requires incision and drainage under local anesthesia with removal of pus and debris. The patient should be instructed on meticulous wound care and sitz baths. Antibiotic therapy is not indicated unless the patient is immunocompromised. Surgical referral is given, particularly with a chronic or recurrent cyst that may require surgical excision and closure.

Clinical Pearls

1. Pilonidal abscesses almost always occur in the midline, but can have sinus tracts extending off the midline.
2. Pilonidal disease is three times more common in men than in women.

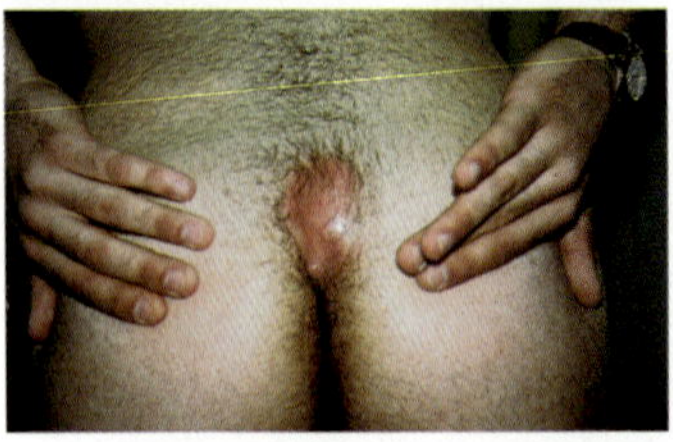

Figure 9.27 Pilonidal Abscess

Redness, fluctuance, and tenderness in the gluteal cleft seen with a pilonidal abscess. (Courtesy of Louis La Vopa, MD.

CHAPTER 10

GYNECOLOGIC AND OBSTETRIC CONDITIONS

Robert G. Buckley
Kevin J. Knoop

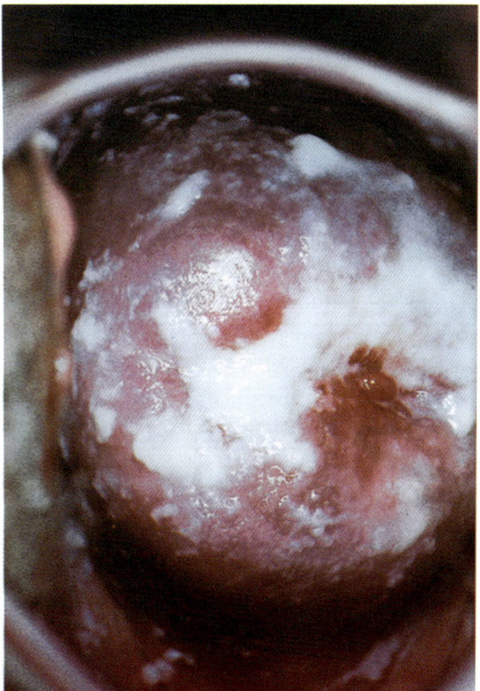

Associated Clinical Features

Candidal vaginitis is characterized by a thick curdy white discharge, (Fig. 10.1) and vulvar discomfort. Intense vulvar erythema, pruritus, or burning are often present. A microscopic slide prepared with 10% potassium hydroxide yielding characteristic branch chain hyphae and spores establishes the diagnosis (Fig. 17.8). The pH of the discharge is less than 4.5. Predisposing factors which should be considered include oral contraceptive, antibiotic, or corticosteroid use; pregnancy; and diabetes. Sexually transmitted diseases are not usually associated with isolated candidal vaginitis.

Trichomonas vaginitis presents as a persistent, thin, copious discharge that is often frothy (Fig. 10.2), green, or foul smelling. The pH of these secretions is greater than 4.5. The amount of vaginal and cervical erythema and inflammation varies considerably; thus the diagnosis depends on the presence of motile flagellates on normal saline wet mount microscopy. Occasionally, multiple petechiae on the vaginal wall (strawberry spots) or cervix (strawberry cervix) are seen.

Bacterial vaginosis (previously termed *Haemophilus,* or *Gardnerella* vaginitis) is characterized by a malodorous, homogeneous discharge (Fig. 10.3) with a pH greater than 4.5 and a transient amine (fishy) odor when mixed with a drop of KOH solution (positive sniff test). Clue cells present on normal saline wet mount establish the diagnosis (Fig. 17.5). Other associated vaginal or abdominal complaints are minimal and, if significant, may represent another disease process.

Differential Diagnosis

Vaginal foreign bodies, especially in prepubescent girls, may present with a heavy white discharge, but would be unaccompanied by vulvar erythema or the microscopic appearance of hyphae. Atrophic vaginitis is commonly found in postmenopausal women and is discriminated from candidal vaginitis by mucosal dryness, atrophy, dyspareunia, and minimal discharge and itching. Other considerations include contact dermatitis, local irritation secondary to tight-fitting underwear, and contact dermatitis from toiletry items.

ED Treatment and Disposition

For *candidal vaginitis,* various regimens of topical antifungal agents are the mainstay of treatment (clotrimazole 1% cream, one applicatorful inserted high into the vaginal vault for 7 nights, clotrimazole, two 100-mg vaginal tablets for 3 nights or one 500-mg vaginal tablet for single-dose treatment). Oral fluconazole (Diflucan, 150 mg as a single dose) is also effective. Nystatin vaginal tablets (100,000 U daily for 2 weeks) are generally considered safe for use in the first trimester of pregnancy.

For *Trichomonas vaginitis* a single, one-time dose of metronidazole (2 g) is generally curative. Alternatively, 250 mg given three times daily can be used for recurrent or refractory cases. Metronidazole is contraindicted in pregnancy and is associated with an Antabuse-like reaction when taken with alcohol. For the pregnant patient, clotrimazole (100-mg vaginal suppositories daily for 7 to 14 days) may provide symptomatic relief.

For *Bacterial vaginosis,* metronidazole (500 mg twice daily for 7 days) is recommended in the nonpregnant patient. Amoxicillin (500 mg tid for 7 days) or clindamycin (300 mg bid) for 7 days is a safe, but less effective, alternative during pregnancy. Treatment for asymptomatic infection or for male sexual partners is not generally recommended.

Clinical Pearls

1. Diabetes mellitus or immunosuppression should be considered in refractory or recurrent cases of candidal vaginitis.
2. A history of balanitis in the sexual partner should be sought and, if present, treated.
3. *Trichomonas* should be considered a sexually transmitted disease. It is generally recommended, therefore, that concomitant culturing for gonorrhea and *Chlamydia* be performed. Serologic testing for syphilis, HIV, and hepatitis B should be considered.
4. Patients treated with metronidazole should abstain from alcohol for the duration of treatment and for at least 24 h after their last dose.

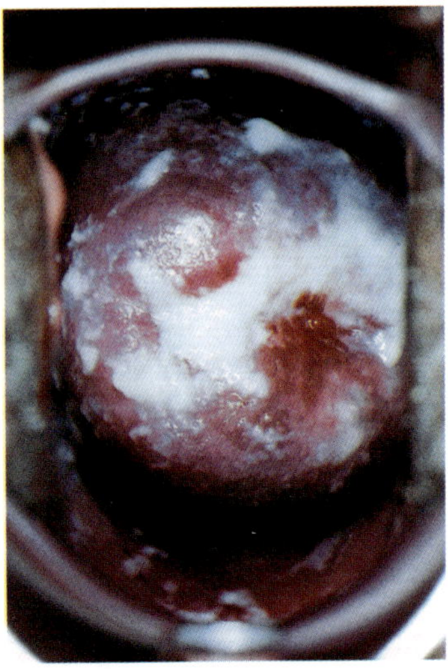

Figure 10.1 Candidal Vaginitis

Thick, curdy white discharge secondary to candidal vaginitis. (Courtesy of Kevin J. Knoop, MS, MD.)

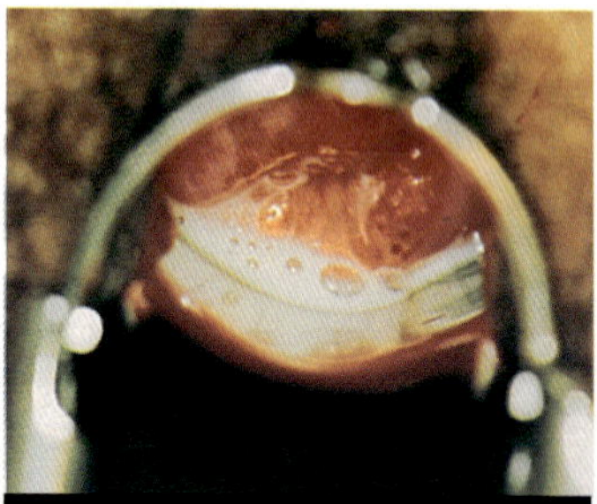

Figure 10.2
Trichomonas Vaginitis

Thin vaginal discharge suggestive of *Trichomonas* vaginitis. (Courtesy of H. Hunter Handsfield: *Atlas of Sexually Transmitted Diseases.* New York, McGraw-Hill, 1992.)

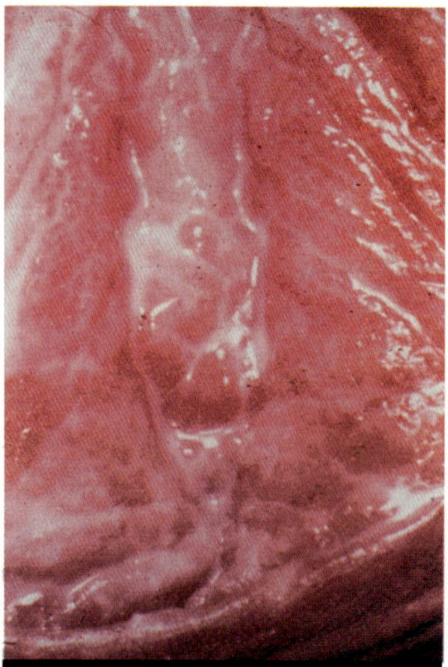

Figure 10.3
Gardnerella Vaginitis

Thin milky white discharge suggestive of *Gardnerella* vaginitis. (Courtesy of Curatek Pharmaceuticals.)

DIAGNOSIS BARTHOLIN'S GLAND ABSCESS

Associated Clinical Features

Bartholin's glands and ducts are located over the lower third of the introitus near the labia minora. A cyst or abscess can result from an obstructed duct which usually occurs secondary to scarring from trauma, delivery, or episiotomy. Infection of the cyst is usually with mixed vaginal or fecal flora (*Escherichia coli*), but may also contain *Neisseria gonorrhoeae* and *Chlamydia trachomatis.* Progressive enlargement and infection leads to increasing pain, swelling, and dyspareunia. A tender, fluctuant cystic mass with surrounding labial edema is easily appreciated on examination (Fig. 10.4).

Differential Diagnosis

Epidermal inclusion cysts and sebaceous cysts of the labia majora may look similar, but are generally smaller. When inflamed or infected, maximal fluctuance generally points toward the external aspect of the labium, as opposed to Bartholin's gland cysts, which point medially. Occlusion and infection of apocrine sweat glands can lead to subcutaneous abscess formation—known as hidradenitis suppurativa. Vulvar hematoma, leiomyoma, lipoma, and fibromas may occasionally be confused with a noninfected Bartholin's cyst. Vulvar cancer usually arises in postmenopausal women and is generally either ulcerated, excoriated, or exophytic.

ED Treatment and Disposition

Simple incision and drainage followed by sitz baths provide the most effective and expeditious relief on an emergency basis. Unfortunately, reocclusion and reaccumulation of cystic swelling are common. Definitive therapy of recurrent Bartholin's gland cysts involves marsupialization by suturing the introital mucosa to the inner cyst wall.

Clinical Pearls

1. Antibiotics, although commonly used, are usually not required.
2. Placement of a Word catheter into the cyst cavity (Fig. 10.5) decreases the incidence of reocclusion, but must be allowed to remain in place for up to 6 weeks to ensure epithelialization of the drainage tract.

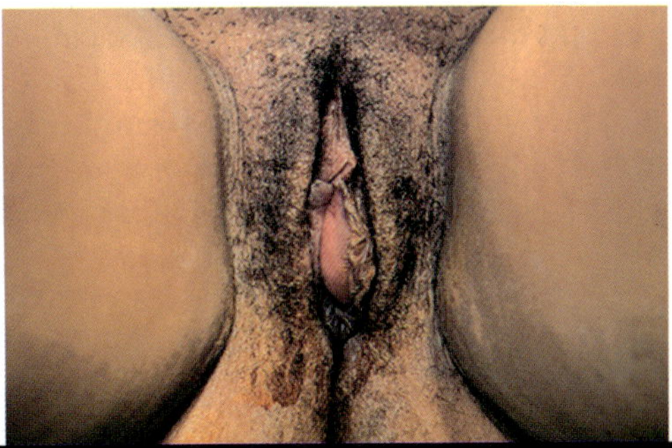

Figure 10.4 Bartholin's Gland Abscess

Typical appearance of a Bartholin's gland abscess with the labial fluctuance pointing medially.

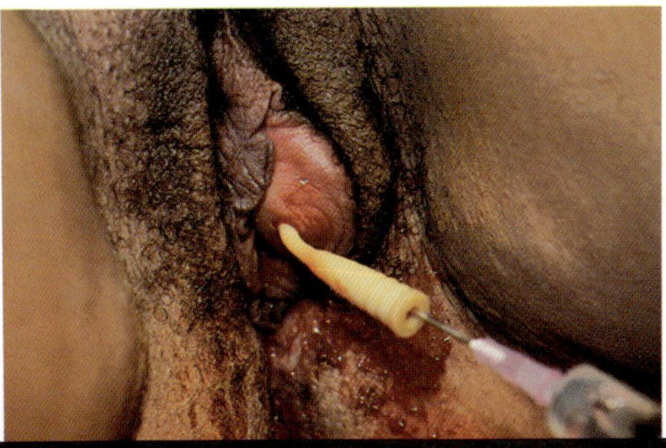

Figure 10.5 Bartholin's Gland Abscess

Insertion and inflation of a Word catheter into the cyst cavity. The free end of the catheter can be tucked into the vagina for long-term placement, allowing for the epithelialization of the incision site. (Figures 10.4 and 10.5 courtesy of the Medical Photography Department, Naval Medical Center, San Diego.)

Associated Clinical Features

Speculum examination reveals a purulent, viscous discharge emanating from the cervical os (Fig. 10.6). A purulent discharge may be seen on a cervical swab. A Gram's stain may reveal either gram-negative intracellular diplococci consistent with *Neisseria* gonorrhoeae (Fig. 17.4) or be nonspecific, consistent with *Chlamydia trachomatis,* a coinfectant with *Gonococcus* about 50% of the time.

Differential Diagnosis

Physiologic cervical mucous discharge at the time of ovulation may occur, but is generally clear, with few WBC's on Gram's stain.

ED Treatment and Disposition

Cultures for *Chlamydia trachomatis* and *Neisseria gonorrhoeae* should be obtained. Ceftriaxone (125 mg as a single intramuscular dose) provides coverage for *Neisseria gonorrhoeae*. Single-dose oral quinolones (ciprofloxacin, 500 mg, or ofloxacin, 400 mg) can be used in penicillin-allergic patients. Doxycycline (100 mg) or ofloxacin (300 mg bid for 7 days or a single 1-g dose of azithromycin) provides coverage for *Chlamydia.* Erythromycin (base 500 mg qid for 7 days) is the alternative for pregnant patients.

Clinical Pearls

1. The discharge of candidal, trichomonal or *Gardnerella* vaginitis is almost never limited solely to the cervix.
2. Mucopurulent cervicitis is almost always secondary to a sexually transmitted disease; thus sexual partners should be treated.
3. Refer all patients for gynecologic follow-up after treatment. Early cervical neoplasia may have a similar appearance.

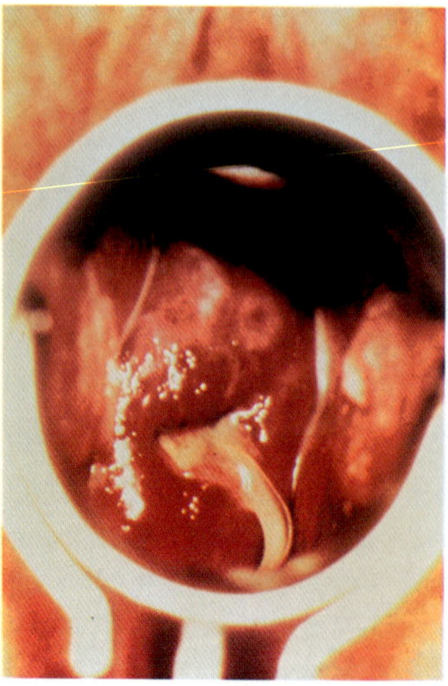

Figure 10.6 Mucopurulent Cervicitis

Viscous, opaque discharge emanating from the cervical os, consistent with mucopurulent cervicitis. The string from an intrauterine device is seen descending through the os in this patient. (Courtesy of Sue Rist, FNP.)

Associated Clinical Features

Spontaneous abortion is associated with vaginal bleeding and abdominal discomfort. Severe pain, heavy bleeding with the passage of clots or tissue (Fig. 10.7), fever, and hypotension may also be present. *Threatened abortion* is diagnosed when mild cramping and vaginal bleeding are not accompanied by the complete or partial extrusion of tissue, cervical dilation, or ectopic pregnancy. Uterine cramping with progressive dilation of the cervix, with or without partial extrusion of the products of conception, indicates the presence of an *inevitable abortion* (Fig. 10.8). In an *incomplete abortion,* some elements of the conceptus have passed, yet retained intrauterine tissue leads to ongoing uterine cramping, cervical dilation, and persistent bleeding.

Differential Diagnosis

Ectopic pregnancy should be considered in all first-trimester females with lower abdominal pain or vaginal bleeding. The presence of frank tissue passage or cervical dilation essentially excludes this diagnosis. Large blood clots or an intrauterine decidual cast (Fig. 10.9), however, may occasionally be mistaken for products of conception.

ED Treatment and Disposition

Intravenous access, fluid resuscitation, cross-matching of blood, and urgent gynecologic consultation should be made in the presence of severe pain, heavy bleeding, or hypovolemia. All tissue should be sent to pathology for definitive identification. Occasionally, patients who initially have an open cervical os will rapidly expel the remaining products of conception, with subsequent resolution of all pain and bleeding. These patients may be discharged from the emergency department with the diagnosis of completed abortion if otherwise clinically stable. Anti-Rh immunoglobulin (RhoGAM) should be administered in all cases of vaginal bleeding in the pregnant patient where the mother is Rh negative and the father is not Rh negative.

Clinical Pearls

1. The passage of large clots usually indicates rapid heavy bleeding.
2. *Completed abortion* is characterized by the passage of tissue, followed by resolution of bleeding and closure of the cervical os.
3. Fever, leukocytosis, pelvic tenderness, and malodorous cervical discharge should suggest *septic abortion.*

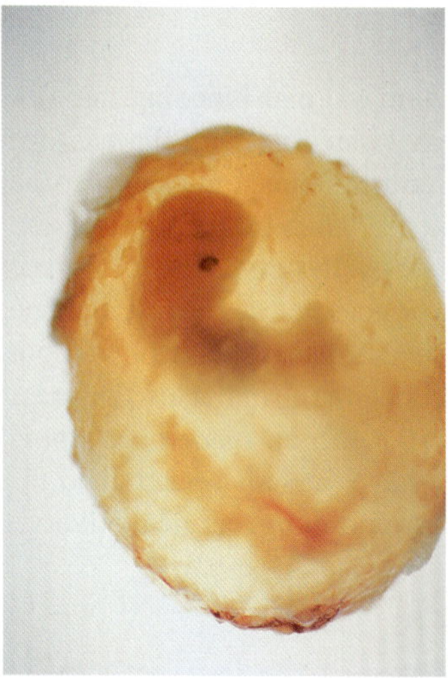

Figure 10.7 Spontaneous Abortion

Passage of tissue in a spontaneous abortion at 4 weeks. (Courtesy of Lawrence B. Stack, MD.)

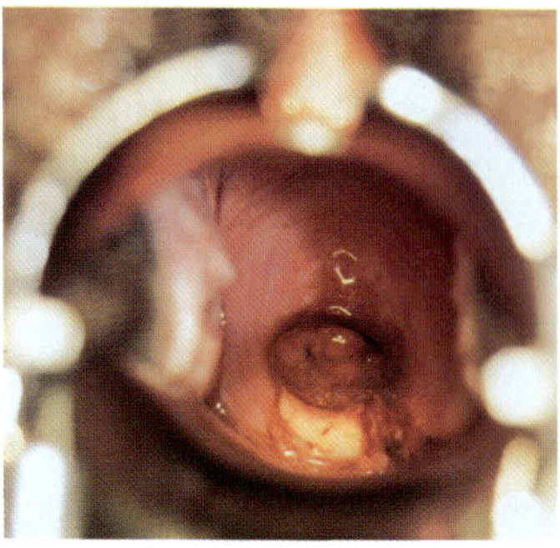

Figure 10.8 Spontaneous Abortion

Dilation of the cervical os with partial extrusion of tissue in the setting of an inevitable abortion. (Courtesy of Robert Buckley, MD.)

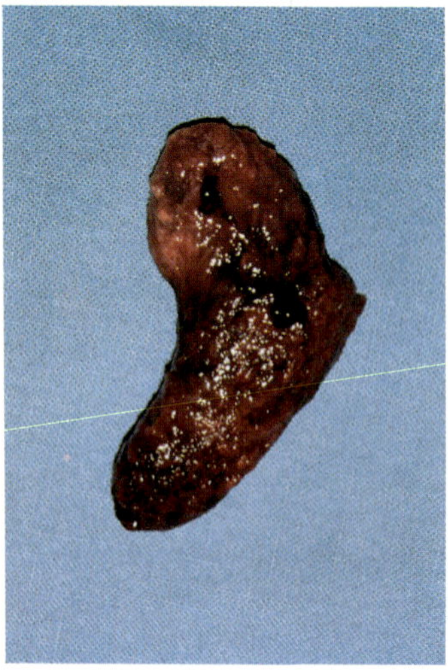

Figure 10.9 Decidual Cast

A decidual cast or organized clot may occasionally be mistaken for products of conception. (Courtesy of the Medical Photography Department, Naval Medical Center, San Diego.)

Associated Clinical Features

A cystocele occurs when there is relaxation and bulging of the posterior bladder wall and trigone into the vagina and is usually due to birth trauma. Patients complain of bulging or fullness over the introitus that is worsened with Valsalva (Fig. 10.10) and relieved with recumbency. It is often associated with urinary incontinence or symptoms of incomplete emptying. Most cystoceles, however, are asymptomatic. Examination reveals a thin-walled bulging of the anterior vaginal wall, which, in severe cases, may pass through the introitus with Valsalva.

Differential Diagnosis

An enterocele may lead to a similar bulging of the anterior vaginal wall but is much less common and is generally limited to those patients who have had a hysterectomy. Rectocele, uterine prolapse, and soft-tissue tumors should also be considered.

ED Treatment and Disposition

Larger cystoceles or those associated with urinary symptomatology, pain, or bothersome bulging should be referred to a gynecologist for further evaluation.

Clinical Pearl

1. Most cystoceles are asymptomatic and are detected incidentally at the time of pelvic examination.

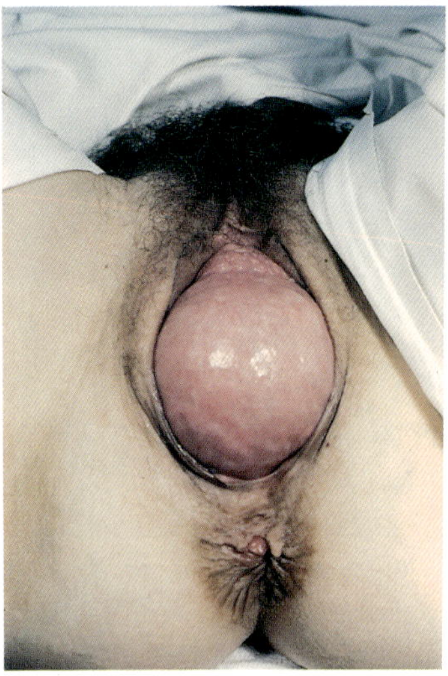

Figure 10.10 Cystocele

Cystocele worsening with Valsalva. (Courtesy of Matthew Backer, Jr., MD.)

Associated Clinical Features

Most small rectoceles are completely asymptomatic, though symptoms of introital bulging, constipation, and incomplete rectal evacuation may occur. Bulging of the introitus can be seen grossly on physical examination (Fig. 10.9) and can become worse with Valsalva (Fig. 10.10). Rectovaginal examination reveals a thin-walled protrusion of the rectovaginal septum into the lower part of the vagina.

Differential Diagnosis

Cystocele, enterocele, uterine prolapse, and soft-tissue tumors should all be easily distinguished by careful inspection.

ED Treatment and Disposition

Supportive measures with hydration, laxatives, and stool softeners are generally all that are needed to relieve the patient's symptoms. Those patients with large symptomatic rectoceles, who do not desire further childbearing, are candidates for posterior colpoperineorrhaphy.

Clinical Pearl

1. A rectocele is the herniation of the rectovaginal wall and is usually due to childbirth.

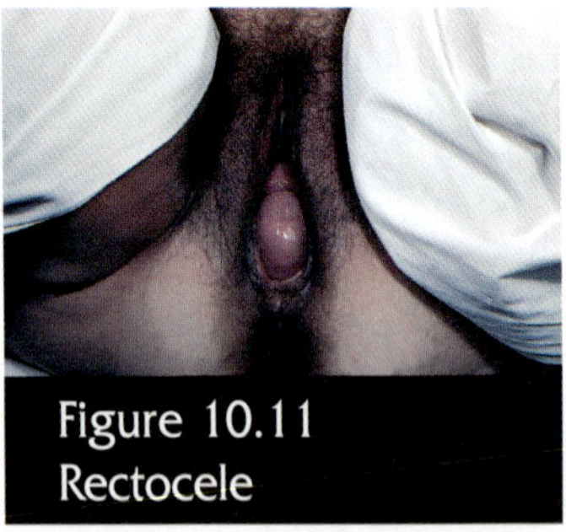

Figure 10.11 Rectocele

Characterized by bulging of the posterior vaginal wall at the introitus. (Courtesy of Matthew Backer, Jr., MD.)

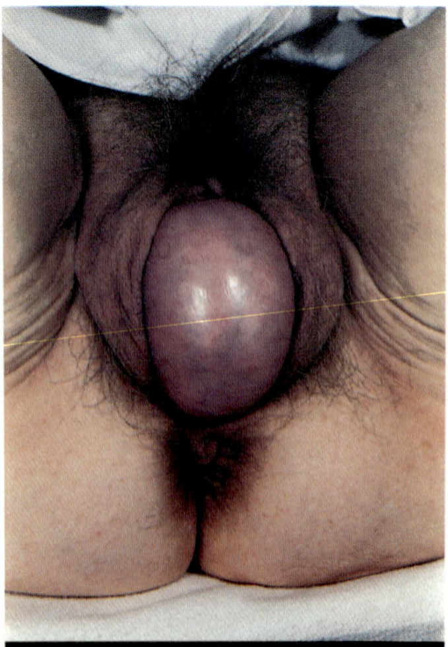

Figure 10.12 Rectocele

Worsening of the rectocele with Valsalva. (Courtesy of Matthew Backer, Jr., MD.)

CHAPTER 11

EXTREMITY TRAUMA

Cathleen M. Vossler
Daniel L. Savitt
Alan B. Storrow

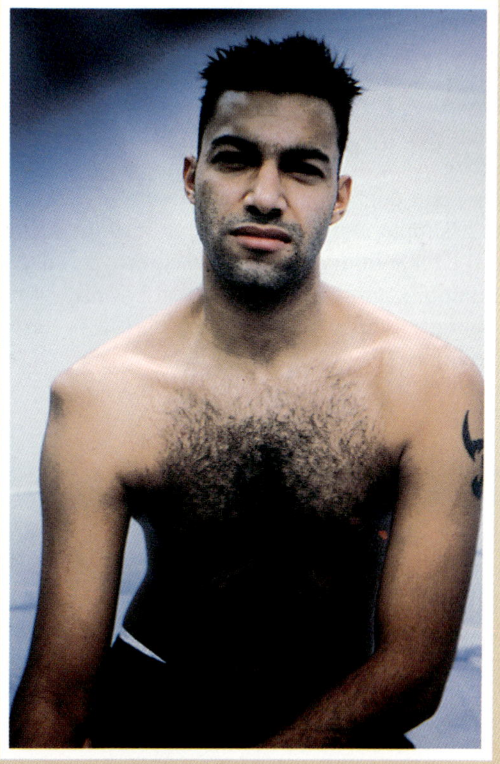

Associated Clinical Features

Injury to the acromioclavicular (AC) joint is a common finding in the ED resulting from direct trauma with an adducted arm, or indirectly from a fall on an outstretched arm with pressure directed to the joint (Fig. 11.1). There are three degrees of injury (Fig. 11.2). A first-degree injury is equivalent to a sprain. There is an incomplete tear of the ligament. Radiographs are negative. A second-degree injury consists of subluxation of the AC joint and disruption of the ligament. Subluxation of the clavicle from the acromion of less than 50% is only evident on stress radiographs. Complete disruption of the AC, coracoacromial, and coracoclavicular ligaments is a third-degree injury. Stress radiographs reveal more than 50% displacement of the clavicle from the acromion. All patients complain of pain at the joint site with moderate to severe amounts of swelling. Stress radiographs are obtained by suspending 5 to 10 lb of weight from each arm and taking a bilateral anteroposterior (AP) shoulder film. The joint space and any subluxation is easily visualized.

Differential Diagnosis

Clavicular fracture, scapular fracture, rotator cuff injury, shoulder dislocation, contusion, or isolated coracoclavicular ligament damage can be confused with AC joint separation.

ED Treatment and Disposition

First- and second-degree injuries are treated with rest, ice, analgesics, and a simple sling, until acute pain with movement is relieved. Third-degree injury treatment is controversial. Many experts advocate immobilization with a sling for 3 weeks, whereas others advocate operative repair. Orthopedic referral is essential for all third-degree injuries.

Clinical Pearls

1. The AC joint stress test is an accurate means of testing for AC joint separation. The patient is instructed to bring the arm across the chest and try to align the opposite shoulder with the elbow. The production of pain over the AC joint confirms the diagnosis.
2. The classic AP stress film indicating a second-degree injury shows distal clavicle-acromion separation of less than one-half the diameter of the clavicle.

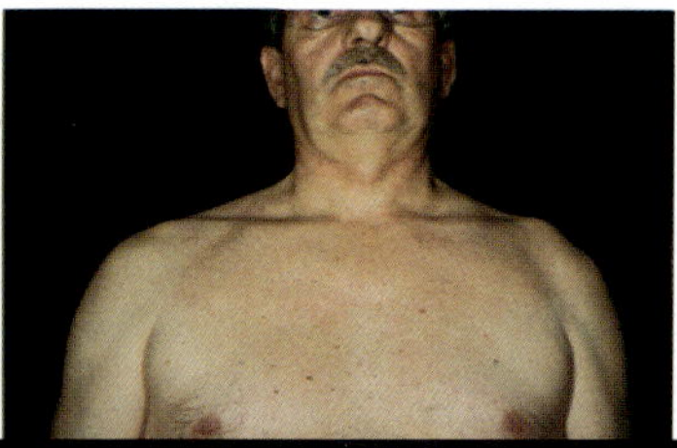

Figure 11.1 Acromioclavicular Joint Separation

Subtle prominence of the left distal clavicle. The upward displacement of the clavicle is due to stretching or disruption of the suspending ligaments. (Courtesy of Frank Birinyi, MD.)

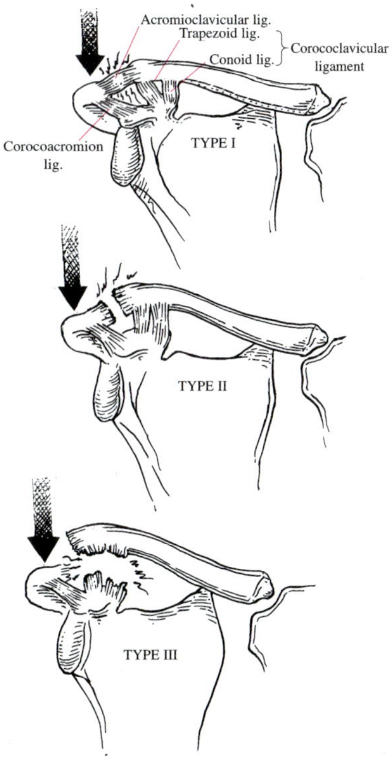

Figure 11.2 Acromioclavicular Joint Injuries

Classification of acromioclavicular joint injuries. (Adapted with permission from Rockwood CA, Green DP, Bucholz RW: *Rockwood and Green's Fractures in Adults,* 3d ed. Philadelphia, JB Lippincott, 1991.)

Associated Clinical Features

Anterior shoulder dislocations are the most common dislocation seen in the ED. They are caused by external rotation and abduction that disrupts the capsule and glenohumeral ligaments. The affected extremity is held in slight abduction and external rotation. Often, the patient supports the dislocated shoulder with the other arm. The acromion becomes prominent and there is a squared-off boxlike appearance to the top of the shoulder. The rounded contour of the deltoid is lost (Fig. 11.3). These patients complain of shoulder pain and refuse to move the shoulder on the affected side. Many patients will appear diaphoretic and pale. A neurologic examination of the upper extremity should be performed to rule out associated injury, most commonly of the axillary nerve (sensation over the deltoid). Radiographic examination is necessary to evaluate for associated fracture (Fig. 11.4). Posterior shoulder dislocations are commonly missed because of subtle radiographic findings (Figs. 11.5 and 11.6). The arm is held internally rotated and adducted. There is no external rotation. On examination, a posterior prominence exists. Posterior dislocations commonly occur during seizures. The Hill-Sachs deformity (an impaction of the humeral head) can occur in a significant percentage (11 to 50%) of these patients.

Differential Diagnosis

Acromioclavicular separation, fracture of the greater tuberosity, humeral fracture, and fracture of the humeral head are commonly mistaken for a shoulder dislocation prior to radiographic examination.

ED Treatment and Disposition

Closed reduction is the treatment of choice and may require conscious sedation. There are many methods to reduce shoulder dislocations, including Stimson, traction-countertraction, and external rotation. Neurovascular and radiographic examination should occur before and after reduction. The patient should be placed in a sling and swathe after reduction. The shoulder should remain immobilized for 2 to 5 weeks (shorter periods for older patients owing to their greater ability to develop shoulder stiffness).

Clinical Pearls

1. Patients with dislocated shoulders usually cannot touch the contralateral shoulder with the hand of the affected side.
2. Relaxation of the pectoral musculature is an excellent aid in shoulder reduction. This can be accomplished by manual massage of the muscle. Some patients can voluntarily relax this muscle when asked to do so (e.g., weightlifters).

3. Luxatio erecta is inferior glenohumeral dislocation. The humeral head is forced below the inferior aspect of the glenoid fossa. These patients present with the arm locked 180 deg overhead.

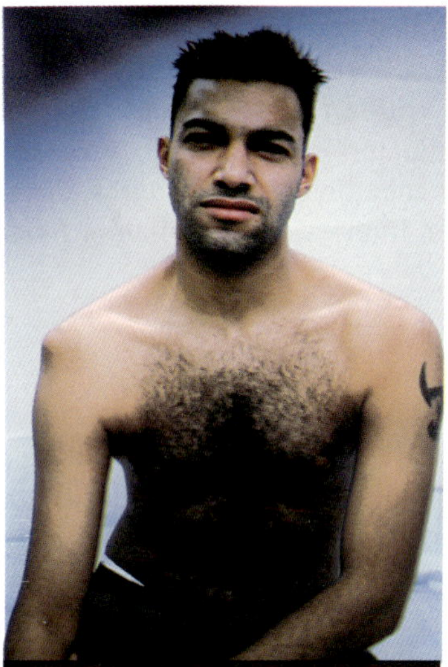

Figure 11.3 Anterior Shoulder Dislocation

This right anterior shoulder dislocation occurred when the patient fell while playing basketball. There is an obvious contour deformity as well as prominence of the acromion. (Courtesy of Kevin J. Knoop, MD, MS.)

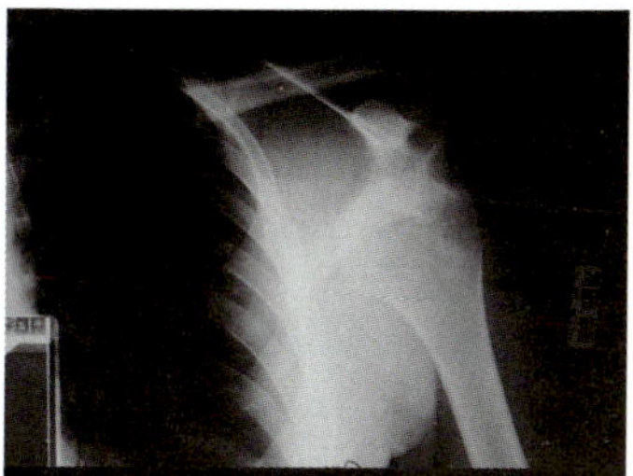

Figure 11.4 Anterior Shoulder Dislocation

Radiographic evaluation of this anterior shoulder dislocation demonstrates that the humeral head is not in the glenoid fossa, but is located anterior and inferior to it. (Courtesy of Kevin J. Knoop, MD, MS.)

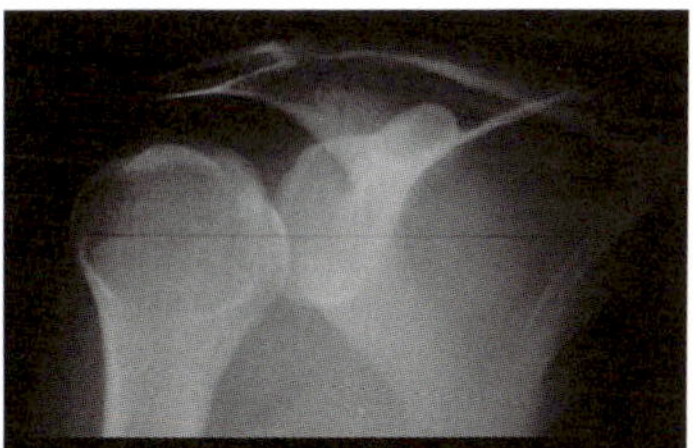

Figure 11.5 Posterior Shoulder Dislocation

AP radiograph of this rare type of shoulder dislocation. Because of internal rotation of the greater tuberosity, the humeral head appears like a dip of ice cream on a cone, thus called the "ice cream cone sign." (Courtesy of Alan B. Storrow, MD.)

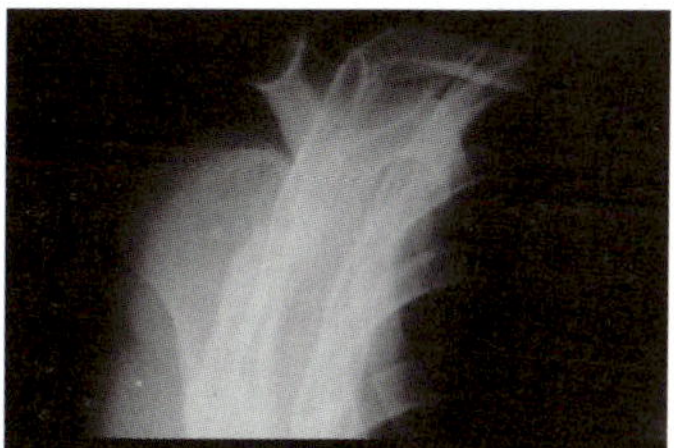

Figure 11.6 Posterior Shoulder Dislocation

A scapular Y view of the same patient confirms the diagnosis. (Courtesy of Alan B. Storrow, MD.)

Associated Clinical Features

Colles' fracture (Fig. 11.7) occurs most commonly from a fall on an outstretched hand. This results in dorsiflexion of the wrist and a transverse fracture of the metaphysis of the radius. There is no intraarticular involvement, and the fracture fragment is displaced dorsally. The original description by Colles was for an isolated radial fracture as described above, though the term is frequently applied to a radial fracture in combination with an ulnar styloid fracture. Patients complain of pain, swelling, tenderness, and decreased range of motion. Associated injuries include carpal fractures, distal radioulnar subluxation, flexor tendon injuries, and median or ulnar nerve injuries.

Differential Diagnosis

Barton's fracture (dorsal rim fracture of the distal radius), Smith's fracture (fracture of the distal radius with volar angulation), Hutchinson's fracture (radial styloid fracture), wrist sprain, Galeazzi's fracture (displaced distal radial fracture with radioulnar subluxation), carpal bone dislocation, radial dislocation, Chauffeur's fracture (a transverse nondisplaced fracture of the radial styloid), and ulnar dislocation can all be confused with a Colles' fracture (Fig. 11.8). Classically, a Colles' fracture results from extension, a Smith's fracture from flexion, and both Hutchinson's and Barton's fractures from a push-off.

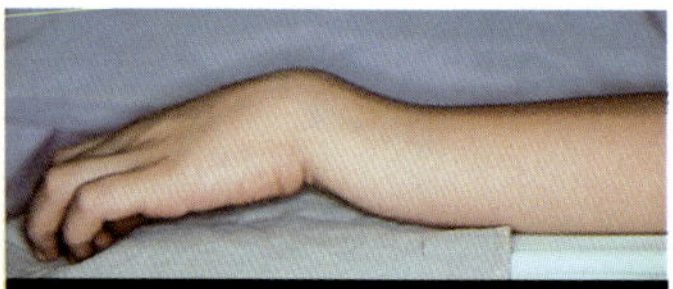

Figure 11.7 Colles' Fracture

The classic dinner fork deformity is demonstrated in this photograph. The distal forearm is displaced dorsally. (Courtesy of Cathleen M. Vossler, MD.)

ED Treatment and Disposition

Nondisplaced fractures require no manipulation and can be casted. Displaced fractures may be reduced by using finger traps for distraction while applying dorsal pressure to the distal fragment. Optimal anesthesia is a regional block. A regional block is accomplished by axillary block of the brachial plexus. Alternative methods of anesthesia include hematoma and Bier blocks. Initial immobilization with a double sugar tong splint with the forearm in 20 deg of supination is adequate. The goals of reduction include restoration of volar tilt and radial inclination, as well as maintaining radial length. Long-term complications include stiffness, malunion, nonunion, and chronic pain. Therefore, all Colles' fractures should be followed up by an orthopedic surgeon.

Clinical Pearls

1. Median nerve function must be evaluated before and after any reduction because of associated paresthesias which occur secondary to tension or pressure on the nerve.
2. Some Colles' fractures are unstable and require more aggressive treatment including external or internal fixation. Colles' fractures with intraarticular involvement, comminution, more than 20 deg of angulation, and more than 1 cm of shortening may be unstable and require fixation. These fractures are more likely to lead to complications such as loss of reduction, joint instability, and arthritis.

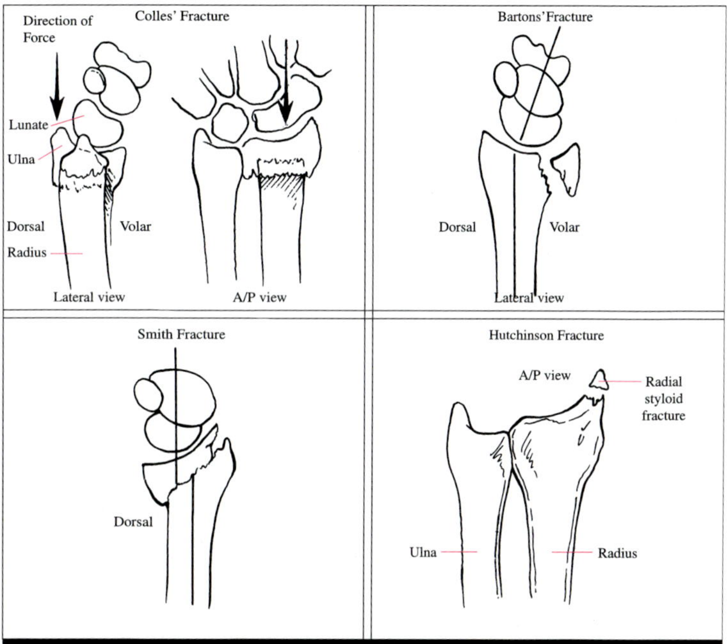

Figure 11.8 Distal Forearm Fractures

These illustrations depict the different types of distal forearm fractures: Colles', Smith's, Barton's, and Hutchinson's. (Adapted from Simon R: *Emergency Orthopedics: The Extremities.* Norwalk, CT, Appleton and Lange, 1987, pp 118–119.)

Associated Clinical Features

Flexor and extensor tendon injury occur from lacerations or wounds to the hand. Tendon rupture can also occur secondary to forces applied to the hand causing avulsion of the bone or rupture of the tendon. Many patients state that they are unable to flex or extend the digit (Fig. 11.9). Tendon function must be checked with any injury to the hand. Accurate assessment of a tendon can be misleading, since a 90% lacerated tendon can still retain function. Partial tendon lacerations can often be identified by testing strength against resistance. Strength against resistance is decreased if a partial tendon laceration exists. It is helpful to evaluate the resting hand. Note the flexor cascade of the fingers. An abnormal resting posture is suspicious for tendon injury. Flexor digitorum profundus and superficialis as well as all individual flexor and extensor tendons should be tested. Ask the patient to extend each digit individually while the other digits are held in place. Suspicion for an extensor tendon laceration should arise if this cannot be done.

Differential Diagnosis

Partial tendon laceration, tendon sheath laceration, tenosynovitis, or acute arthritis may be confused with tendon injury.

ED Treatment and Disposition

Initial wound care should include irrigation, exploration for foreign bodies, debridement, antibiotics, and tetanus prophylaxis if needed. Treatment of a partial tendon laceration requires no repair and is treated with a protective splint. Extensor tendon repair can be performed in the ED after careful irrigation, inspection, and debridement or can be performed later by the consultant. Flexor tendon repair requires immediate orthopedic consultation for operative repair.

Clinical Pearls

1. Wounds should be examined through a full range of motion. A tendon laceration sustained with the finger in flexion will be missed if the finger is examined only in extension secondary to retraction of the tendon.
2. Excellent hemostasis is required for a complete tendon examination. The brief use of a blood pressure cuff or other tourniquet may be necessary.

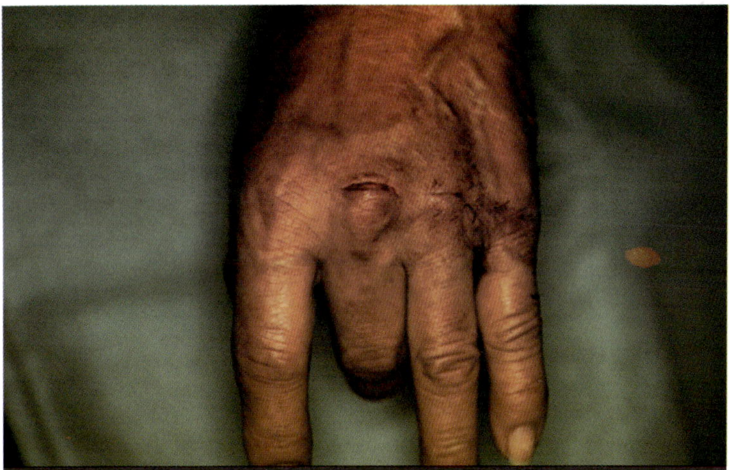

Figure 11.9 Extensor Tendon Laceration

Note the laceration over the third metacarpal head. The inability to extend the long finger is strong clinical evidence of complete extensor tendon disruption. (Courtesy of Kevin J. Knoop, MD, MS.)

Associated Clinical Features

The clenched fist injury classically occurs during a fight when the metacarpophalangeal (MCP) joint contacts human teeth resulting in a laceration in the skin (Fig. 11.10). Many patients will not divulge the true circumstances surrounding the injury; therefore all wounds at the MCP joint are considered a clenched fist injury until proven otherwise. Once these wounds occur, the inoculated organisms are sealed in a warm closed environment allowing rapid spread and destruction. Serious complications can result, including infection, loss of function, and amputation. Most wounds are polymicrobial. Patients who present initially may have little on physical examination, whereas those who present more than 18 h after injury are more likely to have evidence of infection including pain, swelling, erythema, and purulent drainage.

Differential Diagnosis

Abrasions or lacerations secondary to a source other than human teeth can be mistaken for a clenched fist injury.

ED Treatment and Disposition

All wounds should be irrigated, debrided, explored, elevated, and immobilized. Patients should receive antibiotics directed at both oral and skin flora. Tetanus prophylaxis is given if needed. Radiographs should be obtained to evaluate for fractures and any foreign bodies remaining in the wound. These wounds should never be closed initially. All patients require careful follow-up with a hand specialist. Reliable patients who present early, without evidence of infection or significant medical history (e.g., diabetes), and have no involvement of bone, joint, or tendon may be treated on an outpatient basis. They must return in 24 h for a wound check, sooner if any signs of infection develop. Any patient who does not meet these requirements must be hospitalized for IV antibiotics and wound care.

Clinical Pearls

1. Complications include cellulitis, lymphangitis, septic arthritis, abscess formation, osteomyelitis, and tenosynovitis.
2. All wounds need to be examined in full flexion and extension so tendon injuries are not missed. A tendon injury sustained with the fingers flexed will be missed if the hand is only examined in extension due to the retraction of the tendon with extension.

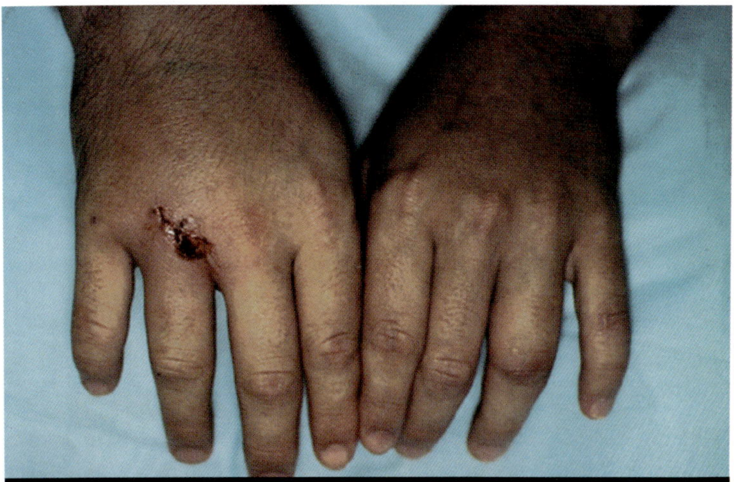

Figure 11.10 Fight Bite

The small lacerations seen in this photograph were sustained from human teeth during a fight. (Courtesy of Lawrence B. Stack, MD.)

Associated Clinical Features

A boxer's fracture is a metacarpal neck fracture of the fifth, and sometimes fourth digit, which commonly occurs after a direct blow to the metacarpophalangeal joints of the clenched fist. The proximal metacarpal bone is angulated dorsally and the metacarpal head is angulated volarly. On physical examination, the "knuckle" is missing and can be palpated on the volar surface (Figs. 11.11 and 11.12). Any associated laceration should be considered secondary to human teeth ("fight bite," see "Clenched Fist Injury" Fig. 11.10).

Differential Diagnosis

Metacarpal head fracture, metacarpal shaft fracture, hematoma, sprain, clenched fist injury, and metacarpophalangeal dislocation are often mistaken for a boxer's fracture until radiographic evaluation is performed.

ED Treatment and Disposition

Prior to reduction, the injury must be evaluated for rotational malalignment. This is easily done by having the patient place all fingers in the palm; all fingers should point to the scaphoid bone (Fig. 11.13). Rotational deformities of greater than 15% require reduction. An ulnar nerve block provides sufficient anesthesia for the fifth metacarpal, but median and radial nerve blocks can be used for the other metacarpals. Hematoma block can be used as an alternative. Once adequate anesthesia is achieved, reduction can be attempted. A nondisplaced nonangulated fracture requires no reduction. Treatment includes ice, elevation, and immobilization in a gutter splint. For reduction, the distal interphalangeal (DIP), proximal interphalangeal (PIP), and metacarpophalangeal (MCP) joints are all held in flexion at 90 deg. Pressure is exerted on the proximal phalanx directed upward to push the metacarpal head dorsally back into position. At the same time, the metacarpal shaft is stabilized with pressure on the dorsum over the shaft. The patient should be splinted with the MCP at 90 deg of flexion. Postreduction radiographs are necessary to ensure adequate reduction. Early follow-up (within 7

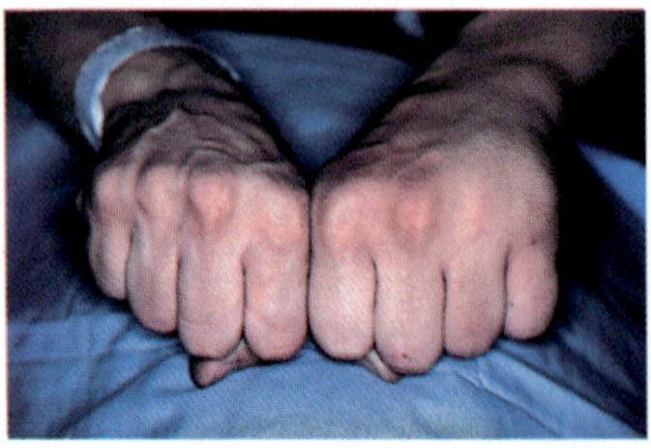

Figure 11.11 Boxer's Fracture

This boxer's fracture occurred when the patient punched a wall with his hand. There is loss of the "knuckle" when the dorsum of the hand is examined, especially noticeable when the patient makes a fist. (Courtesy of Cathleen M. Vossler, MD.)

days) with a hand specialist is essential, since simple splinting may not adequately maintain proper reduction and fractures with higher degrees of angulation and instability may require fixation.

Clinical Pearls

1. Second and third metacarpal neck fractures will not tolerate any angulation and require orthopedic referral for anatomic reduction. Fourth and fifth metacarpal neck fractures can tolerate up to 30 and 50 deg of angulation, respectively, before function is impaired.
2. Subtle malrotation can be recognized by looking at the alignment of the nail beds with the digits flexed. Complications include collateral ligament damage, extensor injury damage, and malposition or clawing of the fingers secondary to incomplete reduction.

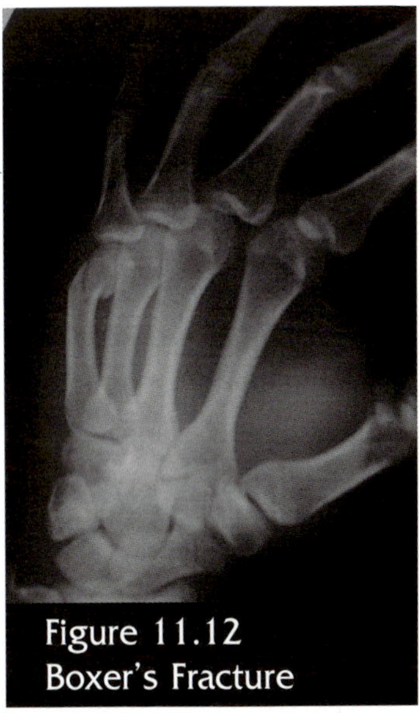

Figure 11.12
Boxer's Fracture

Radiographic examination reveals a fracture through the neck of the metacarpal and volar displacement of the fractured segment. (Courtesy of Cathleen M. Vossler, MD.)

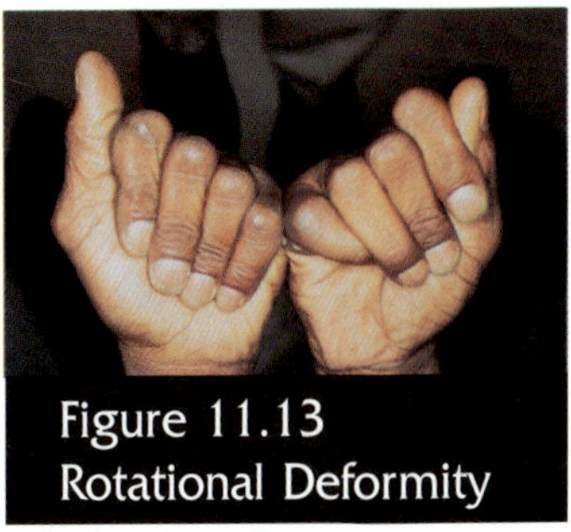

Figure 11.13
Rotational Deformity

Malpositioning of the right fifth digit due to a boxer's fracture. Normally, all the digits point toward a single spot on the scaphoid. (Courtesy of Alexander T. Trott, MD.)

Associated Clinical Features

The boutonnière deformity is a result of injury or disruption to the insertion of the extensor tendon on the dorsal base of the middle phalanx. Common causes of this problem are proximal interphalangeal (PIP) joint contusion, forceful flexion of the PIP joint against resistance, and palmar dislocation of the PIP joint. Initially, a deformity may be absent, but will develop over the course of time if the injury remains untreated. The lateral bands sublux and exert a proximal pull on the middle phalanx. The result is flexion of the PIP joint and extension of the DIP joint (Figs. 11.14 and 11.15). Radiographically, a small fragment of bone may be visualized at the proximal portion of the dorsal aspect of the middle phalanx.

Swan neck deformity occurs as a result of the shortening of interosseous muscles secondary to systemic diseases such as rheumatoid arthritis. The digit is contorted with hyperextension of the PIP and flexion of the distal interphalangeal (DIP) and metacarpophalangeal (MCP) joints (Fig. 11.16).

Differential Diagnosis

Fracture, dislocation, or tendon damage can be mistaken for a boutonnière or swan neck deformity.

ED Treatment and Disposition

When dealing with a closed injury resulting in a boutonnière deformity, immobilization of the PIP joint in extension is adequate. Splinting the MCP and DIP joints is not necessary. The splint should be used for 4 weeks, at which point active range of motion can start. Open injuries must be carefully explored and repaired. Swan neck deformities are treated by splinting the digit to prevent further deformity. Both deformities require referral to a hand specialist.

Clinical Pearls

1. Boutonnière deformity generally develops weeks after the initial injury as the lateral bands contract; therefore, it is frequently missed in the emergency department. Early diagnosis can be made with the proper examination of the finger. The digit should be adequately anesthetized, then examined for range of motion and joint stability.
2. Any injury involving the dorsal PIP surface should be reexamined for development of a boutonnière deformity after 7 to 10 days.
3. Surgical repair may be required for cases where conservative therapy yields inadequate results.

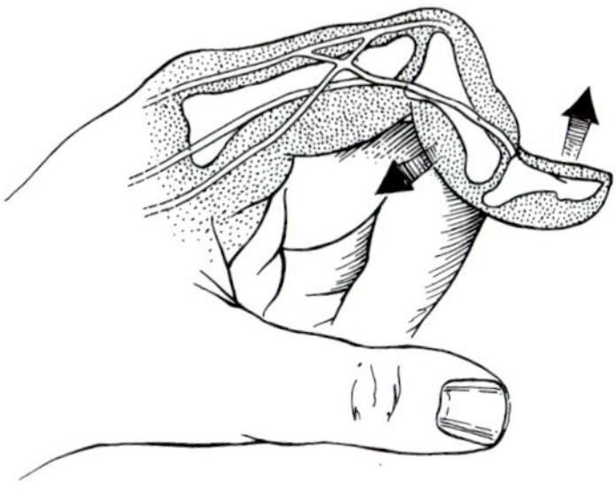

Figure 11.14 Boutonnière Deformity

This depiction of a boutonnière deformity illustrates the rupture of the central slip and the resultant subluxation of the lateral bands. The subluxation exerts a pull on the middle phalanx, resulting in the deformity.

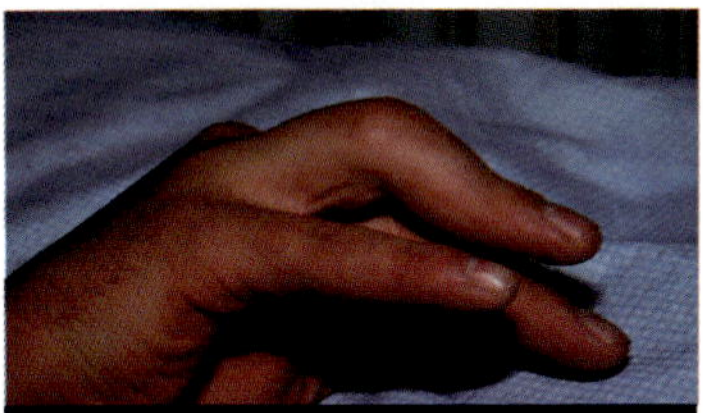

Figure 11.15 Boutonnière Deformity

A boutonnière deformity of the fourth digit. Note the flexion of the PIP joint and the extension of the DIP joint. (Courtesy of E. Lee Edstrom, MD.)

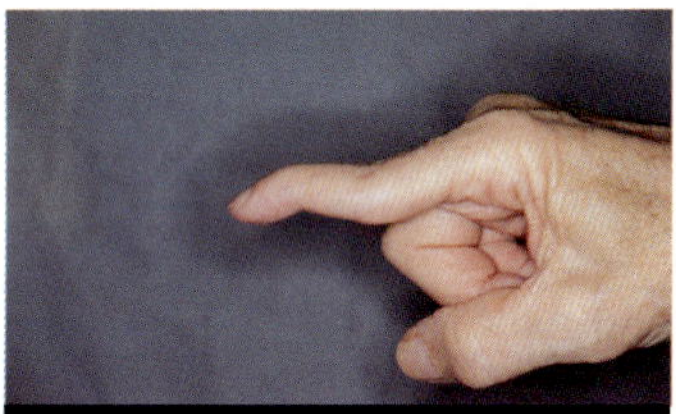

Figure 11.16 Swan Neck Deformity

A swan neck deformity of the index finger. Note the hyperextension of the PIP joint and the flexion of the DIP joint. (Courtesy of Cathleen M. Vossler, MD.)

Associated Clinical Features

Mallet finger commonly occurs after the distal finger, specifically the distal interphalangeal (DIP) joint, is forcibly flexed such as from a sudden blow to the tip of the extended finger. This injury represents complete avulsion or laxity of the extensor tendon from the proximal dorsum of the distal phalanx (Fig. 11.17). The patient presents with an inability to extend the distal phalanx, and it remains in a flexed position (Fig. 11.18). On radiograph, a small chip fragment on the dorsum at the DIP joint may be visualized.

Differential Diagnosis

Intraarticular fracture of the distal phalanx, distal tuft fracture, or extensor tendon laceration can be confused with a mallet finger.

ED Treatment and Disposition

A closed mallet finger without involvement of the joint can be treated by splinting the DIP joint in extension to *mild* hyperextension. True hyperextension is to be avoided. This should be worn for 6 to 8 weeks, at which point active range of motion begins. There is no need to splint the other joints. Motion of the PIP joint should not be blocked with the splint. Hand surgery follow-up is required.

Clinical Pearls

1. During follow-up, some patients exhibit hyperextension of the distal phalanx while out of the splint. This is due to a weakness in the volar plate. These patients should be splinted with the DIP joint in flexion and followed closely.
2. Avulsion of a significant portion of the articular surface (more than one-third) may require open reduction with internal fixation by a hand surgeon.

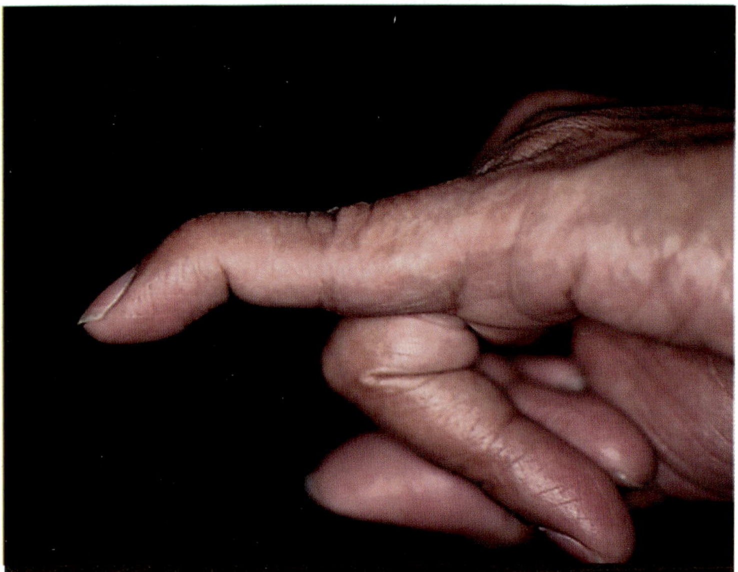

Figure 11.17 Mallet Finger

This photograph depicts a mallet finger. The distal phalanx is held in flexion and the patient is unable to extend it. (Courtesy of Kevin J. Knoop, MD, MS.)

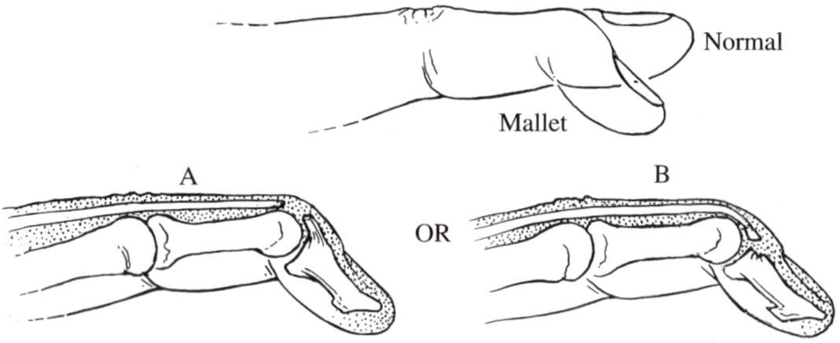

Figure 11.18 Mallet Finger

This illustration demonstrates that the unopposed flexion of the DIP joint is secondary to the complete tear (A) or avulsion (B) of the tendon.

Associated Clinical Features

A subungual hematoma is a collection of blood found underneath the nail, usually occurring secondary to trauma to the distal fingers (Fig. 11.19). They can be quite painful because of pressure beneath the nail. There also can be swelling, tenderness, and a decreased range of motion of the associated finger. Associated injuries include nail bed trauma (Fig. 11.20) and distal tuft fractures.

Differential Diagnosis

A nail bed melanoma may resemble a subungual hematoma and is differentiated from a hematoma by lack of a history of recent trauma and subsequent appearance of the "lesion."

ED Treatment and Disposition

A radiograph should be done to evaluate for possible fracture. If there is no associated nail bed injury and the subungual hematoma covers less than 25%, trephining the nail with a sterile needle is adequate to relieve pain by allowing drainage. Management of larger hematomas is somewhat controversial. Some authors advocate removal of the nail if the hematoma covers more than 50% of the nail or there is an associated fracture. A more recent conservative approach states that removal of the nail is best reserved for those injuries which damage the nail plate and surrounding tissues, regardless of the size of the hematoma or presence of a tuft fracture. In many cases, trephination of the nail is sufficient to relieve pain.

Clinical Pearls

1. Subungual hematomas are a sign of nail bed injury.
2. Subungual hematomas with surrounding nail bed and nail fold injuries require nail removal and evaluation of the nail bed for injury and careful repair if needed.
3. A hand-held, high-temperature, portable cautery device is a good tool for drainage of a subungual hematoma.

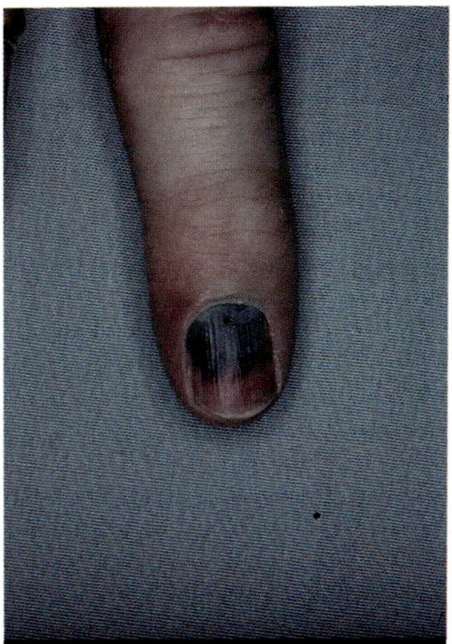

Figure 11.19
Subungual Hematoma

This subungual hematoma occurred after the patient hit his finger with a hammer. The hematoma covers approximately 50% of the subungual area. (Courtesy of Margaret P. Mueller, MD.)

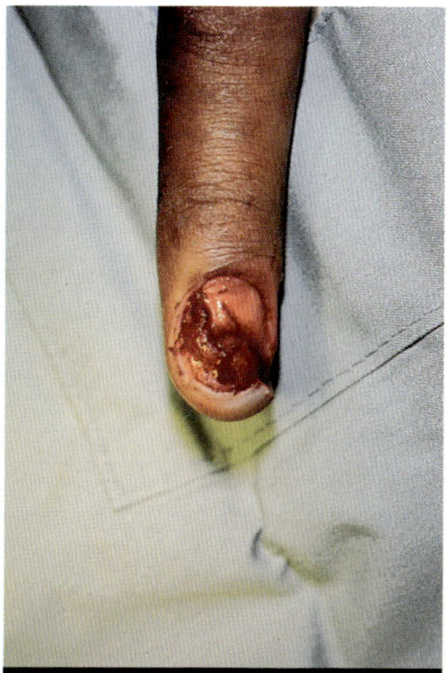

Figure 11.20
Nail Bed Laceration

Bleeding from a nail bed laceration causes a subungual hematoma. This image depicts a nail bed laceration seen after removal of the nail. (Courtesy of Alan B. Storrow, MD.)

Associated Clinical Features

Rupture of the Achilles' tendon occurs most frequently in middle-aged males involved in athletic activities. There are three mechanisms that result in this injury: a direct blow to the tendon, forceful dorsiflexion of the ankle, or increased tension on an already taut tendon. Rupture occurs 2 to 3 cm above its attachment to the calcaneus (Fig. 11.21). Patients complain of a feeling of being hit in the posterior aspect of the lower leg. They may hear or feel a pop. There is weakness when pushing off of the foot; pain, edema, and ecchymoses develop. A Thompson's test can be diagnostic of an Achilles' rupture (Fig. 11.22). The patient should be placed in a prone position; the gastrocnemius muscle should be grasped and squeezed. If the Achilles' tendon is even partially intact, then the ankle will plantar flex; if ruptured, there will be no movement of the ankle.

Differential Diagnosis

Partial Achilles' tendon tear, plantaris tendon rupture, ankle sprain, and partial gastrocnemius muscle rupture have been confused with an Achilles' tendon rupture.

ED Treatment and Disposition

Treatment is either operative or conservative. In either case, the extremity is immobilized without weight bearing for 6 weeks, followed by 6 weeks of partial weight bearing. ED treatment consists of elevation, analgesia, ice, and immobilization with a posterior splint. Orthopedic consultation should be obtained so that a plan of treatment can be chosen. These patients can be discharged home with close orthopedic follow-up or can be admitted for acute repair. Partial tears are generally treated conservatively.

Clinical Pearls

1. Advantages to surgical repair are increased strength and mobility, and a decreased rate of rerupture.
2. Approximately 25% of these injuries are initially misdiagnosed as ankle sprains.
3. These patients maintain the ability to plantar flex the foot in a non-weight-bearing position owing to the action of the tibialis posterior, toe flexor, and peroneal muscles.
4. Palpation of the tendon alone may not detect rupture, as the tendon sheath is often intact.

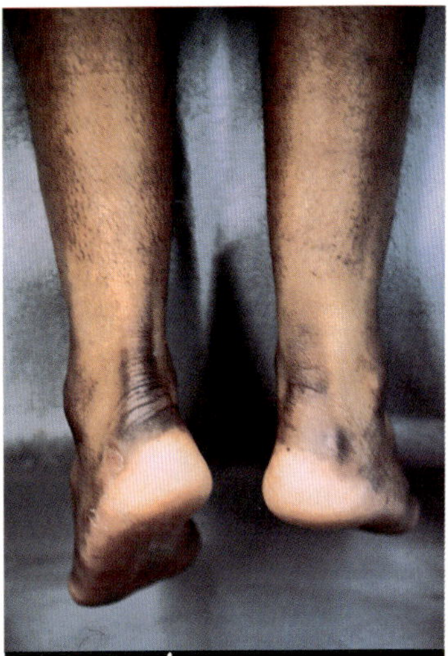

Figure 11.21 Achilles' Tendon Rupture

This photograph depicts a patient with a right Achilles' tendon rupture. Note the loss of the normal resting plantar flexion on the right owing to disruption of the tendon. This is seen with the patient in a non-weight-bearing position. Swelling is also apparent over the site of the tendon injury. (Courtesy of Kevin J. Knoop, MD, MS.)

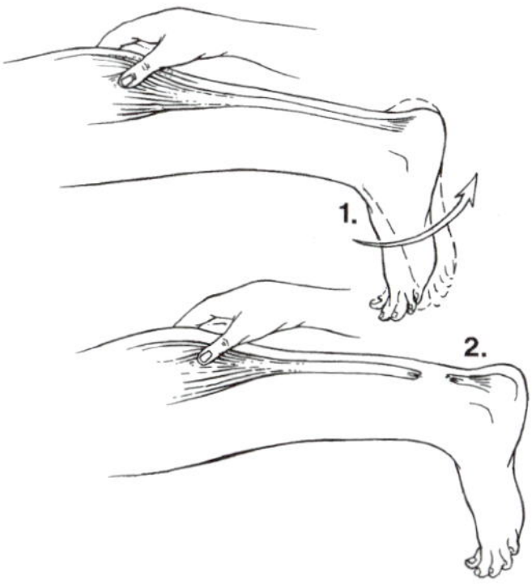

Figure 11.22 Thompson's Test

This illustration demonstrates the Thompson's test where compression of the gastrocnemius-soleus complex normally produces plantar flexion of the foot (1). If the tendon is completely ruptured, then this will not occur (2).

Associated Clinical Features

Patients complain of pain, swelling, decreased range of motion, and tenderness over the lateral aspect of the foot (Fig. 11.23). Fractures of the fifth metatarsal base have been generically referred to as Jones fractures (Fig. 11.23). However, the fractures can be divided into three types, depending on their anatomic location. Treatment is determined by this division.

The classic Jones fracture is a transverse fracture of the fifth metatarsal diaphysis (Fig. 11.24). It occurs when a force is applied to a plantar flexed and inverted foot. It is also referred to as a proximal shaft stress fracture and is usually due to repetitive stress injury. Patients often have prodromal symptoms.

A fracture at the metaphyseal-diaphyseal junction has been termed a pseudo-Jones fracture. It is always an acute injury.

The last type is an avulsion fracture of the fifth metatarsal base caused by sudden inversion of the foot (Fig. 11.25). The avulsion injury is caused by traction on the lateral cord of the plantar aponeurosis.

Differential Diagnosis

Care must be taken to avoid confusing the two sesamoid bones in this area with a fracture. The more common of the two, the os peroneum (present in approximately 15%), lies within the peroneus longus tendon. More rare is the os vesalianum, which lies in the peroneus brevis tendon. Both have smooth, rounded surfaces and usually occur bilaterally. The fifth metatarsal base apophysis might also be confused as a fracture. It usually fuses by 16 years of age, although some fail to fuse.

Other entities to consider include ankle sprain, other metatarsal fractures, and foot dislocations.

ED Treatment and Disposition

A Jones fracture should be splinted and referred to orthopedics for definitive repair. It may heal slowly and cause permanent pain and disability. Surgical treatment is sometimes recommended, particularly since the stress involved with these fractures usually occurs in the sporting activities of young patients.

A pseudo-Jones fracture usually heals without complication, although more slowly than the avulsion fracture. Referral to orthopedics for a walking, or non-weight-bearing, cast according to local preference, is indicated.

The avulsion fracture usually heals rapidly and seldom leads to permanent disability. Most orthopedic physicians treat these patients symptomatically with a short leg walking cast or hard sole shoe for 2 to 3 weeks. Surgery is rarely indicated.

Clinical Pearls

1. It is important to differentiate between the different types of fifth metatarsal base fractures; treatment and disposition are dictated by these categories.
2. The original description of these fractures was by Sir Robert Jones, who personally sustained an injury while dancing. The avulsion fracture is sometimes referred to as the ballet dancer's fracture.
3. The classic Jones fracture has a high incidence of delayed healing and nonunion.

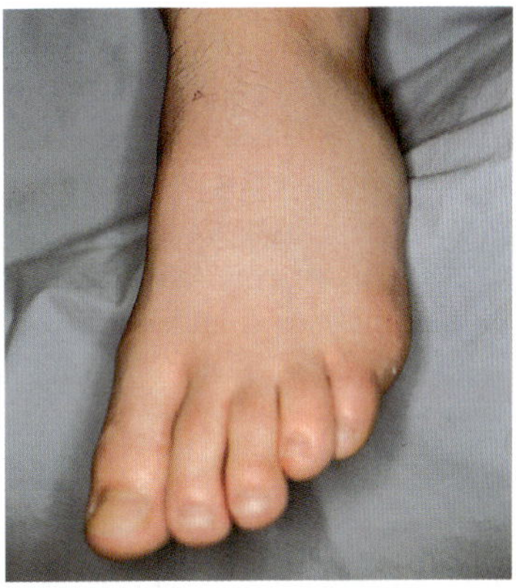

Figure 11.23 Jones Fracture

This patient sustained an injury of the fifth metatarsal and presented with pain and swelling over this site. His radiograph revealed a fracture. (Courtesy of Cathleen M. Vossler, MD.)

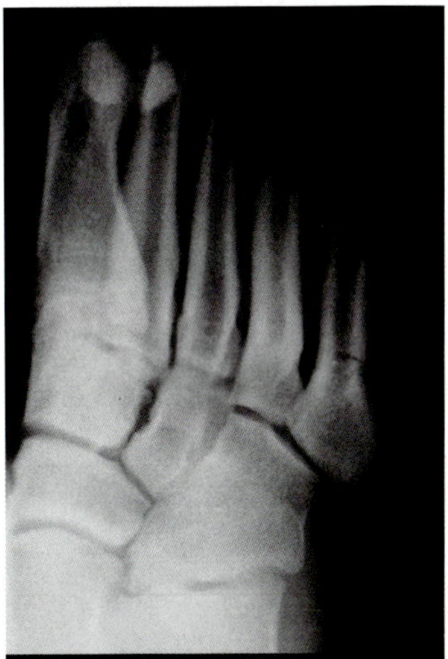

Figure 11.24 Jones Fracture

Radiograph with typical appearance for a diaphyseal fracture of the fifth metatarsal base. (Courtesy of Alan B. Storrow, MD.)

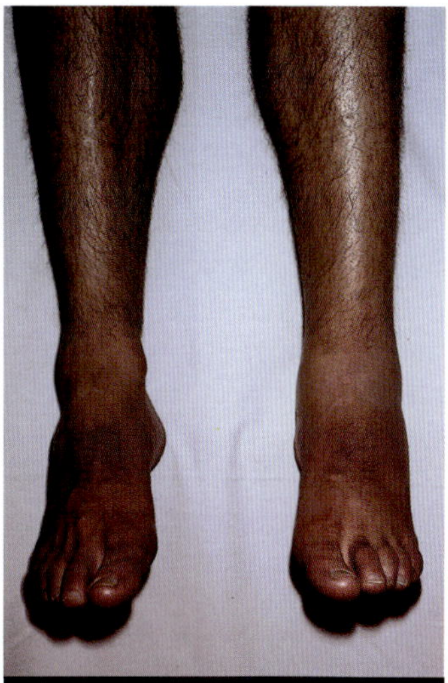

Figure 11.25 Fifth Metatarsal Avulsion Fracture

Radiograph illustrating an avulsion type fracture of the fifth metatarsal base, sometimes referred to as a ballet dancer's fracture. (Courtesy of Alan B. Storrow, MD.)

Associated Clinical Features

Ankle sprains are extremely common problems in the ED. Classification of these injuries based on physical examination and radiography helps guide management and definitive treatment.

The most common mechanism is an inversion stress that injures, in order, the joint capsule, anterior talofibular ligament, calcaneofibular ligament, and posterior talofibular ligament. Since the medial deltoid ligament is quite strong and elastic, serious eversion injuries usually result in avulsion of the medial malleolus or fracture of the lateral malleolus.

A first-degree sprain is defined by a stretch injury, or microscopic damage, to ligaments resulting in pain, tenderness, minimal swelling, and maintenance of the ability to bear weight. A second-degree sprain is defined by a partial tear of the ligamentous structures resulting in pain, swelling (Fig. 11.26), local hemorrhage (Fig. 11.27), and moderate degree of functional loss. A third-degree sprain is a complete tear of the ligament or ligaments and presents with positive stress testing, significant swelling, and an inability to bear weight.

Differential Diagnosis

Malleolar and fifth metatarsal fractures can be confused with ankle sprains prior to radiographs. Any patient with joint pain should have an infectious etiology considered.

ED Treatment and Disposition

First-degree injuries are treated with ice packs, elevation, woven elastic (Ace) wrap, and early mobilization. For patients with mild second-degree sprains, immobilization for 72 h, followed by use of an ankle support has been advocated. More serious second-degree and all third-degree sprains should receive immobilization, ice, and elevation and be referred to orthopedics. In younger patients surgery is an option, although clear recommendations are lacking.

Another option for patients with marked swelling, in whom grading is uncertain, is immobilization, ice, elevation, and a reassessment at 72 h.

Clinical Pearls

1. Ankle injuries are the most common orthopedic problem in emergency medicine.
2. Complications of ankle sprains include instability, persistent pain, recurrent sprains, and peroneal tendon dislocation.
3. The most common eversion injury is a fracture of the lateral malleolus. Since inversion injuries also produce lateral problems, the most common injuries to the ankle involve the lateral side.
4. Both malleoli, the proximal fibula, and the fifth metatarsal should be examined for injury when evaluating a patient with an ankle sprain.

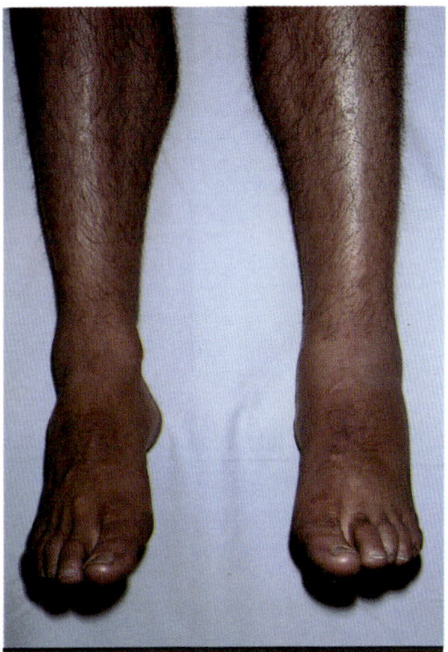

Figure 11.26
Ankle Sprain

Comparison view of a patient with a second-degree left lateral ankle sprain. Note the swelling and asymmetry of the affected area. (Courtesy of Kevin J. Knoop, MD, MS.)

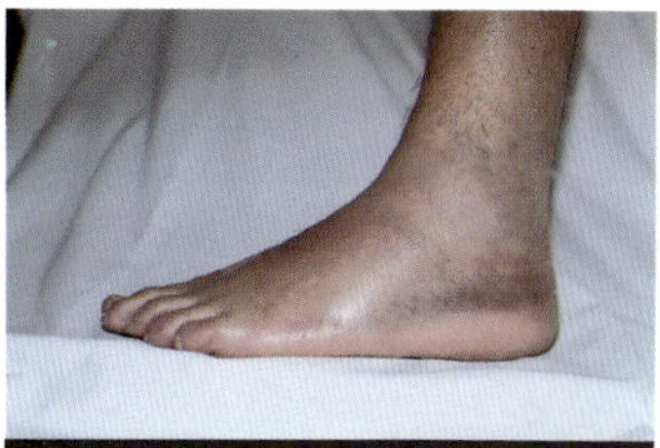

Figure 11.27
Ankle Sprain

Note the dependent ecchymosis and swelling in this patient with a second-degree left lateral ankle sprain. (Courtesy of Lawrence B. Stack, MD.)

CHAPTER 12

EXTREMITY CONDITIONS

Selim Suner
Daniel L. Savitt

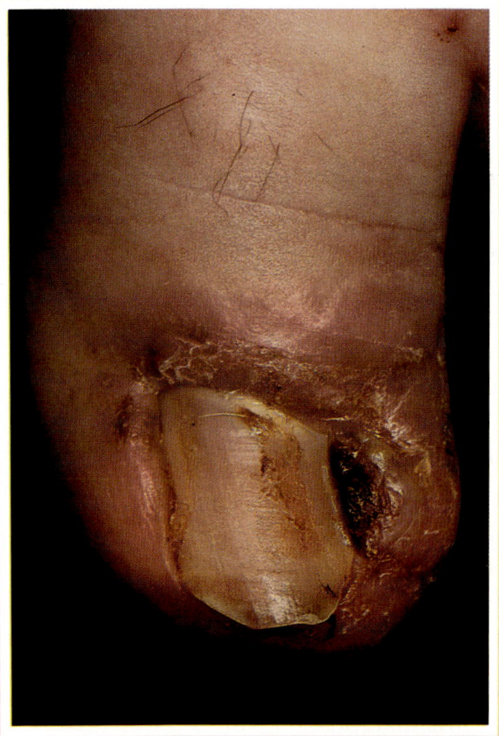

Associated Clinical Features

Cellulitis is infection of the skin or subcutaneous tissues from local invasion, traumatic wounds, or hematogenous dissemination. The local inflammatory response is characterized by erythema with poorly defined borders, edema, warmth, pain, and limitation of movement (Figs. 12.1 and 12.2). Fever and constitutional symptoms may be present and are commonly associated with bacteremia. Trauma, lymphatic or venous stasis, immunodeficiency, and foreign bodies are predisposing factors. There may be enlarged regional lymph nodes. Organisms commonly causing cellulitis are group A beta hemolytic *Streptococcus* and *Staphylococcus aureus* in nonintertriginous skin not associated with an ulcer, gram-negative organisms in intertriginous skin and ulcerations, and *Haemophilus influenzae* in children younger than 3 years. In immunocompromised hosts *Escherichia coli, Klebsiella* species, *Enterobacter* species, and *Pseudomonas aeruginosa* may be the etiologic agents.

Differential Diagnosis

Deep venous thrombosis of the lower extremities, erythema nodosum, septic or inflammatory arthritis, osteomyelitis, herpes zoster, allergic reactions, arthropod envenomation, and burns are included in the differential diagnosis of cellulitis.

ED Treatment and Disposition

Treatment of minor cases commonly consists of immobilization, elevation, analgesia, and oral antibiotics with reevaluation in 48 h. Admission and parenteral administration of antibiotics may be necessary for immunocompromised or toxic appearing patients or those who do not initially respond to outpatient therapy.

Clinical Pearls

1. Aggressive treatment of cellulitis with parenteral antibiotics in immunocompromised patients (e.g., diabetes mellitus) is warranted.
2. Fever is uncommon and associated with bacteremia.
3. Radiography for the presence of foreign body or gas in the tissue should be considered.
4. Leading edge aspirates are of low yield, but may be of help in a toxic-appearing patient.

Associated Clinical Features

This painful condition is the result of impingement and puncture of the medial or lateral nail fold epithelium by the nail plate. Tenderness and swelling of the nail fold is followed by granulation tissue growth causing sharp pain, erythema, and further swelling (Fig. 12.6). If not promptly treated, the granulation tissue becomes epithelialized, preventing elevation of the nail above the medial or lateral nail groove. Often there is secondary bacterial or fungal infection.

Differential Diagnosis

Paronychia, felon, and benign or malignant mass should be considered in the differential diagnosis of an ingrown toenail.

ED Treatment and Disposition

Early: Elevation of the nail out of nail fold and placement of gauze under nail to prevent contact in conjunction with warm soaks is the initial mode of therapy. *Late:* Surgical management involves removal of part of the nail and the inflamed tissue and destruction of the involved nail matrix. In the ED, the lateral portion of the affected nail is removed after digital block followed by packing of the paronychial fold with petroleum gauze or other nonadherent dressing. Dressing changes should be done daily with follow-up by a podiatrist until nail plate growth is complete. The destruction of the nail matrix is required only in patients with recurrent infected ingrown toenails and is not part of the emergency department management, which is designed to prevent injury to the nail matrix.

Clinical Pearls

1. Ingrown toenail is most common in the great toe, is associated with tight-fitting footwear, and may result from improper nail trimming (i.e., cutting the nail too short).
2. Antibiotics are indicated only if cellulitis is suspected or if the patient is a diabetic or has peripheral vascular disease.
3. Use of antibiotics is not a substitute for surgical excision and will result in only transient improvement of symptoms.

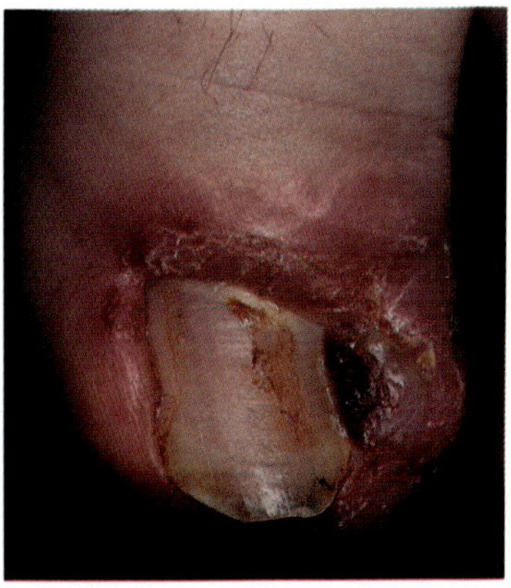

Figure 12.6
Ingrown Toenail

An ingrown toenail on the medial aspect of the left great toe. (Courtesy of Frank Birinyi, MD.)

Associated Clinical Features

Inflammation of lymphatic channels in the subcutaneous tissues is commonly caused by the spread of local bacterial infection. Group A streptococcus is the most frequently implicated agent. Lymphangitis is characterized by red linear streaks (Figs. 12.7 and 12.8) extending from the site of infection (e.g., finger, toe) to regional lymph nodes (e.g., axilla, groin). The lymph nodes are often enlarged and tender. There may be associated peripheral edema of the involved extremity. Lymphangitis may develop within 24 to 48 h of the initial infection.

Differential Diagnosis

Cellulitis, trauma, and superficial thrombophlebitis are in the differential diagnosis of lymphangitis.

ED Treatment and Disposition

Rest, elevation, and immobilization in addition to antibiotics are the mainstays of treatment. Lymphangitis may be treated with oral antibiotics in afebrile patients who are not immunocompromised. Coverage for *Streptococcus* and *Staphylococcus* is appropriate. Toxic-appearing patients require admission for parenteral antibiotics. Any patient sent home with oral antibiotics should be followed up in 24 to 48 h. Patients who subsequently do not show improvement require admission for parenteral antibiotic therapy.

Clinical Pearls

1. Consider *Pasteurella multocida* with cat bites, *Spirillum minus* with rat bites, and *Mycobacterium marinum* in association with swimming pools and aquaria.
2. Chronic lymphangitis may be associated with mycotic, mycobacterial, and filarial infection.
3. In Africa and Southeast Asia, filariasis (*Wuchereria bancrofti*) is the most common etiologic agent.

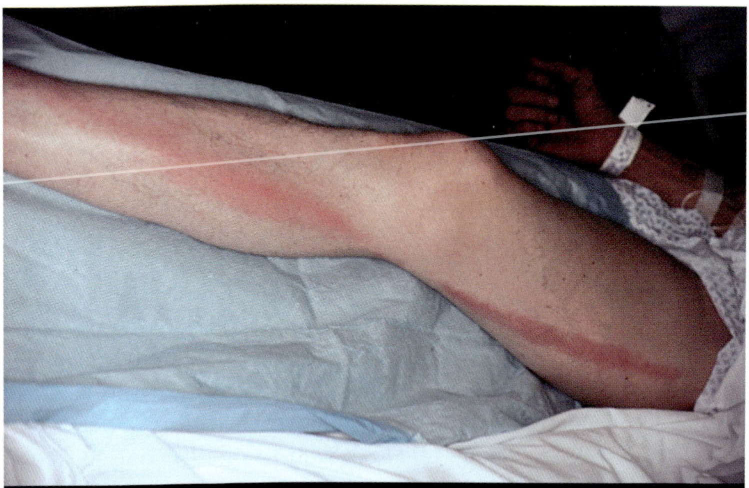

Figure 12.7 Lymphangitis

Severe lymphangitis is seen in the lower extremity. The red streak extends from the ankle to the groin and follows lymphatic channels. The site of infection, in this case, was located on the great toe. (Courtesy of Liudvikas Jagminas, MD.)

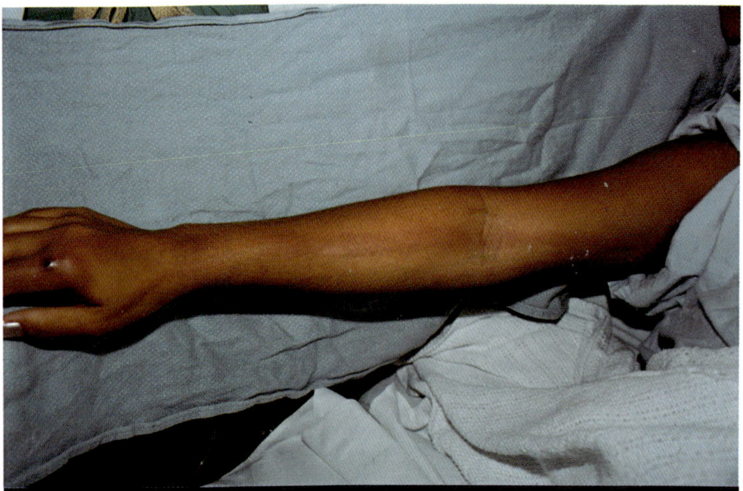

Figure 12.8 Lymphangitis

The lymphangitis extends from the wrist to the upper arm. Lymphangitis in the upper extremity commonly arises from nail biting. (Courtesy of Daniel L. Savitt, MD.)

Associated Clinical Features

Olecranon or patellar bursitis is an inflammatory reaction of the bursa over the olecranon process (Fig. 12.9) or the patella (Fig. 12.10). It is associated with chronic irritation, trauma, or infection. The fluid collection may be infectious (septic bursitis, Fig. 12.11), gouty, or inflammatory. It is most commonly caused by repetitive minor trauma to the joint and is characterized by progressive pain, tenderness, and swelling. There may be erythema, warmth, and limited flexion of the joint secondary to pain. It is critical to differentiate septic from benign inflammation since the signs and symptoms can be similar. Prepatellar bursitis, also termed *housemaid's knee,* involves the prepatellar bursa, which is anterior to the infrapatellar tendon. Characterized by a warm, swollen tender knee, it may result from kneeling. It is important to distinguish this condition from a knee effusion.

Differential Diagnosis

Septic arthritis, crystal synovitis, fracture, and traumatic effusion may all mimic this condition. Aspiration and fluid analysis with Gram's stain, culture, and polarized microscopy are diagnostic in both instances. Synovial fluid with greater than 50,000 WBC, polymorphonuclear neutrophil leukocyte (PMN) predominance, and a positive Gram's stain and culture is associated with septic arthritis. High WBC count and PMN predominance with negative Gram's stain and sterile cultures may be seen in rheumatoid and seronegative arthritides. There are commonly fewer than 50,000 WBCs without PMN predominance and a negative Gram's stain with inflammatory bursitis. Crystals seen under polarized microscopy differentiate this condition from crystalline-induced synovitis.

ED Treatment and Disposition

Rest, bulky dressings, and nonsteroidal anti-inflammatory medications are used to treat both conditions. If bursa is infected, repeated aspirations along with gram-positive antibiotic coverage is the treatment. The rare cases resistant to treatment may require incision and drainage or excision. Most patients can be treated as outpatients with close follow-up.

Clinical Pearls

1. The most important diagnostic dilemma is to differentiate between bursitis and a septic joint.
2. Patients with arthritis, unlike bursitis, will allow passive range of motion of the joint, and joint effusion is usually absent.
3. The olecranon and patellar bursa have a propensity to become infected. Infected bursae may have lower total cell counts than are commonly associated with septic joints.

4. Local steroid injection into the bursa may be used in aseptic bursitis. Complications of steroid injections include infection, local atrophy, bleeding, and tendon rupture.
5. Incision and drainage are not recommended for routine bursitis.

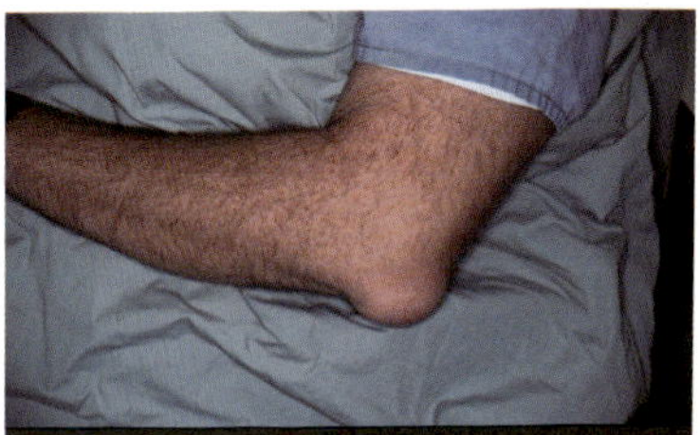

Figure 12.9 Olecranon Bursitis

Olecranon bursitis is evident in this flexed elbow. (Courtesy of Selim Suner, MD, MS.)

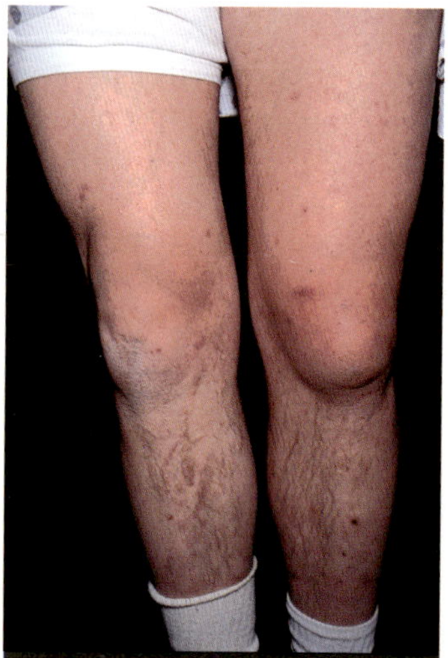

Figure 12.10 Prepatellar Bursitis

Local bursal swelling is evident over the left knee. (Courtesy of Kevin J. Knoop, MD, MS.)

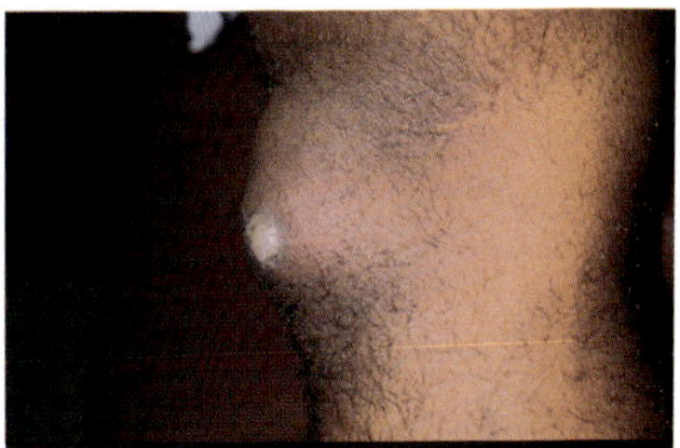

Figure 12.11 Septic Prepatellar Bursitis

This patient with diabetes presented with systemic signs of infection and required operative drainage of this pus-filled bursa. (Courtesy of Alan B. Storrow, MD.)

Associated Clinical Features

Tenosynovitis is inflammation of the tendon and the surrounding synovial sheath characterized by pain and tenderness. Pyogenic flexor tenosynovitis is infection of the tendon sheath from hematogenous origin, puncture wounds, or local extension. Tenosynovitis is characterized by the four signs of Kanavel (described for a finger flexor tendon): mild flexion contracture (Fig. 12.12), fusiform swelling along the volar finger surface, tenderness along the entire tendon sheath especially at the palmar surface of the metacarpophalangeal (MCP) joint, and severe pain with passive extension. Tenosynovitis may be complicated by fibrosis and adhesions leading to stiffness, loss of function, and tendon necrosis from destruction of the blood supply.

Differential Diagnosis

Cellulitis, traumatic injury, lymphangitis, osteomyelitis, septic arthritis, carpometacarpal arthritis, and allergic reactions may mimic some of the signs and symptoms of tenosynovitis.

ED Treatment and Disposition

It is difficult to distinguish infectious and noninfectious etiologies early in the course of the illness. Early (24 to 48 h) management of tenosynovitis, thought to be noninfectious, is accomplished with immobilization and nonsteroidal anti-inflammatory medications. Parenteral antibiotics, rest, immobilization, elevation, compressive dressing, and early consultation with a hand surgeon for incision and drainage within 24 to 48 h are mandated with pyogenic flexor tenosynovitis.

Clinical Pearls

1. *Staphylococcus aureus* is the most common organism but *Streptococcus,* gram-negative, and anaerobic organisms may also be responsible.
2. The most specific sign of tenosynovitis is pain with passive extension of the digit.
3. The abductor pollicis longus (APL) and the extensor pollicis brevis (EPB) (de Quervain's tenosynovitis) and the wrist are the most common sites for tenosynovitis.
4. Finkelstein's test is used to support the diagnosis of de Quervain's tenosynovitis (Fig. 12.13). The patient is instructed to make a fist with the thumb tucked inside the other fingers and the wrist is passively deviated to the ulnar side. Sharp pain along the APL and EPB tendons denotes a positive Finkelstein's test and is strong evidence of de Quervain's tenosynovitis.

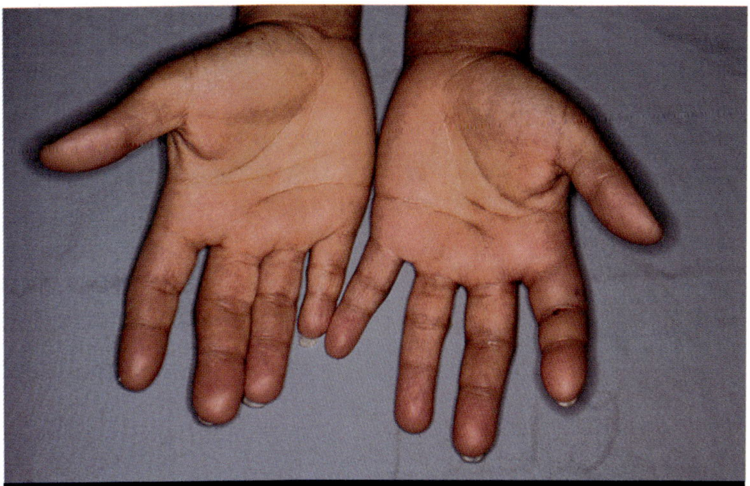

Figure 12.12 Tenosynovitis

Flexor tenosynovitis of the left index finger (after patient sustained a paper cut). Note the flexion and mild swelling of the index finger with the hand in the resting position. (Courtesy of Selim Suner, MD, MS.)

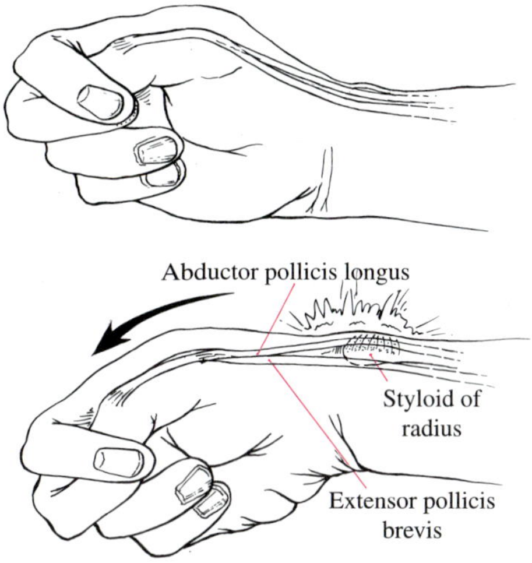

Figure 12.13 Finkelstein's Test

Pain over the radial styloid is elicited with ulnar deviation of the wrist as shown.

Associated Clinical Features

Paronychia is the most common infection seen in the hand and is characterized by infection and pus accumulation along the lateral nail fold. Paronychia may spread to involve the eponychium (Fig. 12.14) at the base of the nail and the opposite lateral nail fold if untreated. *Staphylococcus aureus* is the most frequently implicated organism.

Differential Diagnosis

Felon, dactylitis, herpetic whitlow, and traumatic injury should be considered when making the diagnosis of paronychia.

ED Treatment and Disposition

If recognized early, warm soaks with or without oral antibiotics may be sufficient. After 2 to 3 days, there may be sufficient pus accumulation along the eponychial fold to warrant incision and drainage. After digital block, a longitudinal incision is made along the eponychial fold. If the affected portion begins under the nail, removal of the proximal nail may be necessary. Another technique is elevation of the infected eponychium and lateral nail fold with a number 11 scalpel blade. The incisions should be packed open with gauze (removed in 24 to 48 h). Oral antibiotics should be prescribed, and the finger should be reevaluated in 2 to 3 days.

Clinical Pearls

1. Paronychia is typically associated with nail biting, manicure trauma, and small foreign bodies.
2. Superinfection with fungal agents may occur with immunocompromised patients or neglected paronychia.
3. Damage to the germinal matrix during excision of the nail plate results in nail deformity.
4. It is important to distinguish a paronychia from herpetic whitlow where incision and drainage is contraindicated.

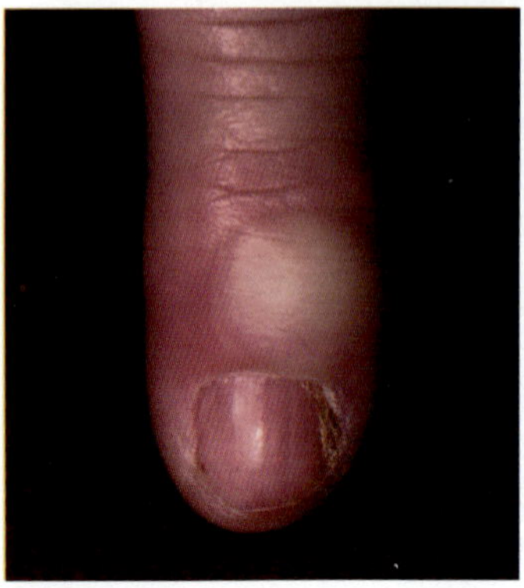

Figure 12.14
Paronychia

A paronychia involving one lateral fold and the eponychium. There is swelling, erythema and tenderness on the dorsum of the distal phalanx. (Courtesy of Frank Birinyi, MD.)

Associated Clinical Features

Digital clubbing results from increase in soft-tissue density at the tips of the fingers, particularly on the dorsum. Associated with the increased tissue mass is enhanced blood flow, excessive curvature of the fingernails, and hyperemic and swollen skin folds around the fingernail (Fig. 12.15). Clubbing may also be seen in the toes. The mechanism underlying clubbing is not known, but it is postulated that the end result is dilatation of the distal digital blood vessels with soft-tissue hypertrophy. Clubbing may be hereditary, idiopathic, or acquired and is associated with multiple medical conditions including carcinoma, intrathoracic sepsis, bacterial endocarditis, cyanotic congenital heart disease, esophageal disorders, cirrhosis, inflammatory bowel disease, pulmonary disorders, atrial myxoma, repeated pregnancies, and pachydermoperiostosis. The incidence of clubbing with each of these conditions is variable. Digital clubbing may be reversible in certain disease processes.

Differential Diagnosis

Hypertrophic osteoarthropathy, infection, and trauma should be considered in the differential diagnosis of clubbing.

ED Treatment and Disposition

Treatment of the underlying condition is indicated. The disposition depends on the underlying diagnosis and condition of the patient.

Clinical Pearls

1. Bone radiographs can be used to diagnose hypertrophic osteoarthropathy. Subperiosteal formation of bone is seen in the distal diaphyses of long bones.
2. Patients rarely observe clubbing in their own fingers even if the fingers are markedly clubbed.

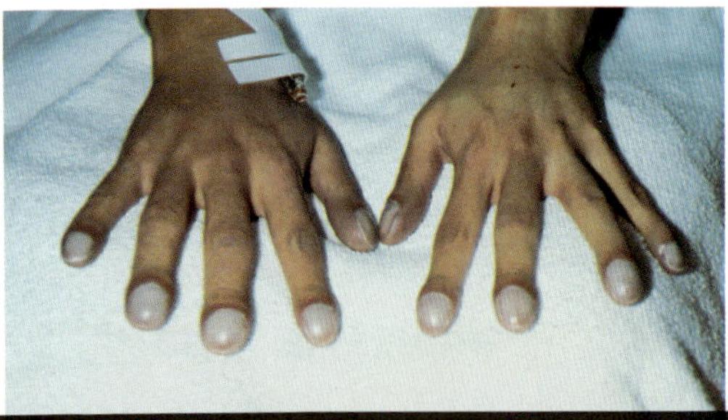

Figure 12.15 Clubbing

Marked digital clubbing can be seen in this patient. Note the hyperemia in the skin folds around the nail. (Courtesy of Alan B. Storrow, MD.)

CHAPTER 13

CUTANEOUS CONDITIONS

Christopher R. Sartori
Michael B. Brooks

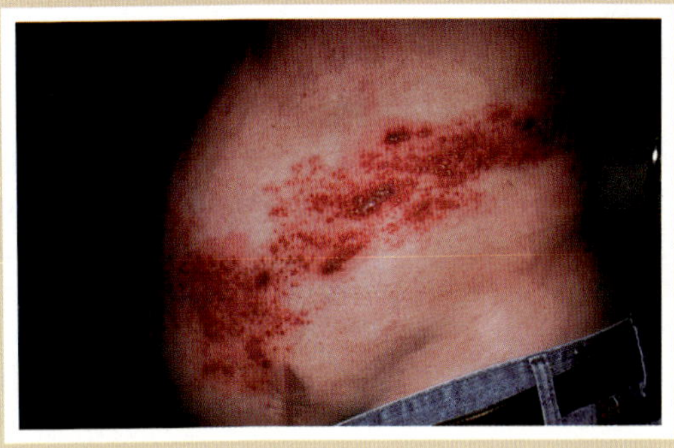

Associated Clinical Features

Considered a hypersensitivity syndrome, erythema multiforme (EM) presents with characteristic target or iris-shaped papules and vesicobullous plaques (Figs. 13.1 and 13.2). These lesions are frequently cutaneous manifestations of a drug reaction or herpes simplex infection. These plaques are usually symmetric, pruritic, and painful, often involving the mucous membranes and extremities including the palms and soles. The milder form of the disease has minimal mucosal involvement, no bullae, and no systemic symptoms. Fever, malaise, and other constitutional symptoms are noted in the severe form of EM, known as Stevens-Johnson syndrome (see next diagnosis).

Differential Diagnosis

The maculopapular presentation may be confused with urticaria or fixed drug eruption, whereas the oral vesicobullous plaques resemble herpetic gingivostomatitis. However, the cutaneous target lesions and their symmetry are typical of EM.

ED Treatment and Disposition

Elimination of any possible etiology (idiopathic cause noted approximately 50%) and supportive measures to allay the burning and itching is basic to treating this disorder. Milder forms of the disease usually resolve spontaneously within 2 to 3 weeks. Corticosteroids are reserved for the severest presentations. Erythema multiforme minor can be treated on an outpatient basis. However, patients with significant systemic illness and additional eruptions involving the mucosal surfaces (Stevens-Johnson syndrome) may require admission and supportive care.

Clinical Pearls

1. Symmetrically distributed target lesions on the extensor surfaces of the extremities and a lack of significant systemic manifestations are classified as erythema multiforme minor.
2. Drug-associated erythema multiforme usually begins within 2 to 3 weeks of initiating therapy. Sulfonamides and penicillins are most often the culprits.
3. Many clinicians empirically treat idiopathic cases with a trial of acyclovir therapy owing to the high incidence of subclinical herpes simplex infections as the cause of the EM.

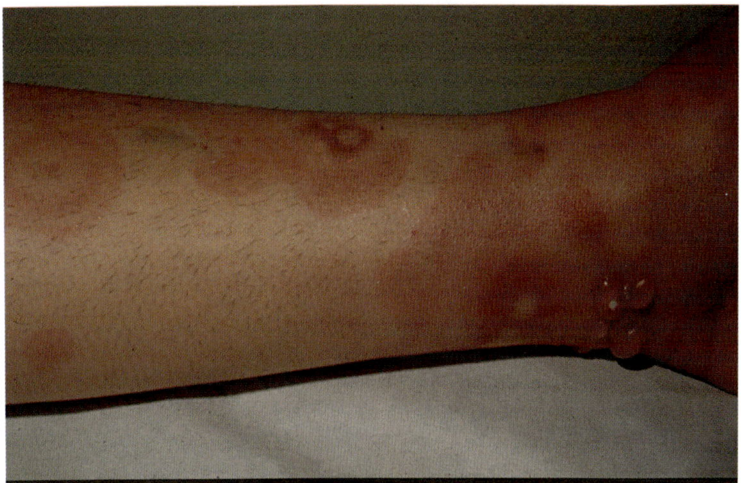

Figure 13.1 Erythema Multiforme

Note the characteristic target eruption, an erythematous macule with central clearing. Distally located on the extremity is a vesicobullous plaque, a common variation in presentation. (Courtesy of Dept. of Dermatology, Wilford Hall USAF Medical Center and Brooke Army Medical Center, San Antonio, TX.)

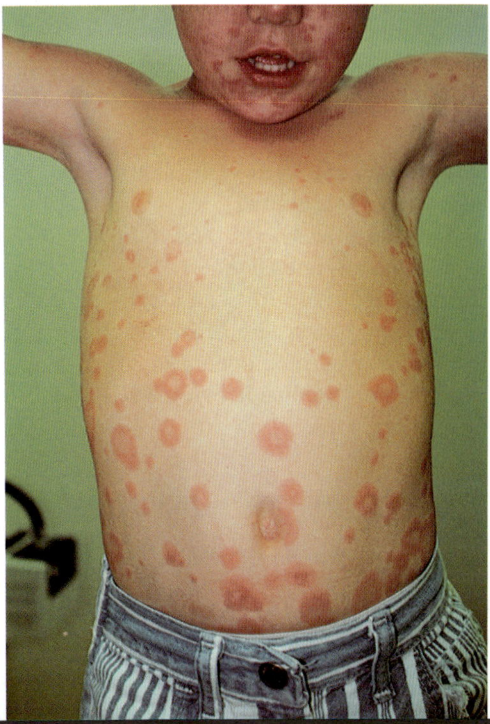

Figure 13.2 Erythema Multiforme

Note the symmetric distribution of the targetoid macules. (Courtesy of Michael Redman, PA-C.)

Associated Clinical Features

Rickettsia rickettsii is transmitted via the bite of an infected tick. Prodromal symptoms of fever, rigors, headache, myalgias, and weakness occur 7 to 10 days after inoculation. The initially blanching macular eruption begins on the distal extremities and somewhat later on the palms and soles (Fig. 13.3). It soon becomes purpuric as it spreads centrally to involve the trunk and abdomen. However, it can also present without obvious cutaneous manifestations.

Differential Diagnosis

Viral exanthems, drug eruptions, necrotizing vasculitis, purpuric bacteremia, and atypical measles syndrome may resemble RMSF.

ED Treatment and Disposition

Tetracycline or chloramphenicol is required for this potentially fatal illness. Tetracycline is the drug of choice, yet it should be avoided in pregnant or lactating females and children younger than 8 years of age. Mildly ill patients may be treated with oral antibiotics on an outpatient basis as long as close follow-up can be arranged. More severely ill patients should be admitted because their care can be complicated by circulatory collapse and coma. Approximately 20% of untreated patients will die.

Clinical Pearls

1. Systemic manifestations of RMSF may present without obvious cutaneous manifestations.
2. Palmar and plantar petechiae in a severely ill patient should be treated as RMSF until proved otherwise.
3. Most cases occur between April and October, with the highest incidence occurring in the Southeast and South-Central states.
4. Atypical measles syndrome occurs in individuals vaccinated with a measles virus vaccine between 1963 and 1968 and subsequently exposed to the virus.

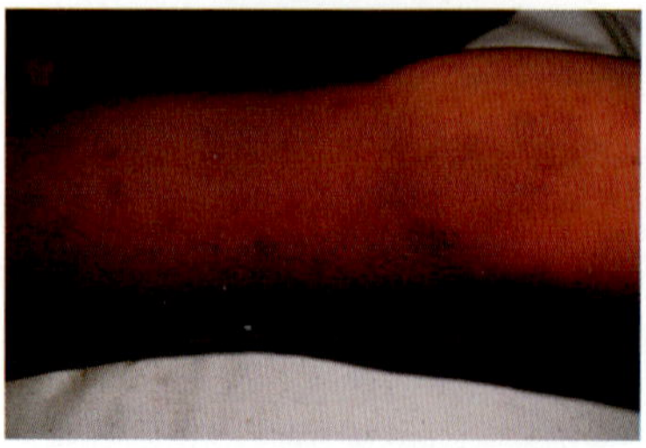

Figure 13.3 Rocky Mountain Spotted Fever

This acral exanthem is characterized by erythematous macules which soon progress to petechiae. (Courtesy of Dept. of Dermatology, Wilford Hall USAF, and Brooke Army Medical Centers, San Antonio, TX.)

Associated Clinical Features

Disseminated gonococcus (GC) is a systemic infection with septic vasculitis following the hematogenous dissemination of the organism *Neisseria gonorrhoeae.* The spectrum of disease varies from skin lesions alone to skin lesions with tenosynovitis or septic arthritis. The initial lesion is an erythematous macule that evolves into a necrotic, purpuric vesicopustule (Fig. 13.4). These purpura are few in number, asymmetric, and predominantly distal in location.

Differential Diagnosis

The purpura may resemble meningococcemia, staphylococcal septicemia, necrotizing vasculitis, or endocarditis with emboli. Infectious arthritis or tenosynovitis must be considered when the patient presents with joint complaints. It is important to obtain Gram's stain of the contents of the vesicopustule, as well as all other body sites and fluids. Biopsy of the vesicopustule is helpful in distinguishing this entity from necrotizing vasculitis and embolic phenomenon.

ED Treatment and Disposition

Ceftriaxone is the agent of choice for initial management. Therapy consists of intravenous or intramuscular ceftriaxone or cefotaxime until symptoms either improve or resolve, followed by an additional 7 days of orally administered ciprofloxacin or cefuroxime. Hospitalization is recommended for noncompliant patients or cases noted to have an associated septic arthritis.

Clinical Pearls

1. The most common symptom of disseminated GC is arthralgia of one or more joints, primarily involving the hands or knees.
2. Skin lesions develop in up to 70% of cases and will resolve within 4 days regardless of antibiotics.
3. The initial erythematous macule of disseminated GC evolves into a necrotic, purpuric vesicopustule.
4. The purpura of septic vasculitis (of whatever bacterial etiology) tend to be fewer in number, asymmetric, and distal in location.

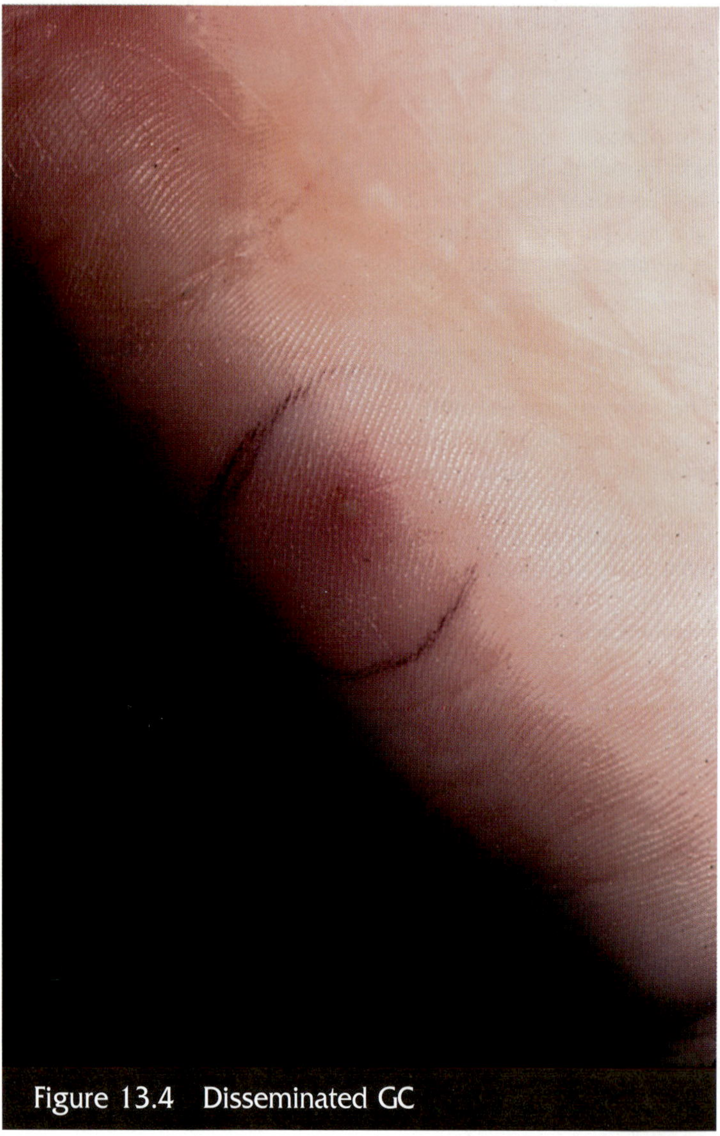

Figure 13.4 Disseminated GC

Here involving the hypothenar eminence of the hand is the characteristic, asymmetric, purpuric vesicopustule of disseminated GC. (Courtesy of Dept. of Dermatology, Wilford Hall USAF Medical Center and Brooke Army Medical Center, San Antonio, TX.)

Associated Clinical Features

Infective endocarditis is an illness characterized by fever, valve destruction, and peripheral embolization manifested by rare, usually distal purpura. *Streptococcus viridans* is the most common causative organism. Janeway lesions (Fig. 13.5) occur in 5% of cases and consist of nontender, small, erythematous macules on the palms or soles. Osler's nodes (Fig. 13.6) occur in 10% of cases and consist of transient, tender, purplish nodules on the pulp of the fingers and toes. Splinter hemorrhages are black, linear discolorations beneath the nail plate (Fig. 13.7). They are present in 20% of cases and are more suggestive of subacute bacterial endocarditis (SBE) if present at the proximal or middle nail plate. Murmurs, retinal hemorrhages, septic arthritis, and significant embolic episodes such as pulmonary embolism or stroke may also be present.

Differential Diagnosis

Meningococcemia, gonococcemia, staphylococcal septicemia, and necrotizing vasculitis must all be considered in the differential diagnosis. Biopsy of the purpura is helpful in distinguishing this condition from septic vasculitis and necrotizing vasculitis. Echocardiogram can aid in the diagnosis.

ED Treatment and Disposition

Antibiotics must be appropriate for the infectious agent; however, therapy is often required before the diagnosis is confirmed or the infecting organism is known. All toxic patients require admission, as do all febrile patients who have prosthetic valves or who are intravenous drug abusers. These patients should receive gentamicin with nafcillin or vancomycin empirically pending the blood culture results. Patients with rheumatic or congenital valve abnormalities may receive streptomycin with penicillin or vancomycin.

Clinical Pearls

1. Janeway lesions, Osler's nodes, and splinter hemorrhages in a febrile patient with a murmur are virtually diagnostic of infective endocarditis.
2. Rheumatic heart disease is the most common predisposing factor, with the mitral valve being the most common site of damage.
3. Congenital heart disease, intravenous drug abuse, and prosthetic heart valves are additional predisposing factors to the development of infective endocarditis.

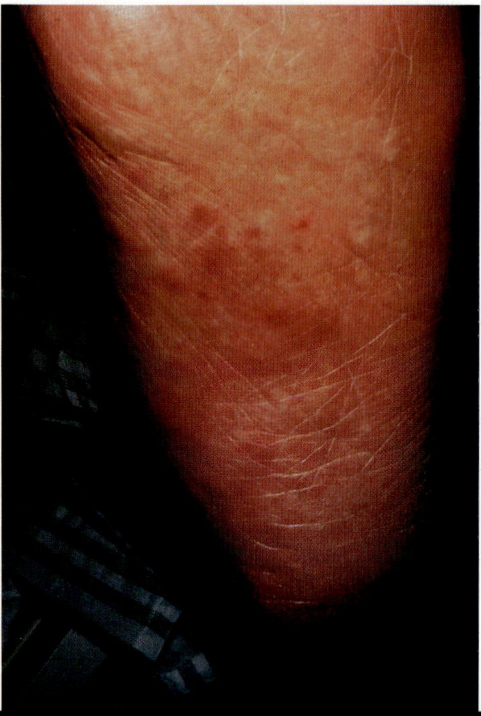

Figure 13.5 Janeway Lesions

Peripheral embolization to the sole resulting in a cluster of erythematous macules known as Janeway lesions. (Courtesy of Dept. of Dermatology, Wilford Hall USAF Medical Center and Brooke Army Medical Center, San Antonio, TX.)

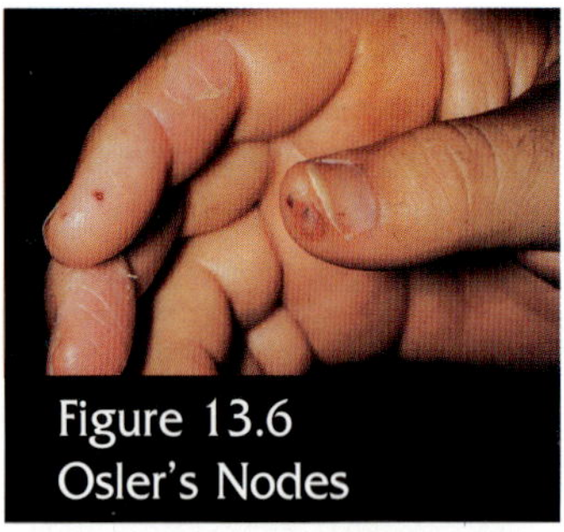

Figure 13.6 Osler's Nodes

Subcutaneous, purplish, and tender nodules in the pulp of the fingers known as Osler's nodes. (Courtesy of the Armed Forces Institute of Pathology, Bethesda, MD.)

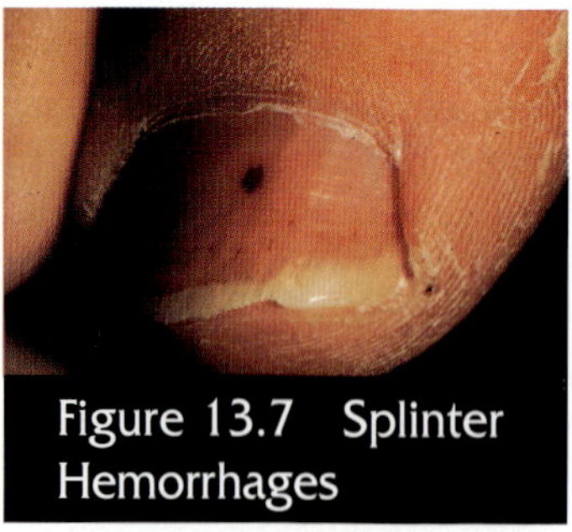

Figure 13.7 Splinter Hemorrhages

Note the splinter hemorrhages along the distal aspect of the nail plate due to emboli from subacute bacterial endocarditis. (Courtesy of the Armed Forces Institute of Pathology, Bethesda, MD.)

Associated Clinical Features

Herpes zoster is a dermatomal, unilateral reactivation of the varicella-zoster virus. Pain, tenderness, and dysesthesias usually precede the eruption composed of umbilicated, grouped vesicles on an erythematous, edematous base (Fig. 13.8). The vesicles may become purulent or hemorrhagic. Nerve involvement may actually occur without cutaneous involvement. Ophthalmic zoster (Fig. 2.15) involves the nasociliary branch of the fifth cranial nerve and presents with vesicles on the nose and cornea. Ramsay-Hunt syndrome is a herpes zoster infection of the geniculate ganglion that presents with decreased hearing and facial palsy.

Differential Diagnosis

The most likely differential diagnosis is herpes simplex infection, which is usually recurrent. Herpes zoster recurs in fewer than 5% of immunocompetent patients. The eruption may resemble contact dermatitis, localized cellulitis, or grouped insect bites. The prodromal pain must be differentiated from potential pleural, cardiac, or abdominal origin. Tzank smear of the floor of a vesicle demonstrating multinucleated giant cells makes the diagnosis of a herpes family infection (Fig. 13.9). Cultures may be necessary to distinguish herpes zoster forms.

ED Treatment and Disposition

Uncomplicated cases of herpes zoster can be managed with supportive care, especially pain control. Admission to the hospital for intravenous acyclovir is usually reserved for complicated cases involving multiple dermatomal distribution or the ophthalmic branch of the trigeminal nerve, disseminated disease, or immunocompromised patients. Acyclovir or famciclovir hasten the healing and decreases the pain if started within 72 h of appearance of the vesicles. These agents have also been shown to reduce the duration of post herpetic neuralgia. Herpes zoster keratitis requires immediate opthalmologic consultation to avoid any potential vision loss.

Clinical Pearls

1. Dermatomally grouped, umbilicated vesicles on an erythematous base are diagnostic of herpes zoster.
2. The thorax is the most common area involved, followed by the face (trigeminal nerve).
3. The nonimmune or immunocompromised should avoid lesional contact from prodrome until reepithelialization, since the crusts can contain the varicella-zoster virus.
4. An infected patient is able to transmit chicken pox, but not herpes zoster, to a nonimmune individual.

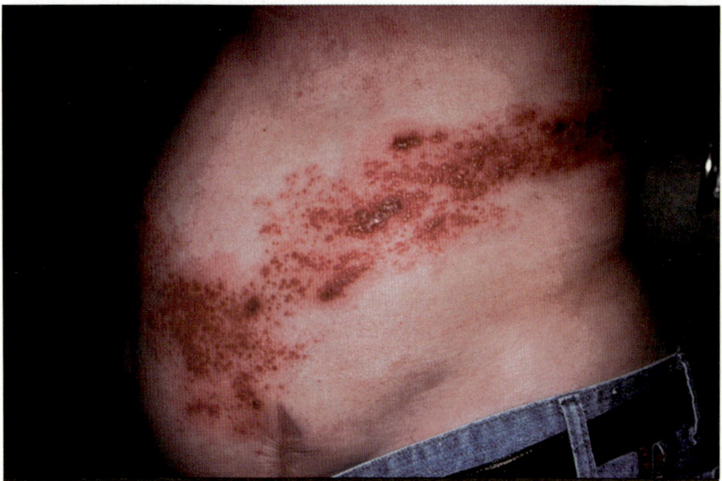

Figure 13.8 Herpes Zoster

This eruption consists of a dermatomal distribution of umbilicated vesicles on an erythematous base. Note the occasional cluster of hemorrhagic vesicles. Tzank smear is positive. (Courtesy of Dept. of Dermatology, Wilford Hall USAF Medical Center and Brooke Army Medical Center, San Antonio, TX.)

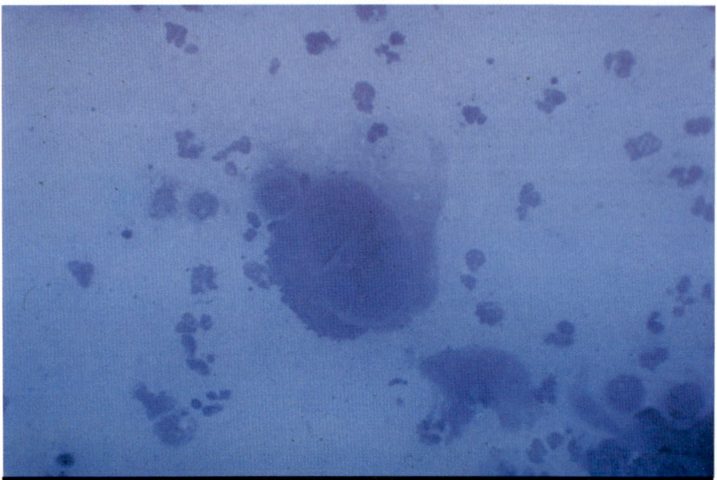

Figure 13.9 Tzank Smear

A Tzank smear of both the roof and floor of a herpetic vesicle demonstrating a multinucleated giant cell. (Courtesy of Dept. of Dermatology, Wilford Hall USAF Medical Center and Brooke Army Medical Center, San Antonio, TX.)

Associated Clinical Features

Herpetic whitlow is a painful herpes simplex infection of the distal finger characterized by edema, erythema, vesicles, and/or pustules grouped on an erythematous base (Fig. 13.10). Fever, lymphangitis, and regional adenopathy often accompany the lesion.

Differential Diagnosis

Paronychia, felon, and contact dermatitis must be differentiated from this contagious illness. A Tzank smear of the floor of the vesicle demonstrating multinucleated giant cells makes the diagnosis.

ED Treatment and Disposition

Acyclovir in addition to analgesics and antipyretics are useful. To be most effective, acyclovir must be started within 72 h of the appearance of the eruption. Topical antibiotic ointments help prevent secondary infection and may speed healing.

Clinical Pearls

1. Grouped, umbilicated vesicles on an erythematous base are diagnostic of a herpes family infection.
2. Wear protective gloves; herpetic whitlow is an occupational hazard in the medical and dental professions.

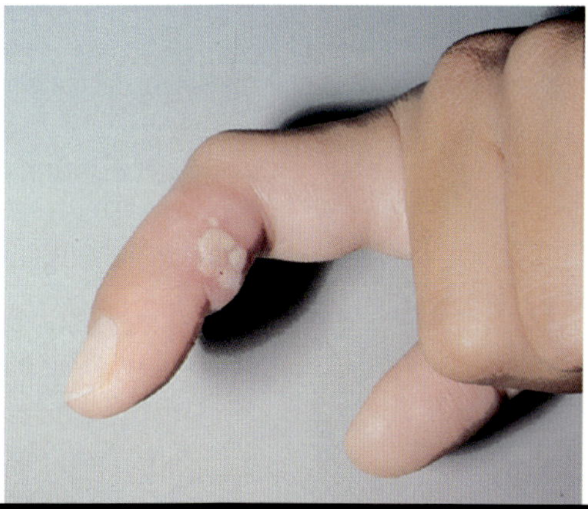

Figure 13.10 Herpetic Whitlow

Note the cluster of vesicles on an erythematous base located at the distal finger. Tzank smear is positive. (Courtesy of Lawrence B. Stack, MD.)

Associated Clinical Features

Erysipelas is a group A streptococcal cellulitis involving the skin to the level of the dermis. The plaque is typically erythematous, edematous, and painful with an elevated, well demarcated border (Fig. 13.11). The associated edema tends to make the plaque appear shiny. Erysipelas frequently occurs on the face and lower extremities.

Differential Diagnosis

Other significant illnesses, such as deep venous thrombosis, thrombophlebitis, and necrotizing fasciitis, must be ruled out.

ED Treatment and Disposition

All infections require rest, elevation, heat, and antibiotics. Mild presentations may be treated on an outpatient basis with oral dicloxacillin or erythromycin in penicillin-allergic patients. More severe illness or toxicity requires hospitalization and intravenous antibiotics.

Clinical Pearls

1. The well demarcated, tender, shiny, erythematous plaque is diagnostic of erysipelas.
2. This same shiny, erythematous plaque on the face of a febrile child may be caused by *Haemophilus influenzae,* necessitating intravenous chloramphenicol or a cephalosporin.

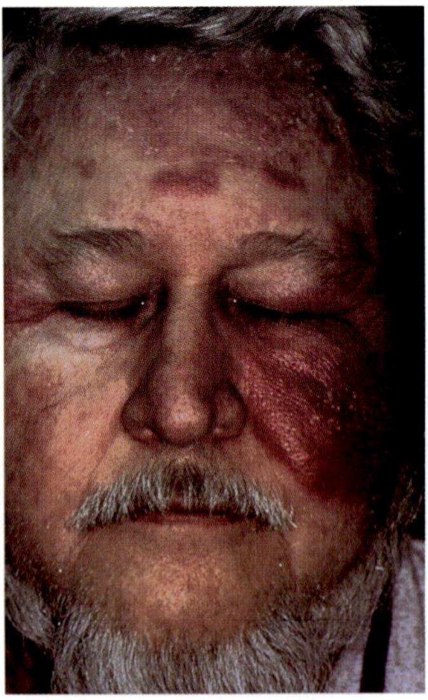

Figure 13.11
Erysipelas

Note the well demarcated, edematous, erythematous, shiny plaque. (Courtesy of Dept. of Dermatology, Wilford Hall USAF Medical Center and Brooke Army Medical Center, San Antonio, TX.)

Associated Clinical Features

Hot tub folliculitis is a pruritic, follicular, pustular eruption confined to the hair follicle and is secondary to a cutaneous infection with *Pseudomonas aeruginosa* (Fig. 13.12). Headache, sore throat, earache, and fever may accompany the pustules, which usually localize to the trunk and proximal extremities.

Differential Diagnosis

Other forms of folliculitis (including those caused by *Staphylococcus aureus*), acne, and miliaria rubra are usually considered in the differential diagnosis.

ED Treatment and Disposition

The folliculitis usually involutes in 7 to 10 days without treatment. Acetic acid compresses and local wound cleansing may speed recovery. In addition, the hot tub or source of exposure must be decontaminated to avoid recurrent exposure.

Clinical Pearls

1. Pruritic pustules confined to the hair follicles of the trunk and proximal extremities is diagnostic of folliculitis.
2. This most commonly occurs in individuals who use hot tubs, whirlpools, or saunas.
3. This may also result from contact with chemicals (exfoliative beauty aids) or repetitive physical trauma (friction from tight clothing).

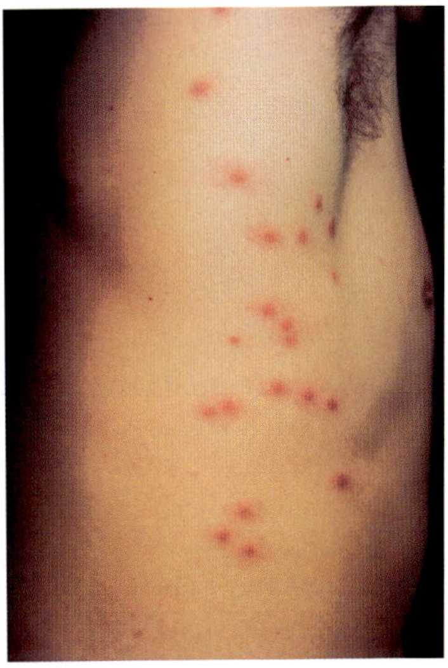

Figure 13.12 Hot Tub Folliculitis

Note the pustules localized to the hair follicles of the trunk and proximal extremity. (Courtesy of Jeffrey S. Gibson, MD.)

Associated Clinical Features

Pityriasis rosea is a mild inflammatory, exanthematous, papulosquamous eruption. The pathognomonic finding is an oval salmon-colored papule with a central collarette of scale. It primarily occurs on the trunk with the long axis of the oval papule following the lines of cleavage in a Christmas tree–like distribution (Fig. 13.13). A herald patch, consisting of a much larger plaque with central clearing and scales, frequently precedes the exanthematous phase by 1 to 2 weeks (Fig. 13.14). The eruption usually lasts 4 to 6 weeks and is frequently pruritic.

Differential Diagnosis

This must be differentiated from the secondary lesions of syphilis, tinea versicolor, and some drug eruptions.

ED Treatment and Disposition

Symptomatic treatment is usually all that can be offered to the patient. Antihistamines may alleviate the associated pruritus. Ultraviolet light has also been used with some success.

Clinical Pearls

1. A salmon-colored papule with central scale, negative KOH examination for hyphae, and negative serologic testing for syphilis makes the diagnosis of pityriasis rosea.
2. It frequently appears very atypical in dark-skinned individuals (acral, face, and genital location).

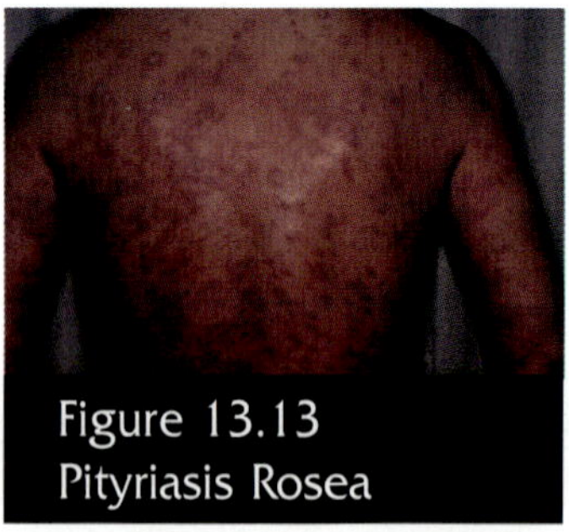

Figure 13.13
Pityriasis Rosea

An exanthematous, papulosquamous eruption with the long axis of the oval papules following the lines of cleavage in a Christmas tree–like distribution. (Courtesy of Dept. of Dermatology, Wilford Hall USAF Medical Center and Brooke Army Medical Center, San Antonio, TX.)

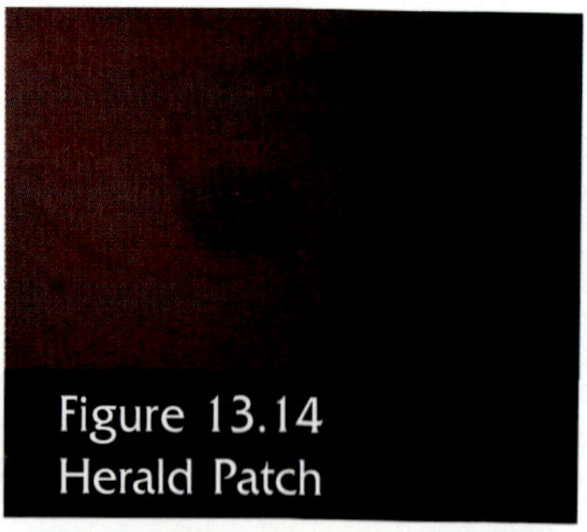

Figure 13.14
Herald Patch

A herald patch precedes the exanthematous phase: a larger, oval, salmon-colored patch with a central collarette of scale. (Courtesy of Dept. of Dermatology, Wilford Hall USAF Medical Center and Brooke Army Medical Center, San Antonio, TX.)

Associated Clinical Features

Borrelia burgdorferi is the tick-borne spirochete responsible for Lyme borreliosis, and erythema chronicum migrans (ECM) is the pathognomonic rash of Lyme disease occuring early in the infection. The initial prodromal symptoms of fever, myalgias, arthralgias, and headache are followed by a macule or papule progressing to a plaque at the site of the bite. This plaque expands its red, raised border as it clears centrally, leading to an annular appearance (Fig. 3.15). The plaque may burn and is rarely pruritic.

Differential Diagnosis

This annular plaque may resemble a fixed drug eruption, tinea corporis, urticaria, or the herald patch of pityriasis rosea. The multiple, secondary annular papules and plaques that may rarely form can resemble secondary syphilis. However, the Lyme-related eruption spares the palms and soles.

ED Treatment and Disposition

The duration of antibiotic treatment (10 to 30 days) depends on the severity of the symptoms. Tetracycline or doxycycline are the drugs of choice. Pregnant or lactating females and children younger than 8 years of age should be treated with penicillin or amoxicillin. Erythromycin is a suitable alternative. Patients with minimal symptoms may be treated on an outpatient basis. Those patients with significant toxicity and complications require admission, supportive care, and parenteral antibiotics.

Clinical Pearls

1. An annular plaque arising at the site of a tick bite in a patient with systemic symptoms should be treated as Lyme disease until proved otherwise.
2. Stage I of Lyme disease consists of constitutional symptoms and the characteristic rash of ECM.
3. Stage II of Lyme disease consists of neurologic (aseptic meningitis, encephalitis, bilateral Bell's palsy) and cardiac (myocarditis, conduction blocks) manifestations.
4. Stage III of Lyme disease consists of an asymmetric, episodic, oligoarticular arthritis.

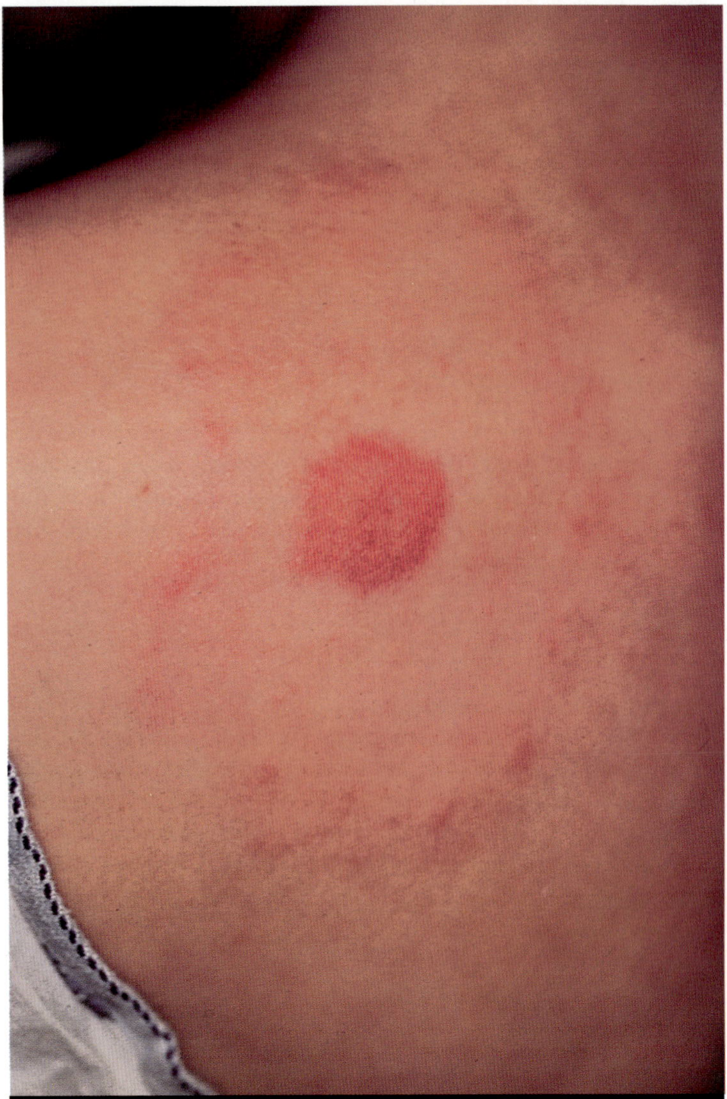

Figure 13.15 Erythema Chronicum Migrans

This pathognomonic eruption of Lyme disease forms at the site of the tick bite. The initial plaque expands its well defined border and clears centrally, forming an annular appearance. (Courtesy of David W. Munter, MD.)

Associated Clinical Features

Tinea corporis includes all dermatophyte infections excluding the scalp, face, hands, feet, and groin. The dermatophytosis is pruritic and consists of well circumscribed scaly plaque with a slightly elevated border and central clearing (Fig. 13.16). This annular configuration is most commonly found on the trunk and neck. Skin scrapings viewed with a KOH preparation exhibit septate hyphae.

Tinea faciale is a dermatophyte infection of the facial skin. It commonly appears as a well circumscribed erythematous patch (Fig. 13.17). Tinea manus is a dermatophyte infection of the hands (Fig. 13.18).

Differential Diagnosis

Pityriasis rosea, secondary syphilis, psoriasis, seborrheic dermatitis, and tinea versicolor are all usually considered in the differential diagnosis. A KOH examination of the scale demonstrating hyphae confirms the diagnosis.

ED Treatment and Disposition

Small, localized plaques may be treated with a topical antifungal cream. Extensive or resistant infection requires systemic griseofulvin or ketoconazole. It is important to treat for 2 weeks beyond the point of clinical cure to ensure successful eradication of the fungus.

Clinical Pearls

1. The scale is usually located at the leading edge of erythema and provides the best yield for scraping as part of the KOH examination.
2. If it scales, scrape it and look for hyphae.

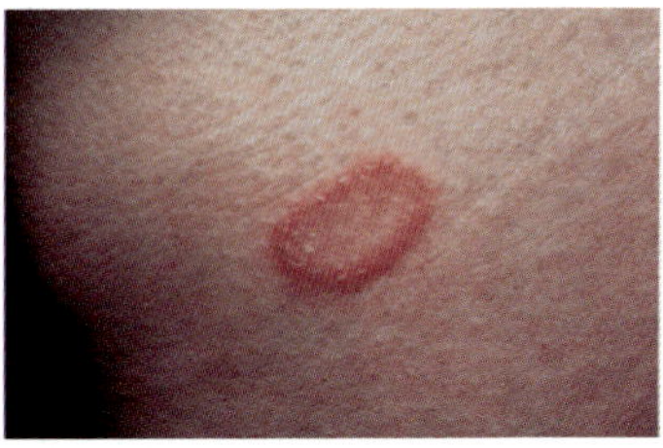

Figure 13.16
Tinea Corporis

This dermatophytosis is known as ringworm, a well defined, pruritic, scaly plaque with a raised border and central clearing (annular). KOH preparation is positive. (Courtesy of Dept. of Dermatology, Wilford Hall USAF Medical Center and Brooke Army Medical Center, San Antonio, TX.)

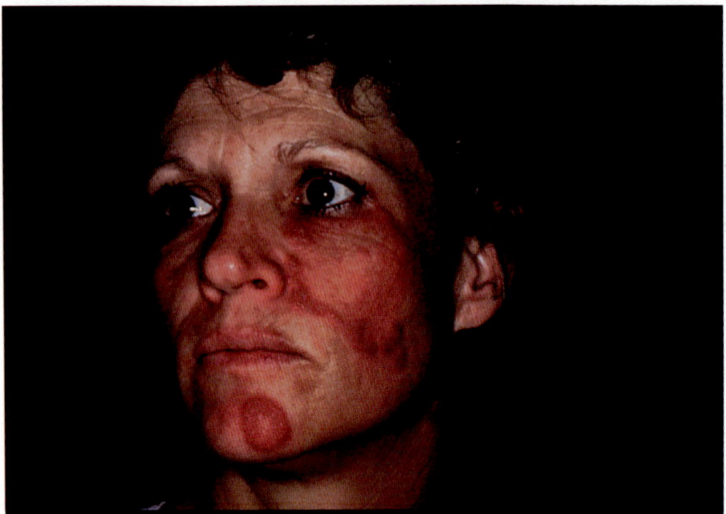

Figure 13.17 Tinea Faciale

Note the sharply marginated, polycyclic, scaly plaque with central clearing localized to the face. KOH preparation is positive. (Courtesy of Dept. of Dermatology, Wilford Hall USAF Medical Center and Brooke Army Medical Center, San Antonio, TX.)

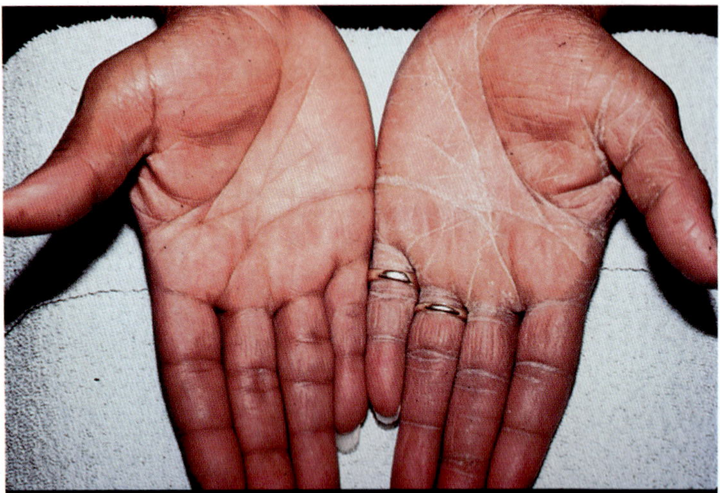

Figure 13.18 Tinea Manus

When this dermatophytosis involves the hands, it is usually unilateral. Note the diffuse hyperkeratosis of the palm of the left hand. KOH preparation is positive. (Courtesy of Dept. of Dermatology, Wilford Hall USAF Medical Center and Brooke Army Medical Center, San Antonio, TX.)

Associated Clinical Features

Tinea cruris, or "jock itch," is a pruritic dermatophytosis of the intertriginous areas, usually excluding the penis and scrotum. The scaly, erythematous plaque spreads peripherally with central clearing (Fig. 13.19). The borders of the plaque are well defined.

Differential Diagnosis

Erythrasma, *Candida albicans,* seborrheic dermatitis, and psoriasis are usually considered in the differential diagnosis. A KOH examination of the scale demonstrating hyphae confirms the diagnosis.

ED Treatment and Disposition

Initial treatment consists of topical antifungal medications. Griseofulvin or ketoconazole are reserved for resistant cases. It is important to treat for 1 week beyond the point of clinical cure to ensure successful eradication of the fungus. Decreasing the amount of perspiration by using topical powders may help prevent recurrences.

Clinical Pearls

1. A less well defined, pruritic, intertriginous plaque which typically involves the scrotum is usually erythrasma. It is caused by *Nocarelia minutissimus* and is treated with topical erythromycin.
2. If it scales, scrape it and look for hyphae.

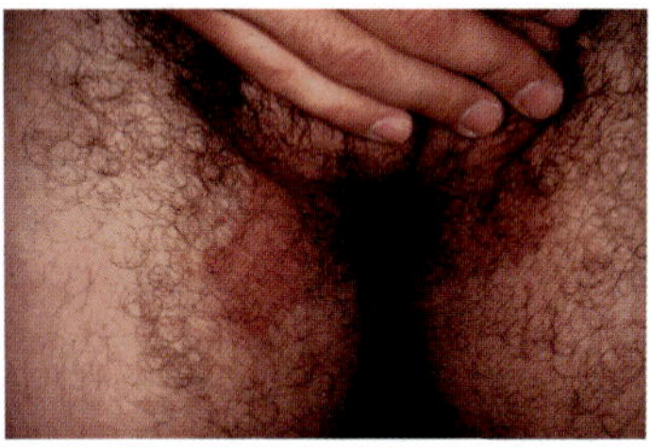

Figure 13.19
Tinea Cruris

This dermatophytosis is commonly called jock itch. Note that the erythematous, scaly plaque with its well defined border does not involve the skin of the scrotum or penis. KOH preparation is positive. (Courtesy of Dept. of Dermatology, Wilford Hall USAF Medical Center and Brooke Army Medical Center, San Antonio, TX.)

Associated Clinical Features

Tinea pedis, or "athlete's foot," is a pruritic dermatophytosis. It consists of erythema and scaling of the sole, maceration, occasional vesiculation, and fissure formation between and under the toes (Fig. 13.20). These pruritic, painful fissures may become secondarily infected with gram-negative organisms. Frequently the toenails are also affected.

Differential Diagnosis

Foot eczema, psoriasis, and Reiter's syndrome are considered in the differential diagnosis. A KOH examination of the scale demonstrating hyphae confirms the diagnosis.

ED Treatment and Disposition

Topical antifungal creams are the initial treatment of choice. Antibiotics may be used to treat secondary infection. Griseofulvin, then ketoconazole, are used for chronic or resistant cases. It is important to treat for 1 week beyond the point of clinical cure to ensure successful eradication of the fungus.

Clinical Pearls

1. If it scales, scrape it and look for hyphae.
2. Macerated areas may become secondarily infected by bacteria.

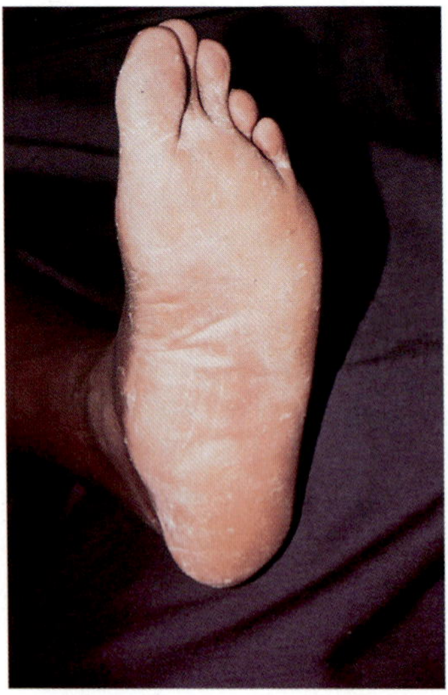

Figure 13.20
Tinea Pedis

This diffuse, pruritic, scaling hyperkeratosis of the sole of the foot extending to the interdigital spaces is known as athlete's foot. KOH preparation is positive. (Courtesy of Dept. of Dermatology, Wilford Hall USAF Medical Center and Brooke Army Medical Center, San Antonio, TX.)

Associated Clinical Features

Tinea capitis is scalp ringworm, or a dermatophytosis of the scalp. It presents as a pruritic, erythematous, scaly plaque with broken or missing hairs frequently referred to as "gray patch" or "black dot" ringworm (Fig. 13.21). This may develop into a kerion. A kerion is a delayed-type hypersensitivity reaction to the fungus where the initial erythematous, scaly plaque becomes boggy with inflamed, purulent nodules and plaques (Fig. 13.22). The hair follicle is frequently destroyed by the inflammatory process in a kerion leading to a scarring alopecia.

Differential Diagnosis

Various inflammatory follicular conditions, such as folliculitis, impetigo, psoriasis, alopecia areata, and seborrheic dermatitis, may resemble tinea capitis. The diagnosis is made by a KOH examination of a scraping of the area revealing hyphae and spores.

ED Treatment Disposition

Systemic griseofulvin is usually required for several weeks to successfully treat tinea capitis. Systemic antibiotics and corticosteroids are usually added when treating a kerion. Selenium sulfide lotion used as a shampoo may actually decrease the duration of the infection. It is important to treat for 2 weeks beyond the point of clinical cure to ensure successful eradication of the fungus. Ketoconazole is reserved for resistant cases.

Clinical Pearls

1. Tinea capitis is a disease of childhood; it is rare in immunocompetent adults.
2. It is epidemic in many African American communities.
3. The KOH scrape is aided by using a disposable urethral brush or similar device.

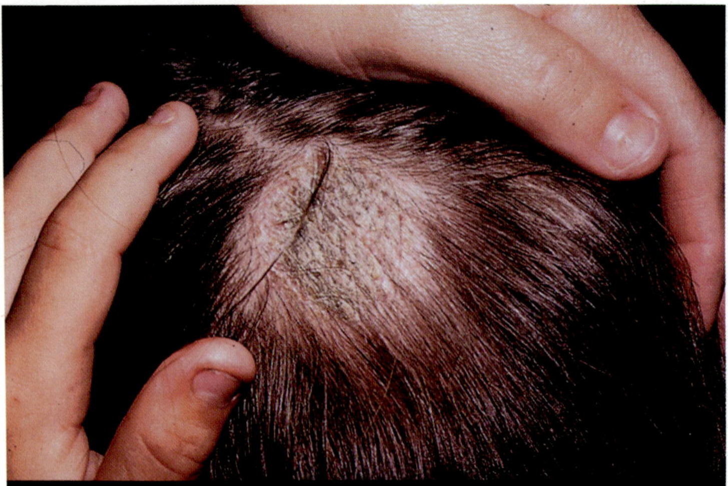

Figure 13.21 Tinea Capitis

This dermatophytosis is characterized by a pruritic, circular area of hair loss covered by adherent scales. KOH preparation is positive. (Courtesy of Dept. of Dermatology, Wilford Hall USAF Medical Center and Brooke Army Medical Center, San Antonio, TX.)

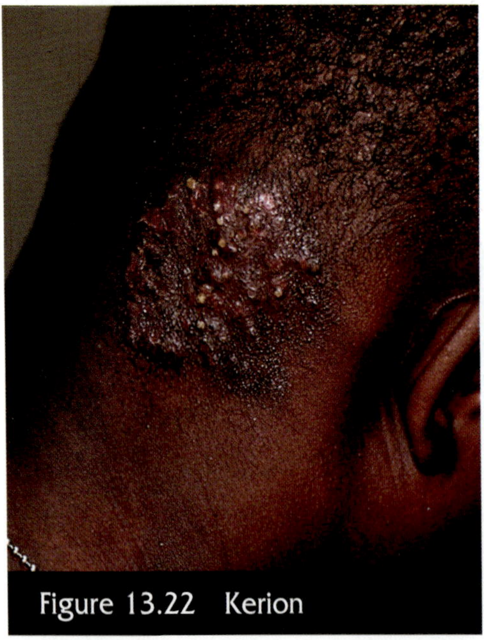

Figure 13.22 Kerion

This collection of boggy, inflamed, purulent nodules and papules is the result of a delayed-type hypersensitivity reaction to the fungus. Scarring alopecia will follow as a result of the actual destruction of the hair follicle. (Courtesy of Dept. of Dermatology, Wilford Hall USAF Medical Center and Brooke Army Medical Center, San Antonio, TX.)

Associated Clinical Features

Onychomycosis is an invasion of the nails by any fungus. Four clinical subtypes are noted. *Distal subungual* presents as discolorations of the free edge of the nail with hyperkeratosis leading to a subungual accumulation of friable keratinaceous debris (Fig. 13.23). *White superficial* consists of sharply outlined white areas on the nail plate which leave the surface friable. *Proximal subungual* presents as discolorations which start proximally at the nail fold. *Candidal onychomycosis* encompasses the entire nail plate, leaving the surface rough and friable.

Differential Diagnosis

Psoriasis and various other nail dystrophies such as distal onycholysis caused by excessive water exposure or drugs must be differentiated from this fungal infection. Pseudomonal nail infection is characterized by the subungual accumulation of green debris. A KOH examination of the keratinaceous debris demonstrating hyphae confirms onychomycosis.

ED Treatment and Disposition

The most common treatment consists of oral griseofulvin. Candidal infections require oral ketoconazole. Toenail onychomycosis is very difficult to eradicate. Recently, itraconazole has shown promise as a drug for curing toenail onychomycosis.

Clinical Pearls

1. All that causes the nail plate to separate from the nail bed is not necessarily fungus.
2. If it scales, scrape it and look for hyphae.

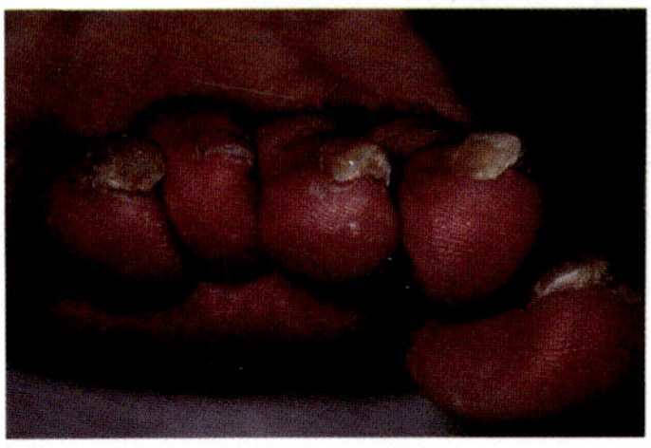

Figure 13.23 Onychomycosis

Note that multiple nail beds have been invaded by the fungus, leading to chronic hyperkeratosis and subungual accumulation of friable keratinaceous debris. (Courtesy of Dept. of Dermatology, Wilford Hall USAF Medical Center and Brooke Army Medical Center, San Antonio, TX.)

Associated Clinical Features

Tinea versicolor is a chronic, superficial fungal infection that involves the trunk and extremities, with little or no involvement of the face. Finely scaling brown macules are present in fair-skinned patients, whereas scaly hypopigmented macules are often noted in dark-skinned patients (Fig. 13.24). These sharply demarcated macules are intermittently pruritic.

Differential Diagnosis

Pityriasis rosea, secondary syphilis, and some drug eruptions must all be considered in the differential diagnosis. A KOH examination of a scraping of the area revealing hyphae and spores makes the diagnosis (Fig. 17.8).

ED Treatment and Disposition

Treatment consists of short applications of selenium sulfide lotion, topical antifungal creams, or topical ketoconazole. Resistant cases require oral ketoconazole. Ultraviolet exposure is required to regain any lost pigment.

Clinical Pearls

1. If it scales, scrape it and look for hyphae.
2. Clinically active areas or areas colonized with the fungus may be identified by the orange fluorescence noted on Wood's light examination.

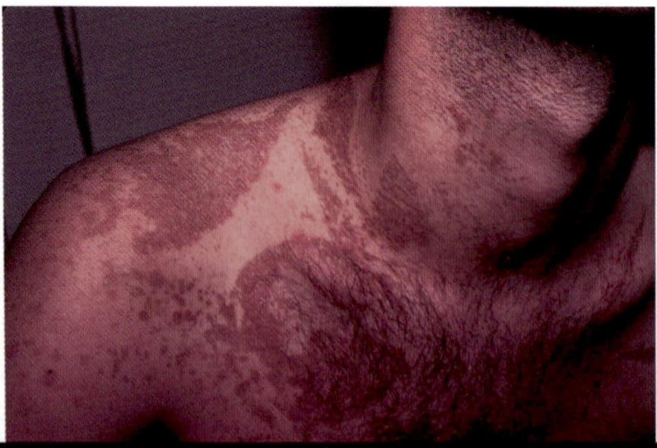

Figure 13.24 Tinea Versicolor

This chronic superficial fungal infection leads to the formation of multiple well defined, scaly, hypopigmented macules on the trunk and extremities. (Courtesy of Dept. of Dermatology, Wilford Hall USAF Medical Center and Brooke Army Medical Center, San Antonio, TX.)

Associated Clinical Features

Basal cell carcinoma is a malignancy of the basal cell layer of the epidermis, presenting as a translucent, pearly papule with central ulceration and rolled borders with fine superficial telangiectasias (Fig. 13.25). It is most frequently located on the head, neck, and upper trunk. The patient frequently notes easy bleeding of the papule with poor to nonhealing. There are several variants of basal cell carcinomas. Pigmented basal cell carcinoma consists of a brownish-black, firm nodule with irregular surface and central ulceration (Fig. 13.26). Superficial multicentric basal cell carcinoma is psoriasiform in nature, consisting of a flat, erythematous, scaly translucent plaque without central ulceration or raised border (Fig. 13.27).

Differential Diagnosis

Pigmented basal cell carcinoma resembles nodular melanoma. Superficial multicentric basal cell carcinoma resembles psoriasis, tinea corporis, and squamous cell carcinoma in situ.

ED Treatment and Disposition

Excisional surgery, cryosurgery, or electrosurgery are recommended forms of treatment. If there is a potential for disfigurement, radiation therapy is usually instituted instead of surgery. Prompt dermatologic consultation must be arranged when evaluating any suspicious lesion.

Clinical Pearls

1. Basal cell carcinoma is the most common form of skin cancer.
2. This malignancy forms in the epidermis that has developing hair follicles; therefore, it is not found on the vermilion border of the lips or the genital mucosal membranes.
3. The pearly, rolled, telangiectatic border with central ulceration is diagnostic of basal cell carcinoma.
4. Despite being locally invasive, basal cell carcinoma does not metastasize.

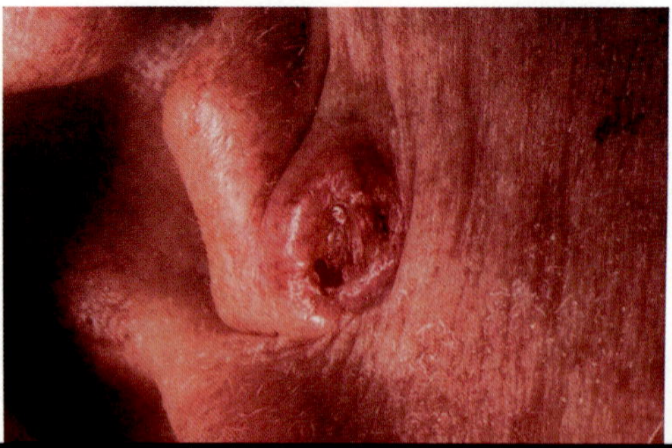

Figure 13.25 Basal Cell Carcinoma

Nodular basal cell carcinoma consists of a firm, centrally ulcerated (rodent ulcer) nodule with a raised, rolled, pearly, telangiectatic border. (Courtesy of Dept. of Dermatology, Wilford Hall USAF Medical Center and Brooke Army Medical Center, San Antonio, TX.)

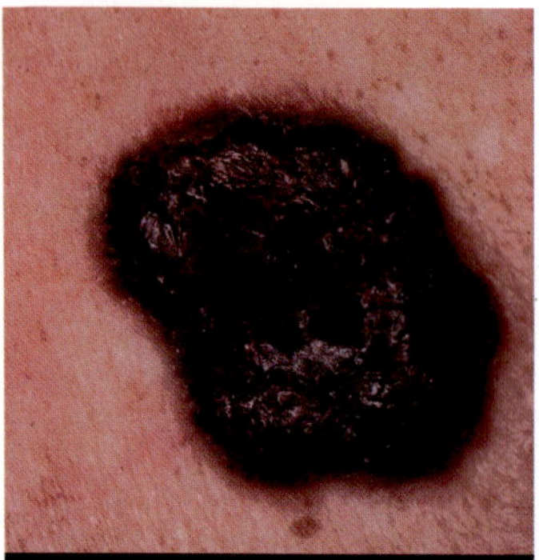

Figure 13.26
Basal Cell Carcinoma

This pigmented basal cell carcinoma consists of a firm, translucent, brownish-black, ulcerated nodule with an irregular surface and asymmetry of its border. (Courtesy of Dept. of Dermatology, Wilford Hall USAF Medical Center and Brooke Army Medical Center, San Antonio, TX.)

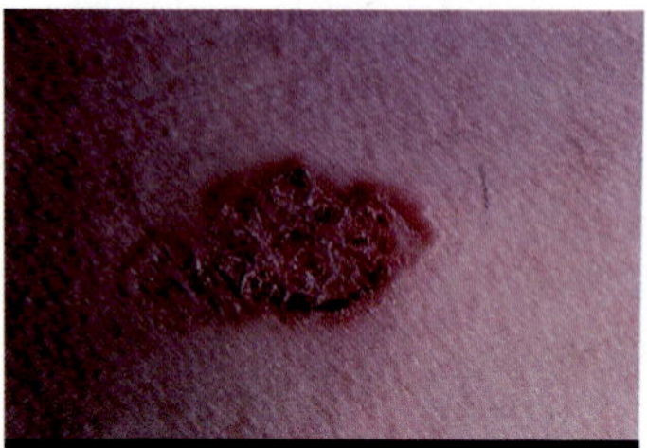

Figure 13.27
Basal Cell Carcinoma

Superficial multicentric basal cell carcinoma is frequently psoriasiform in nature. Note the flat, erythematous, scaly plaque with its elevated, irregular border. (Courtesy of Dept. of Dermatology, Wilford Hall USAF Medical Center and Brooke Army Medical Center, San Antonio, TX.)

Associated Clinical Features

Squamous cell carcinoma varies from erythematous, hyperkeratotic, sharply demarcated plaques to elevated, ulcerative nodules (Fig. 13.28). It may be sun-induced or related to ionizing radiation or industrial carcinogens. Bowen's disease is actually an in situ squamous cell carcinoma consisting of a firm, solitary, erythematous macule or plaque with fine scale and a well defined border. It resembles the superficial multicentric variety of basal cell carcinoma. Erythroplasia of Queyrat consists of the same in situ plaque localized to the penis. Invasive squamous cell carcinoma is characterized by a discrete elevated plaque or nodule with thick keratotic scale and ulceration.

Differential Diagnosis

Squamous cell carcinoma must be differentiated from a benign lesion such as tinea corporis, psoriasis, impetigo, wart, seborrheic keratosis, or keratoacanthoma (Fig. 13.29).

ED Treatment and Disposition

Excisional surgery is required, with radiation therapy utilized in potentially disfiguring cases. All suspicious lesions require prompt dermatologic consultation.

Clinical Pearls

1. Squamous cell carcinoma is the second most common type of cutaneous malignancy.
2. This malignancy develops more commonly in fair-skinned people with a significant history of sun exposure.
3. Most lesions are found on the lips or other sun-exposed areas.
4. A rapidly evolving (2 to 4 weeks) nodule or plaque with a dense hyperkeratotic core is a keratoacanthoma. It is closely related to squamous cell carcinoma and frequently occurs at a site of trauma. Treatment is the same.

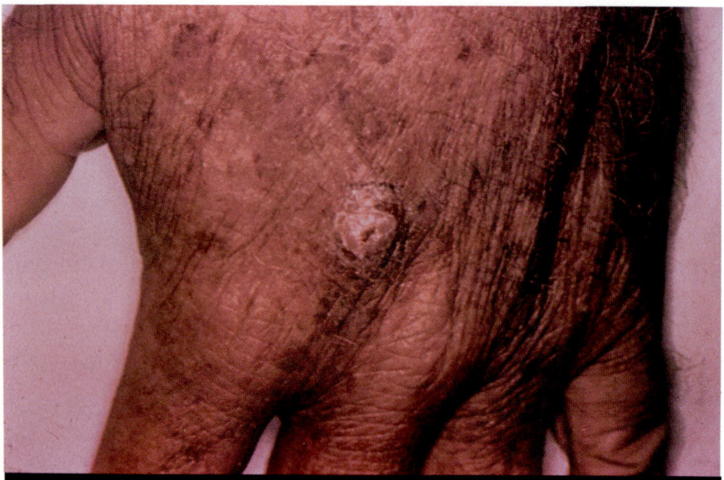

Figure 13.28 Squamous Cell Carcinoma

Note the single erythematous, scaly plaque on the dorsal aspect of this sun-exposed hand. (Courtesy of Dept. of Dermatology, Wilford Hall USAF Medical Center and Brooke Army Medical Center, San Antonio, TX.)

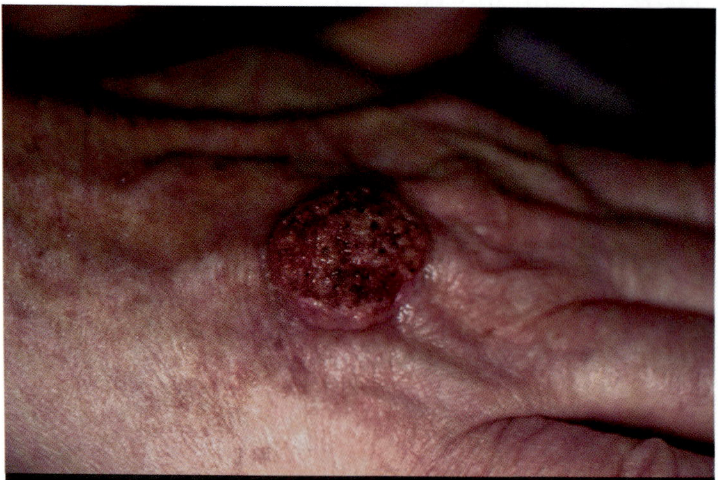

Figure 13.29 Keratoacanthoma

This rapidly evolving neoplasm consists of an erythematous nodule with a hyperkeratotic core. It most closely resembles a squamous cell carcinoma, although it is a benign epithelial neoplasm. Biopsy serves to differentiate these two conditions. (Courtesy of Dept. of Dermatology, Wilford Hall USAF Medical Center and Brooke Army Medical Center, San Antonio, TX.)

Associated Clinical Features

Melanoma is a malignancy involving the melanocytes of the epidermis. Asymmetry, an irregular border, a mottled display of color, a diameter greater than 5 to 6 mm, and an elevation or distortion of the surface are five signs that a lesion may be a melanoma (Fig. 13.30). Melanoma may or may not occur in sun-exposed areas.

Differential Diagnosis

Lentigo maligna is characterized by a single, flat, frecklelike macule with an irregular border, usually on the face (Fig. 13.31). This melanoma in situ is often confused with a solar lentigo or a seborrheic keratosis. Superficially spreading melanoma is the most common form of melanoma. It usually presents as a brown macule with irregular borders and variegation in color. Nodular melanoma usually starts as a papule which becomes an elevated nodule with irregular borders and variegation in color (Fig. 13.32). It must be differentiated from a hemangioma, angiokeratoma, or pigmented basal cell carcinoma. Acral lentiginous melanomas are often mistaken for plantar warts or subungual hematomas; they are flat, pigmented, irregularly bordered macules of the palms, soles, and subungual areas (Fig. 13.33).

ED Treatment and Disposition

Melanoma must be surgically excised with adequate margins. Prompt dermatologic consultation is required of all suspicious lesions because the prognosis of melanoma correlates directly with early detection and treatment.

Clinical Pearls

1. Prognosis of melanoma is most dependent on the depth of invasion, therefore, early detection and treatment are essential.
2. Only 20% of melanomas arise from preexisting moles, so the appearance of a new mole, especially after the age of 30, is particularly significant.

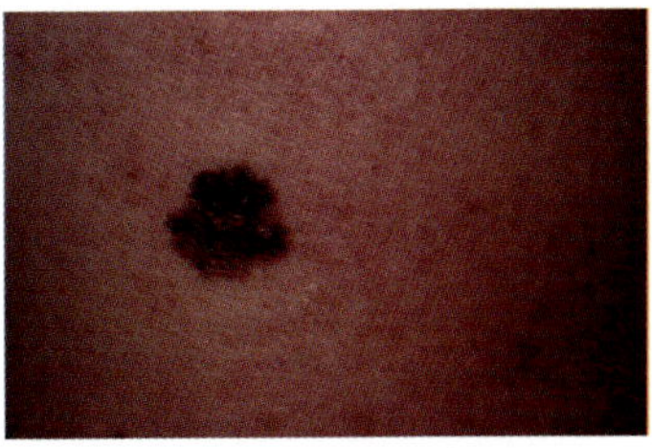

Figure 13.30
Melanoma

Note the asymmetry, irregular border, and focal hyperpigmentation in this melanoma. (Courtesy of Dept. of Dermatology, Wilford Hall USAF Medical Center and Brooke Army Medical Center, San Antonio, TX.)

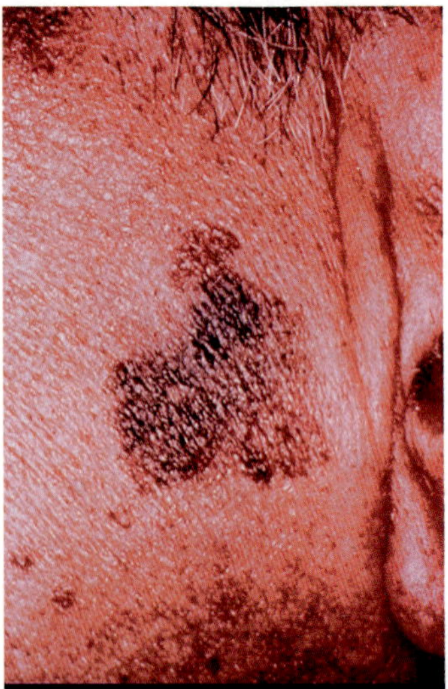

Figure 13.31 Lentigo Maligna Melanoma

This long-lived melanoma in situ has now invaded the dermis, forming a black nodule classified as lentigo maligna melanoma. (Courtesy of Dept. of Dermatology, Wilford Hall USAF Medical Center and Brooke Army Medical Center, San Antonio, TX.)

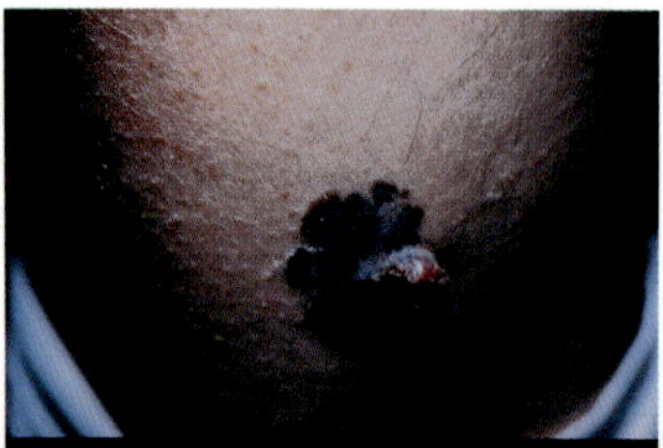

Figure 13.32 Nodular Melanoma

This melanoma has progressed to an exophytic tumor which was deeply invasive histopathologically. (Courtesy of Dept. of Dermatology, Wilford Hall USAF Medical Center and Brooke Army Medical Center, San Antonio, TX.)

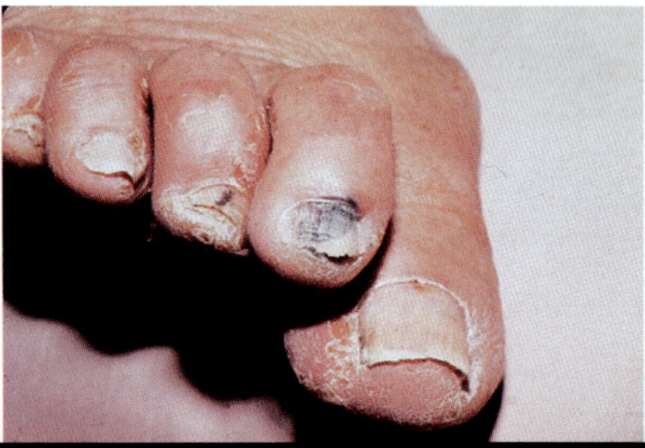

Figure 13.33 Acral Lentiginous Melanoma

The finding of a pigmented, irregularly bordered macule involving the proximal nail fold is called Hutchinson's sign. It represents melanoma of the nail matrix and is therefore classified as an acral lentiginous melanoma. (Courtesy of Dept. of Dermatology, Wilford Hall USAF Medical Center and Brooke Army Medical Center, San Antonio, TX.)

Associated Clinical Features

Exanthematous drug eruptions are an adverse hypersensitivity reaction to a drug. This symmetric, pruritic, morbilliform, blanching, erythematous eruption is the most frequent of cutaneous drug eruptions (Fig. 13.34). The initially pruritic macules or papules usually become confluent and may progress to an exfoliative dermatitis.

Differential Diagnosis

Viral exanthem, secondary syphilis, atypical pityriasis rosea, and scarlet fever must all be considered in the differential diagnosis. A serologic test for syphilis, antistreptolysin O titer, and a good history are usually sufficient to make the diagnosis. Severe drug eruptions may be accompanied by eosinophilia, lymphadenopathy, and liver function abnormalities.

ED Treatment and Disposition

The eruption may resolve despite the drug's continued use. The drug should be discontinued if considered to be the cause of the rash. It may take as long as 2 weeks for the eruption to fade after discontinuation of the causative drug. Symptomatic management includes antihistamines and topical corticosteroids.

Clinical Pearls

1. Drug eruptions are usually symmetric and pruritic as opposed to viral eruptions, which are usually asymmetric and asymptomatic.
2. Mononucleosis patients taking amoxicillin or AIDS patients taking sulfa drugs frequently experience this reaction.

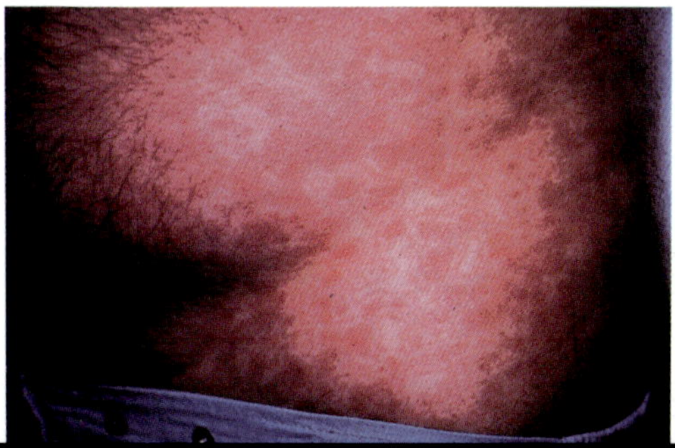

Figure 13.34 Exanthematous Drug Eruptions

This symmetric, morbilliform, blanching eruption was the result of allopurinol. With time, the eruption may become confluent, leading to an exfoliative dermatitis. (Courtesy of Dept. of Dermatology, Wilford Hall USAF Medical Center and Brooke Army Medical Center, San Antonio,

Associated Clinical Features

Urticaria is a vascular reaction localized to the skin composed of transient, erythematous, edematous, pruritic papules or plaquelike wheals (Figs. 13.35 and 13.36). It tends to favor the covered areas (back, chest, buttocks). Angioedema is a circumscribed edema of the dermis and subcutaneous tissues that usually affects the distensible tissues (lips, eyelids, earlobes). It is usually nonpruritic. There are countless causes of urticaria; the most common being food, medications, and underlying infection. Cholinergic urticaria involves micropapular lesions induced by exercise or heat. Dermatographism presents as linear hives at the site of skin stroking. Cold urticaria can be diagnosed with the ice cube test, and solar urticaria occurs in areas exposed to sunlight. Urticaria may also occur as a result of exposure to pressure, heat, and water. Hereditary angioedema is an autosomal dominant disorder with systemic manifestations secondary to edema of the subcutaneous and mucosal tissues of the respiratory and gastrointestinal tract, in addition to the face and extremities (Fig. 13.37). Mortality rates approach 30%, usually from airway obstruction. There is also an acquired form of angioedema secondary to an underlying malignancy, usually lymphoreticular. Angiotensin converting enzyme inhibitor use is a frequent cause of angioedema.

Differential Diagnosis

Bacterial or viral exanthems, erythema multiforme, and drug eruptions must be considered in the differential diagnosis of urticaria. Edema of any etiology (congestive heart failure, glomerulonephritis, chronic liver disease) must be differentiated from the soft-tissue swelling associated with angioedema.

ED Treatment and Disposition

This involves the identification and elimination of any potential etiology. Antihistamines can be effective for urticaria, often requiring both H_1 and H_2 blockers and steroids for stubborn cases. Life-threatening attacks of hereditary angioedema do not respond well to antihistamines, epinephrine, or steroids. Admission for supportive care and active airway management is the mainstay of treatment. Danazol may be utilized for prophylactic management.

Clinical Pearls

1. Both urticaria and angioedema are acute and evanescent.
2. Urticaria is pruritic and responsive to antihistamines, epinephrine, and steroids.
3. Angioedema is only rarely pruritic and minimally responsive to epinephrine, and may require danazol for long-term treatment.

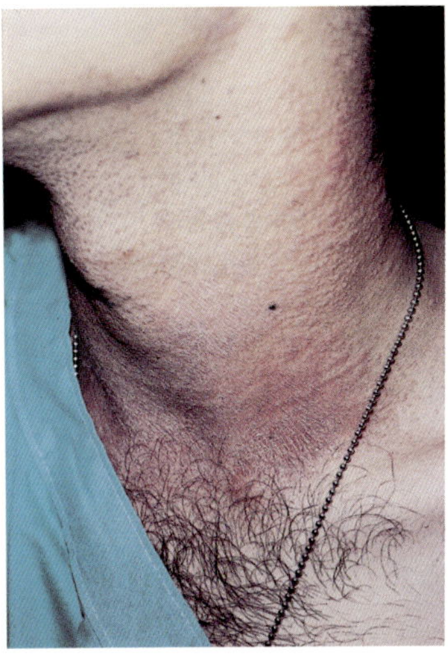

Figure 13.35 Urticaria

Note the edematous papules and wheals covering the skin of the neck. (Courtesy of Alan B. Storrow, MD.)

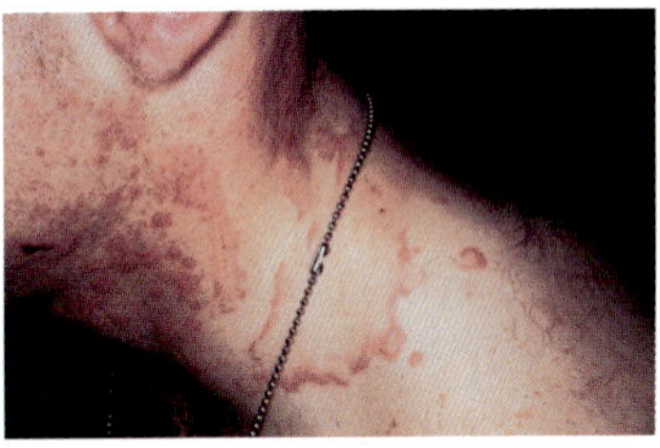

Figure 13.36 Urticaria

This picture demonstrates that the urticarial eruptions may be quite large, forming edematous plaques with central clearing. (Courtesy of Dept. of Dermatology, Wilford Hall USAF Medical Center and Brooke Army Medical Center, San Antonio, TX.)

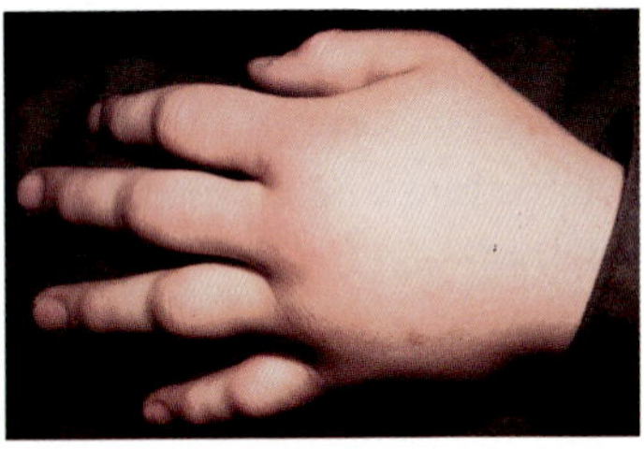

Figure 13.37 Angioedema

This is an example of hereditary angioedema. Note the circumscribed edema of the subcutaneous tissues of the hand, without the presence of urticaria. (Courtesy of Dept. of Dermatology, Wilford Hall USAF Medical Center and Brooke Army Medical Center, San Antonio, TX.)

Associated Clinical Features

Dyshidrotic eczema is a papulovesicular plaque involving the epidermis of the fingers, palms, and soles. The dermatosis initially consists of pruritic, deep-seated vesicles grouped in clusters (Fig. 13.38). Scaling and painful fissure formation are late complications, as is secondary bacterial infection. Spontaneous remissions and recurrent attacks are usually the rule.

Differential Diagnosis

Acute contact dermatitis must be considered in the differential diagnosis of the acute eruption. Psoriasis and dermatophytosis are considered in the differential diagnosis of the chronic eruption.

ED Treatment and Disposition

Burow's wet dressings should be utilized during the early vesicular stage. High-potency topical steroids are used in all stages of the eruption. Systemic corticosteroids should be avoided except for the most severe cases. Antihistamines treat the pruritus. Dicloxacillin or erythromycin are used to treat secondary bacterial infections. Minimal exposure to water and generous emolliation also hasten healing.

Clinical Pearls

1. Deep-seated, tapioca-like vesicles on the sides of the digits followed by scaling and fissure formation is typical of this disease.
2. Dyshidrotic eczema is frequently associated with psychosocial stressors.
3. The "id reaction," due to fungal infections and drug eruptions, may have similar clinical presentations.

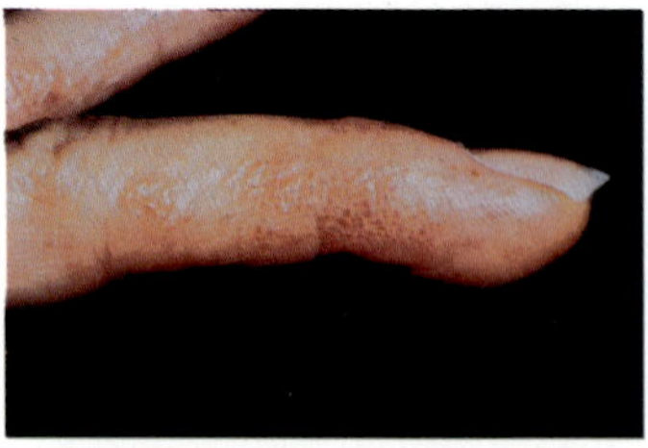

Figure 13.38 Dyshidrotic Eczema

Note the cluster of deep-seated vesicles along the sides of the fingers. Scaling and painful fissure formation may also occur. No overlying erythema is present. (Courtesy of Dept. of Dermatology, Wilford Hall USAF Medical Center and Brooke Army Medical Center, San Antonio, TX.)

Associated Clinical Features

Allergic contact dermatitis is an acute or chronic delayed-type hypersensitivity reaction caused by contact exposure to a variety of agents. The acute form is characterized by multiple, closely grouped vesicles with exudative erosions and crust formation on a well defined erythematous, edematous base (Figs. 13.39 and 13.40). Subacute contact dermatitis consists of dry, scaly patches with areas of desquamation, whereas the chronic form consists of hyperkeratosis and pigmentation. All forms of allergic contact dermatitis are pruritic.

Differential Diagnosis

Atopic dermatitis, nummular eczema, impetigo, and dermatophytosis are included in the differential diagnosis. If it scales, scrape it and look for hyphae to differentiate a dermatophytosis. A positive patch test is diagnostic of an allergic contact dermatitis. Contact exposure of the skin to the allergen leading to erythema and vesicle formation is considered a positive test.

ED Treatment and Disposition

Identify and remove any potential allergen. Antihistamines relieve the pruritus. Topical corticosteroids treat the underlying inflammation. Systemic corticosteroids should be avoided except for the most severe cases.

Clinical Pearls

1. Well defined, pruritic areas of erythema superimposed with exudative vesicles and a recent history of exposure to a specific allergen are diagnostic of allergic contact dermatitis.
2. Poison ivy and oak are the most common causes of allergic contact dermatitis.
3. When treating with topical ointments, a worsening of the dermatitis may signify an allergic reaction to the medication.

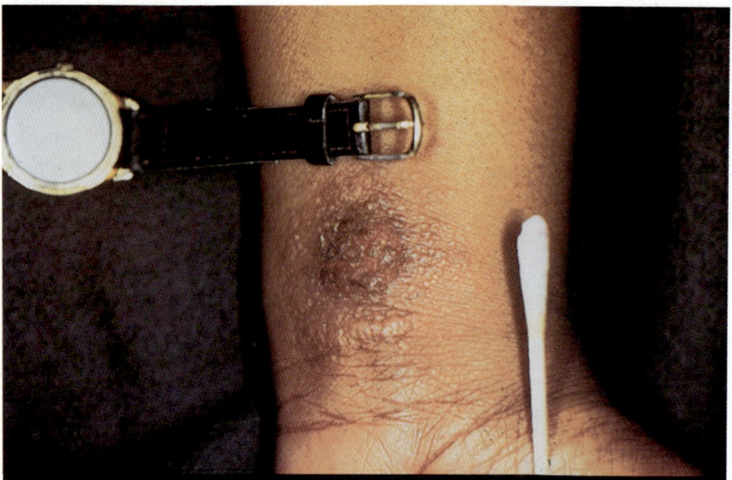

Figure 13.39 Contact Dermatitis

Note that the erythematous, edematous base of the eruption corresponds to the posterior surface of the watch. Superimposed on the erythematous base are multiple vesicles with exudate and crust. (Courtesy of Dept. of Dermatology, Wilford Hall USAF Medical Center and Brooke Army Medical Center, San Antonio, TX.)

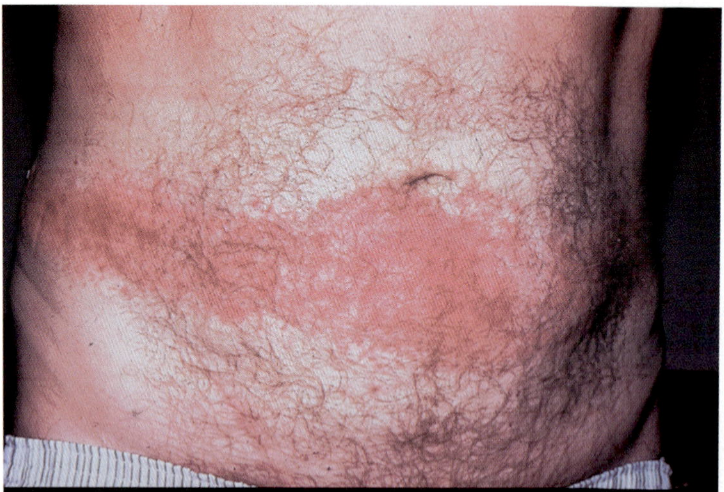

Figure 13.40 Contact Dermatitis

Another example of how the eruption involves only the surface of the skin exposed to the irritant. In this case the irritant is the elastic band of the underwear. Note the linear, well demarcated nature of the eruption, which is classic for contact dermatitis. (Courtesy of Dept. of Dermatology, Wilford Hall USAF Medical Center and Brooke Army Medical Center, San Antonio, TX.)

PART II

SPECIALTY AREAS

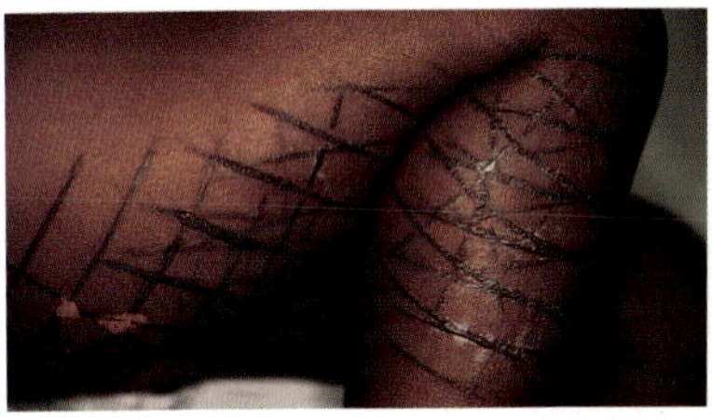

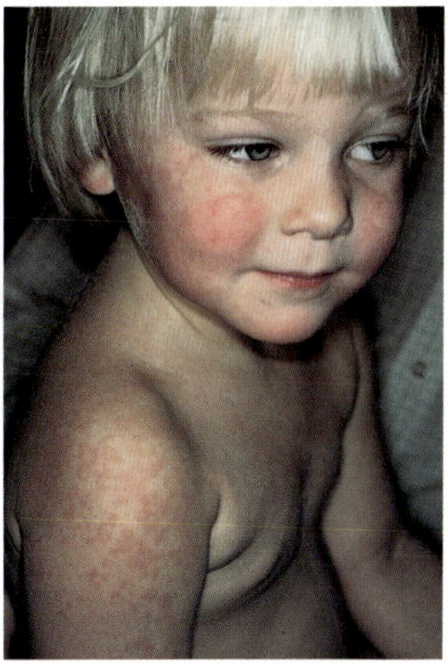

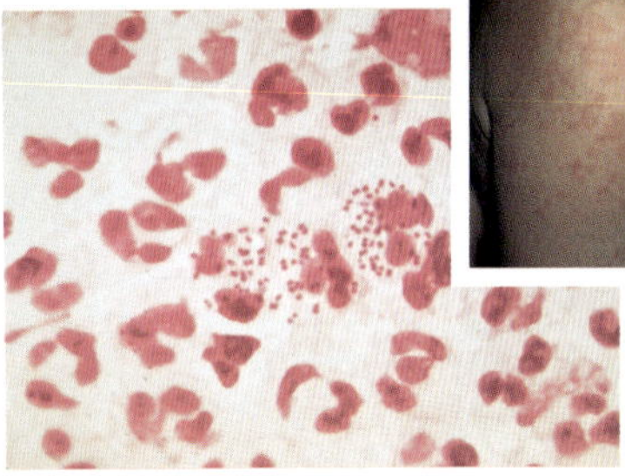

CHAPTER 14

PEDIATRIC CONDITIONS

Javier A. Gonzalez del Rey
Richard M. Ruddy

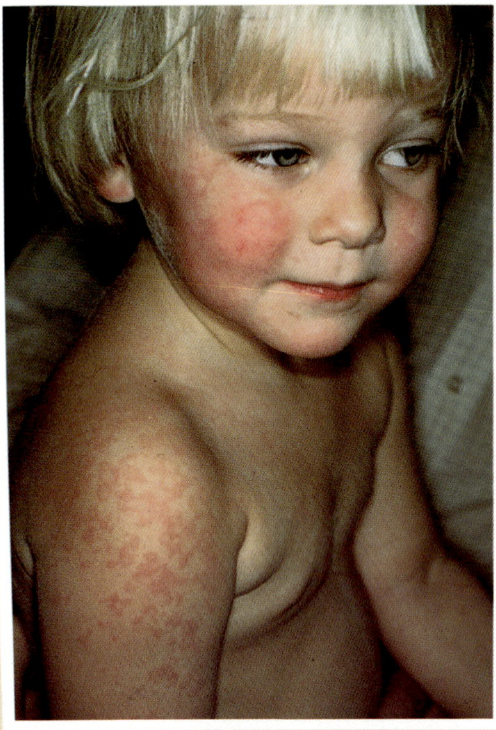

Associated Clinical Features

This benign, self-limiting eruption of unknown etiology in newborns is characterized by small, erythematous macules 2 to 3 cm in diameter (Fig. 14.1) with 1- to 3-mm, firm, pale yellow or white papules or pustules in the center. This rash usually presents within the first 2 to 3 days of life. Each individual lesion usually disappears within 4 or 5 days. New lesions may occur during the first 2 weeks of life. Wright-stained slide preparations of the scraping from the center of the lesion demonstrate numerous eosinophils.

Differential Diagnosis

Transient neonatal pustular melanosis, newborn milia, miliaria, herpes simplex, and impetigo of the newborn should be considered.

ED Treatment and Disposition

As this condition is self-limiting, no therapy is indicated in the setting of a well-appearing newborn with normal activity and appetite. In cases in which impetigo, *Candida,* or herpes infections are suspected, a smear from the center of the lesion and culture may be necessary to make a final diagnosis.

Clinical Pearl

1. Erythema toxicum is the most common rash of the newborn (up to 50% of full terms). The lesions may be present anywhere on the body but tend to spare the palms and soles.

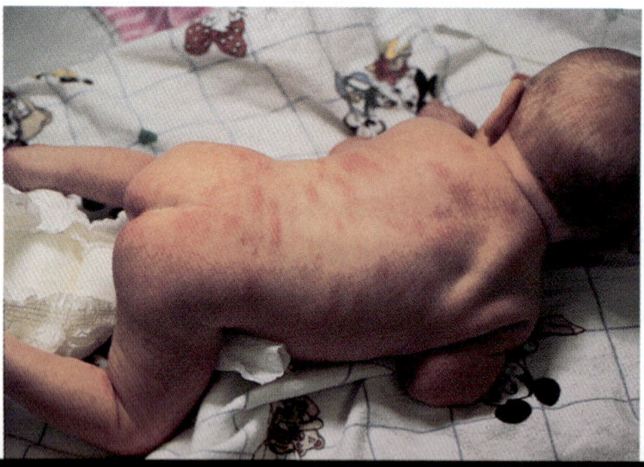

Figure 14.1 Erythema Toxicum

Newborn infant with diffuse macular rash of erythema toxicum. (Courtesy of Kevin J. Knoop, MD, MS.)

Associated Clinical Features

Physiologic jaundice (Fig. 14.2) is observed in 25 to 50% of term newborns. Most cases are self-limited and generally without sequelae. The physiologic ($<$12 mg/dL) jaundice of the newborn usually peaks between the second and fourth day. In preterm infants this peak occurs later. Physiologic jaundice is believed to be a combination of factors including an increase of bilirubin production following breakdown of fetal red blood cells associated with a temporary decrease in conjugation of these by-products by the immature newborn liver. Risk factors for unconjugated hyperbilirubinemia include maternal diabetes, prematurity, drugs, polycythemia, traumatic delivery with cutaneous bruising or hematoma, and breastfeeding. Most infants with jaundice have no disease, but a careful history and organized approach is necessary to identify pathologic causes when these patients present to the ED. Kernicterus is a condition resulting from a severe form of unconjugated hyperbilirubinemia and is associated with mental retardation, deafness, seizures, choreoathetosis, and a multitude of other irreversible neurologic abnormalities.

Differential Diagnosis

Jaundice within the first 24 h of life is usually associated with sepsis, erythroblastosis fetalis, and bleeding disorders or hemorrhage (traumatic delivery with cutaneous bleeding or hematomas). Physiologic jaundice first appears on the second or third day. Any patient presenting with jaundice after the third day of life should be carefully evaluated for the possibility of sepsis. Late-onset jaundice could be suggestive of septicemia, breast milk jaundice, galactosemia, hemolytic anemias, drug-induced hyperbilirubinemia, pyloric stenosis or duodenal atresia, Crigler-Najjar, or Gilbert's disease.

ED Treatment and Disposition

Initial laboratory work-up should include blood type and Coombs' test, complete blood count with smear for red cell morphology and reticulocyte count, and indirect and direct bilirubin. Other studies may be ordered according to the clinical presentation and history. Initial management should ensure adequate hydration and treatment of the underlying condition. Correct acidosis, since bilirubin precipitates in acid media. In cases of physiologic jaundice the level of serum bilirubin at which to start phototherapy is not clearly defined. The traditional approach is to initiate phototherapy to maintain bilirubin level below 20 mg/dL. Exchange transfusion is considered if the serum level remains elevated (22 to 28 mg/dL) despite appropriate phototherapy.

Clinical Pearls

1. Physiologic jaundice in the presence of a good hemoglobin level is orange in color. It is often visible when the bilirubin level exceeds 8 mg/dL. Jaundice associated with anemia is usually lemon in color.
2. Bilirubin levels should be modified for prematurity, sepsis, low birth weight, and other risk factors when phototherapy or exchange transfusion is considered.

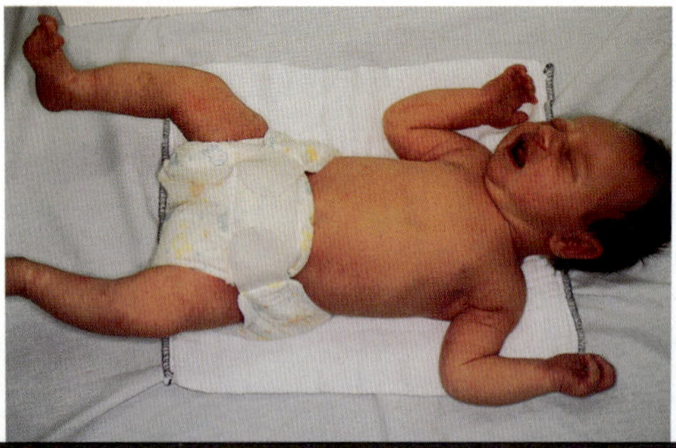

Figure 14.2 Neonatal Jaundice

Newborn with yellowish hue to skin consistent with jaundice. (Courtesy of Kevin J. Knoop, MD, MS.)

Associated Clinical Features

Neonatal mastitis is most common in full-term females, particularly in their second or third week of life. Clinically it manifests as swelling, induration, and tenderness of the affected breast with or without erythema or warmth (Fig. 14.3). In some cases purulent discharge may be obtained from the nipple. Bacteremia and fever are rare. This infection is usually caused by *Staphylococcus aureus,* coliform bacteria, or group B streptococcus. If treatment is delayed, it may progress rapidly with involvement of subcutaneous tissues and subsequent toxicity and systemic findings.

Differential Diagnosis

In the initial stages, neonatal mastitis may mimic mammary tissue hypertrophy owing to maternal passive hormonal stimulation. Minor trauma, cutaneous infections, and duct blockage may precede this infection.

ED Treatment and Disposition

Institution of treatment is important to avoid cellulitic spread and breast tissue damage. In cases of mild cellulitis and no fluctuation, nipple discharge culture and antibiotic coverage (semisynthetic penicillin or first-generation cephalosporins) completes the treatment. Adjustment of coverage may be done once results of cultures or Gram's stain are available, especially in the presence of gram-negative bacilli. If no organism is seen initially, semisynthetic penicillin and an aminoglycoside or cefotaxime should be used. In cases of toxicity or subcutaneous spreading, a complete sepsis work-up should be performed, and hospitalization is usually indicated. In cases of palpable fluctuation, prompt surgical incision and drainage should be performed by a surgeon to avoid further damage of the mammary tissue. Recovery is usually in 5 to 7 days.

Clinical Pearl

1. Consider mastitis in the neonate with edema, induration, and tenderness of the breast tissue. Erythema and fluctuation to palpation ensue if treatment is delayed.

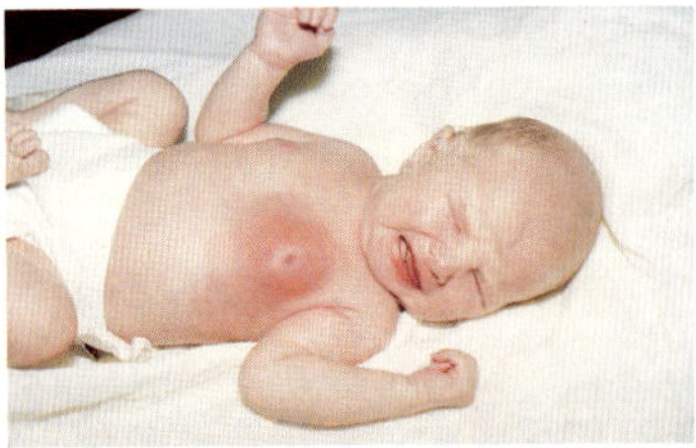

Figure 14.3 Neonatal Mastitis

Neonate with left-sided breast swelling, erythema, and purulent discharge. (Courtesy of Raymond C. Baker, MD.)

Associated Clinical Features

Erythema infectiosum is a viral infection caused by parvovirus B19. It is characterized by an eruption that presents initially as an erythematous malar blush followed by an erythematous maculopapular eruption on the extensor surfaces of extremities, that evolves into a reticulated, lacy, mottled appearance (Fig. 14.4). It may present with low-grade fever, malaise, general aches, arthritis, or arthralgias.

Differential Diagnosis

Morbilliform eruptions may be caused by viruses such as measles, rubella, roseola, and infectious mononucleosis. Bacterial infections (i.e., scarlet fever), drug reactions, and other skin conditions such as guttate psoriasis, papular urticaria, and erythema multiforme are included in the differential.

ED Treatment and Disposition

There is no specific treatment. Once the rash appears, the patient is no longer contagious. It is important to educate the patient and family about the possible risk of B19 virus as a cause of hydrops fetalis or fetal deaths early in pregnancy and the issue of an aplastic crisis in patients with hematologic problems such as sickle cell disease, hereditary spherocytosis, other hemolytic anemias, or immunosuppressed host.

Clinical Pearl

1. Classically this infection begins with the intense redness of both cheeks ("slapped-cheek appearance"). Although the eruption tends to disappear within 5 days of the initial presentation, recrudescences may occur with exercise, overheating, and sunburns as a result of cutaneous vasodilatation.

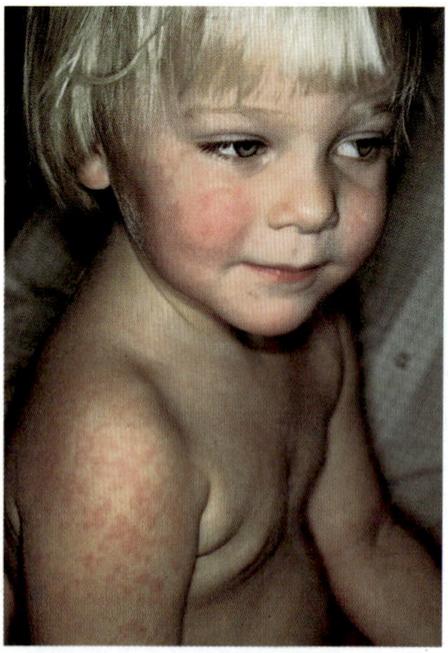

Figure 14.4
Fifth Disease

Toddler with the classic slapped-cheek appearance of fifth disease caused by parvovirus B19. Also note the lacy reticular macular rash on the shoulder and upper extremity. (Courtesy of Anne W. Lucky, MD.)

Associated Clinical Features

The typical presentation of roseola infantum is that of a child with a 2- or 3-day history of fever and irritability. This is followed by rapid defervescence and the appearance of an erythematous morbilliform eruption (Fig. 14.5). It has been associated with various viral agents such as parvovirus, echovirus, and other enteroviruses. Most recently it has been associated with herpesvirus 6.

Differential Diagnosis

Morbilliform eruptions may be caused by common viruses such as measles, rubella, parvovirus B19, or infectious mononucleosis. Bacterial infections (e.g., scarlet fever), drug reactions, and other skin conditions such as guttate psoriasis, papular urticaria, and erythema multiforme may be included in the differential.

ED Treatment and Disposition

Like most viral infections, only supportive therapy is necessary. Special attention should be paid to maintaining fluid intake, fever control for patient's comfort, and parental education about the benign self-limiting characteristics of this illness.

Clinical Pearls

1. The presence of mild eyelid edema with posterior cervical adenopathy in the febrile child without a source may be early indicators for the diagnosis of roseola. Once the fever ends and the rash appears, the diagnosis is clinically confirmed.
2. Rashes *during* the febrile course of an illness are not roseola.

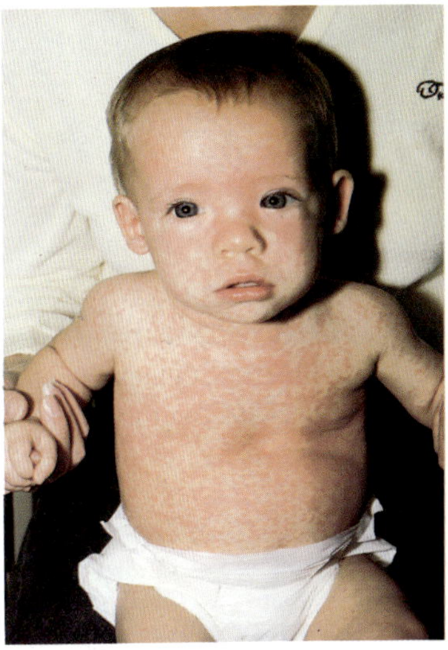

Figure 14.5 Roseola Infantum (Exanthem Subitum)

Toddler with maculopapular eruption of roseola. (Courtesy of Raymond C. Baker, MD.)

Associated Clinical Features

Impetigo is a bacterial infection of the skin produced by *Streptococcus pyogenes* and *Staphylococcus aureus.* It begins as small vesicles or pustules with a very thin roof that rupture easily with the release of a cloudy fluid and the subsequent formation of a honey-colored crust (Figs. 14.6 and 14.7). Often the lesions spread rapidly and coalesce to form larger ones.

Differential Diagnosis

Second-degree burns, cutaneous diphtheria, herpes simplex infections, nummular dermatitis, and kerion may present with crusts and be confused with impetigo.

ED Treatment and Disposition

Since these lesions are contagious, good hand washing and personal hygiene should be discussed with the patient and family. Antibiotic coverage should be directed against the organisms mentioned above. Effective oral agents include erythromycin, first-generation cephalosporins, cloxacillin, or amoxicillin with clavulanic acid. Topical agents such as mupirocin ointment have been proved to be as effective as oral antibiotics.

Clinical Pearls

1. A red, weeping surface and the presence of moist, thin vesicles with honey-colored crusts makes the diagnosis of impetigo.
2. Inflicted cigarette burns may resemble the lesions of impetigo.

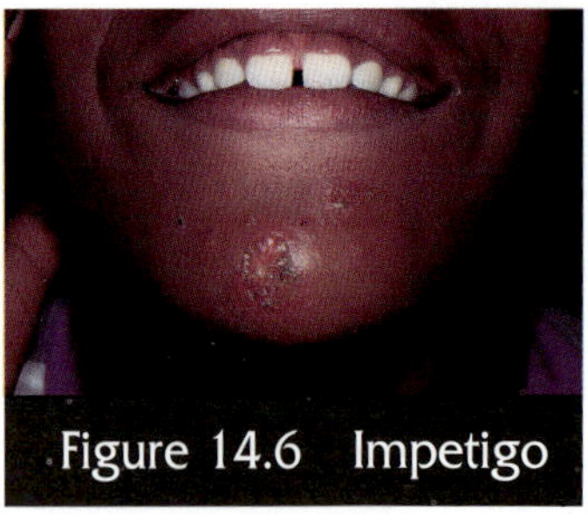

Figure 14.6 Impetigo

Young girl with crusting impetiginous lesions on her chin. (Courtesy of Michael J. Nowicki, MD.)

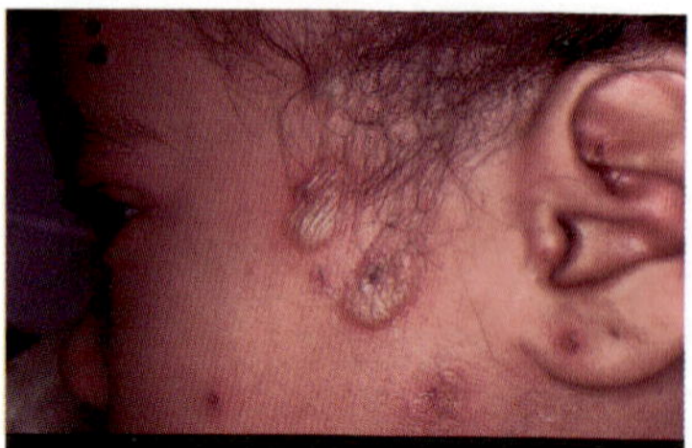

Figure 14.7 Bullous Impetigo

A child with impetiginous lesions on the face. Note the formation of bullae. (Courtesy of Anne W. Lucky, MD.)

Associated Clinical Features

A kerion consists of inflammatory boggy nodules with pustules caused by an exaggerated host delayed hypersensitivity response to infections with either *Microsporum canis* or *Trichophyton tonsurans*. These lesions usually remain localized to one area (Fig. 14.8). It appears 2 to 8 weeks after the initial fungal infection and resolves over 4 to 6 weeks. If untreated, scarring and hair loss may occur.

Differential Diagnosis

Bacterial pyoderma is commonly mistaken for kerion but yields a purulent discharge when aspirated. The diagnosis should be made on clinical appearance.

ED Treatment and Disposition

Topical agents have no role in the treatment of tinea capitis or kerion. Griseofulvin for 4 to 6 weeks is the treatment of choice. Ketoconazole has also been used. Viable spores can be eradicated by adding selenium sulfide shampoo (2.5%) to this therapy. In cases of severe inflammatory reaction, prednisone combined with griseofulvin ensures a rapid resolution of the infection and immunogenic reaction. Incision should be avoided to prevent scar tissue.

Clinical Pearl

1. If a kerion happens to be aspirated or incised, only serosanguineous fluid is obtained.

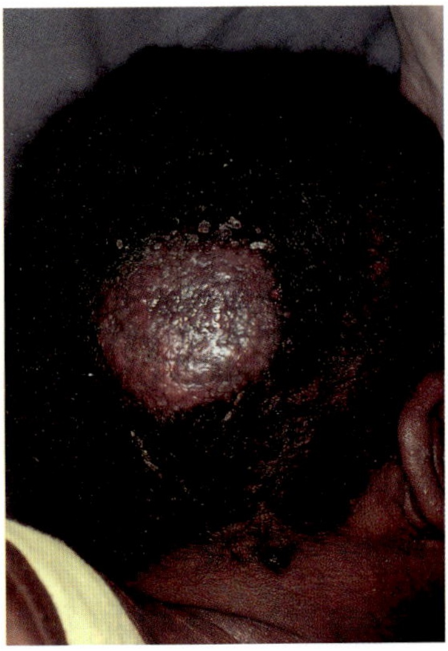

Figure 14.8 Kerion

Occipital boggy swelling with hair loss consistent with kerion. (Courtesy of Anne W. Lucky, MD.)

Associated Clinical Features

Chickenpox results from a primary infection with varicella virus and is characterized by a generalized pruritic vesicular rash (Fig. 14.9), fever, and mild systemic symptoms. The skin lesions have an abrupt onset, develop in crops, and evolve from papules to vesicles (rarely bullae) and finally to crusted lesions within 48 h. The classic lesions are teardrop vesicles surrounded by an erythematous ring (dewdrop on a rose petal) (Fig. 14.10). Secondary bacterial infection of these lesions can occur causing cellulitis, which may be severe. Other complications from varicella include encephalitis, pancreatitis, hepatitis, pneumonia, arthritis, or meningitis. Cerebritis (ataxia) may develop and is usually self-limiting.

Differential Diagnosis

Although several illnesses can present with vesiculobullous lesions, the typical varicella is seldom confused with other problems. Common viral infections that manifest with vesicular rashes include herpes simplex, herpes zoster, coxsackie, influenza, and echovirus infections or vaccinia. On occasions it can be confused with papular urticaria.

ED Treatment and Disposition

Most patients do not develop any complications. Treatment should be symptomatic and directed to pruritus and fever control (avoid salicylates due to association with Reye's syndrome). Oral acyclovir given within 24 h of the onset of the illness may result in a modest decrease in the duration of symptoms and in the number and duration of skin lesions. Acyclovir is not recommended routinely for treatment of uncomplicated varicella in an otherwise healthy child. In the immunocompromised host, VZIG (varicella zoster immunoglobulin) and intravenous acyclovir are effectively used.

Clinical Pearl

1. Skin lesions in varicella present in successive crops so that papules, vesicles, and crusted lesions may be present at any one time. The earliest lesions may begin at the hairline on the nape of the neck.

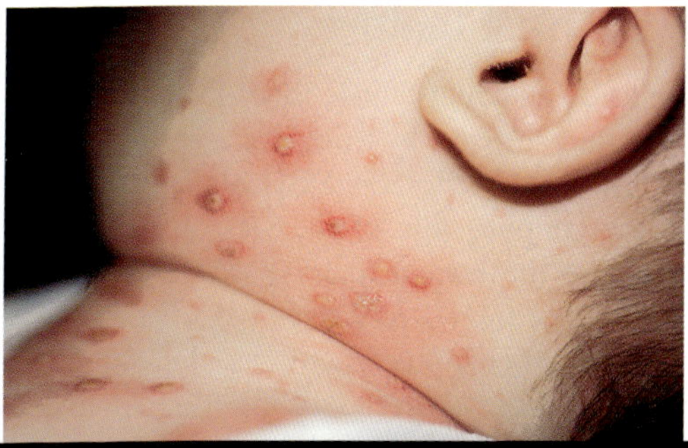

Figure 14.9 Varicella (Chickenpox)

Multiple umbilicated cloudy vesicles of varicella. (Courtesy of Lawrence B. Stack, MD.)

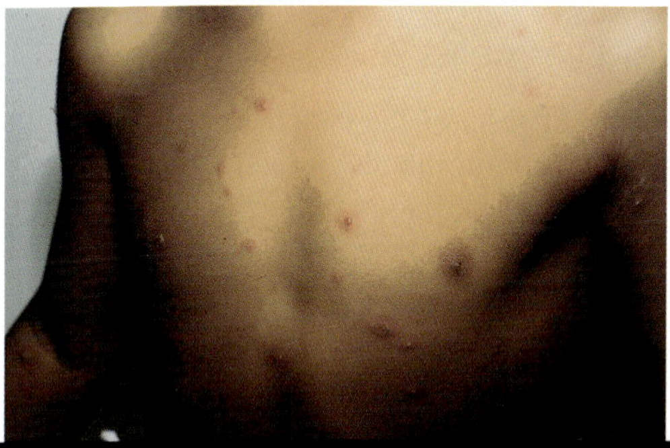

Figure 14.10 Varicella (Chickenpox)

Vesicles in different stages of maturation. Note the clear vesicle on an erythematous base ("dewdrop in a rose petal") in the center of the chest. (Courtesy of Judith C. Bausher, MD.)

Associated Clinical Features

Measles presents as an acute febrile illness with a 3- to 4-day prodromal period characterized by cough, coryza, and conjunctivitis associated with fever (101° to 104°F), chills, and malaise. Koplik's spots, the pathognomonic sign of measles, appear as 1- to 3-mm white elevations on the buccal mucosa (Fig. 14.11, see also Fig. 6.23). They usually present 1 to 2 days before the development of the characteristic erythematous maculopapular rash. This rash appears during the third or fourth day of the illness. It usually begins around the hairline, behind the earlobes, and spreads downward (Fig. 14.12). It tends to fade in the same order it appears. Most cases recover without complications; others may develop otitis media, croup, pneumonia, encephalitis, and rarely subacute sclerosing panencephalitis (SSPE), a very late complication.

Differential Diagnosis

The differential diagnosis of the characteristic rash is vast and includes exanthem subitum; rubella; infections caused by echovirus, coxsackie and adenoviruses; toxoplasmosis; infectious mononucleosis; scarlet fever; Kawasaki disease; drug reactions; Rocky Mountain spotted fever, or meningococcemia.

ED Treatment and Disposition

Supportive therapy includes bedrest, antipyretics, and adequate fluid balance. Complications should be treated according to the presentation. Current available antiviral compounds are not effective. The use of gamma globulins and steroids in SSPE is limited. Passive immunization is effective for prevention and attenuation of measles if given within 5 days of the initial exposure. During outbreaks, measles vaccine (MMR) is given earlier than 15 months and may need to be repeated. A second dose is recommended after the primary series for those born after 1956. This is given at age 11 or 12 years or by entry to junior high school.

Clinical Pearls

1. The classic presentation includes a prodromal phase (fever, hacking cough, coryza, and conjunctivitis), Koplik's spots followed by an abrupt temperature rise, and the rash that spreads in a caudal distribution.
2. Examination of the oral mucosa to identify Koplik's spots may diagnose measles early if performed in all children with an acute febrile illness.

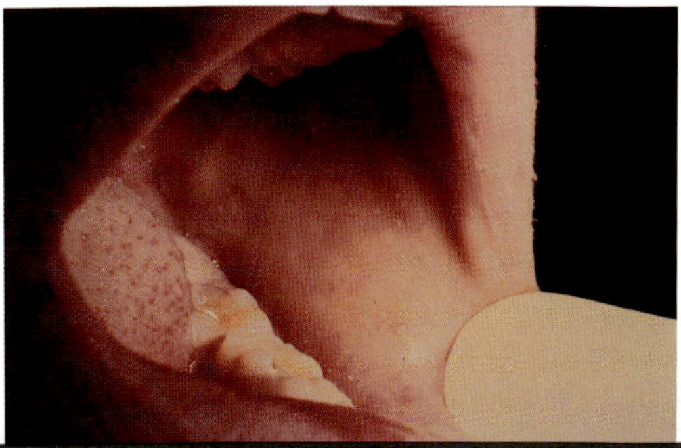

Figure 14.11 Koplik's Spots

Tiny white dots (Koplik's spots) are seen on the buccal mucosa. (Courtesy of Lawrence B. Stack, MD.)

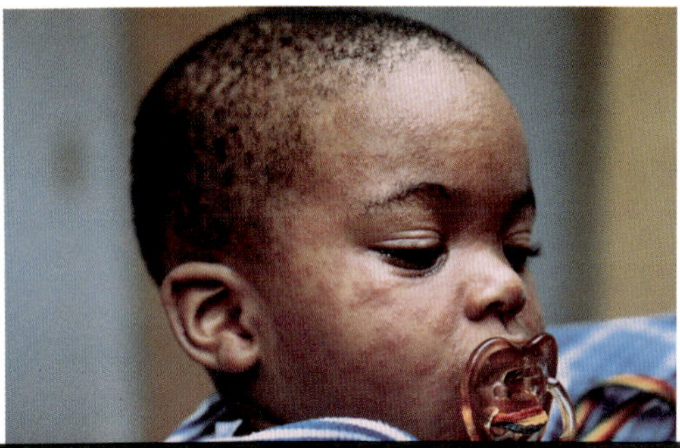

Figure 14.12 Measles

School-age child with morbilliform rash on face consistent with measles. (Courtesy of Javier A. Gonzalez del Rey, MD.)

Associated Clinical Features

Hand, foot, and mouth disease is a seasonal (summer-fall) viral infection caused by coxsackievirus A16. It is characterized by fever, malaise, and anorexia over 1 to 2 days, followed by oral lesions (small, red macules that evolve into small vesicles 1 to 3 mm in diameter) in the posterior oropharynx (Fig. 14.13). This enanthem is then followed by a superficial, nonloculated vesicular eruption on the hands and feet (3 to 7 mm) (Figs. 14.14 and 14.15). These may also be present on the buttocks, face, and legs.

Differential Diagnosis

Herpes simplex, varicella, varicella zoster, influenza, echovirus infections, vaccinia, and other coxsackieviruses should all be considered.

ED Treatment and Disposition

Supportive therapy, especially fluid maintenance and fever control for the patient's comfort are the mainstays of treatment. The duration and characteristics of the illness should be discussed with the parents. In the majority of cases the course is self-limited and the prognosis excellent. On rare occasions, secondary complications such as myocarditis, pneumonia, and meningoencephalitis may occur.

Clinical Pearl

1. The individual lesions are usually seen on the palms, fingertips, and soles. Oral cavity lesions appear as discrete oval erosions and most are classically seen in the posterior oropharynx and soft palate.

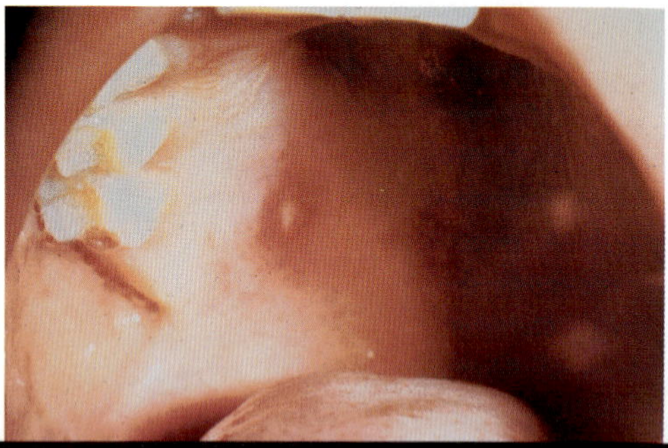

Figure 14.13 Hand, Foot, and Mouth Disease

Discrete vesicular erosions on the posterior oropharynx and soft palate secondary to coxsackievirus. (Courtesy of James F. Steiner, DDS.)

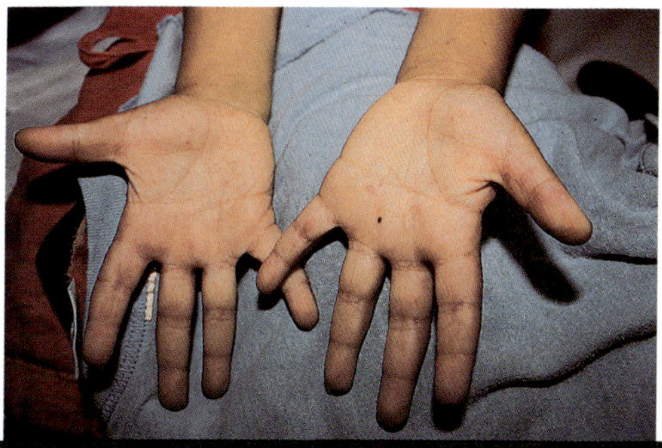

Figure 14.14 Hand, Foot, and Mouth Disease

Erythematous vesicular rash scattered on the palms consistent with coxsackievirus. (Courtesy of Michael J. Nowicki, MD.)

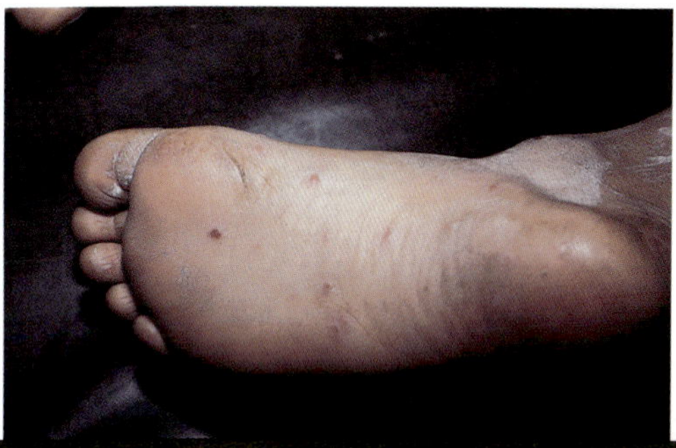

Figure 14.15 Hand, Foot, and Mouth Disease

Vesicular rash of the feet consistent with coxsackievirus. (Courtesy of Raymond C. Baker, MD.)

Associated Clinical Features

Herpetic gingivostomatitis is a viral infection commonly seen in infants and children caused by herpes simplex. Patients usually present with fever, malaise, cervical adenopathy, and pain in the mouth and throat on attempting to swallow. Vesicular and ulcerative lesions appear throughout the oral cavity. The gingiva becomes very friable and inflamed, especially around the alveolar rim. Increased salivation with foul breath may be present. Although fever disappears in 3 to 5 days, children may have difficulty eating for 7 to 14 days. Sometimes, autoinoculation produces vesicular lesions on the fingers (herpetic whitlow) (Fig. 14.16).

Differential Diagnosis

Vincent's angina, aphthous stomatitis, erythema multiforme, Behçet's disease, and other viral infections such as herpangina and hand, foot, and mouth disease (coxsackieviruses) should be considered.

ED Treatment and Disposition

No specific treatment is available. In immunocompromised patients, acyclovir should be considered. In the normal host, fluid balance should be maintained throughout the illness. Because of ulcerative lesions, avoidance of citrus juices or spicy food prevents pain on swallowing. Clear fluids, ice pops, and ice cream may be used in small children. Not infrequently, admission for IV hydration is necessary. Adequate fever control is also necessary for patient comfort and to avoid an increase in fluid losses. Pain control may be achieved by using mixtures of antihistamine (diphenhydramine elixir) and antacids (1:1) applied to lesion with Q-tips. In small children local application of viscous lidocaine (Xylocaine) should be avoided since patients may develop toxic plasma levels due to an altered absorption from an inflamed oral mucosa.

Clinical Pearl

1. Most of these lesions are in the anterior two-thirds of the oral cavity. Posterior lesions sparing the gingiva are most commonly seen in coxsackie infections.

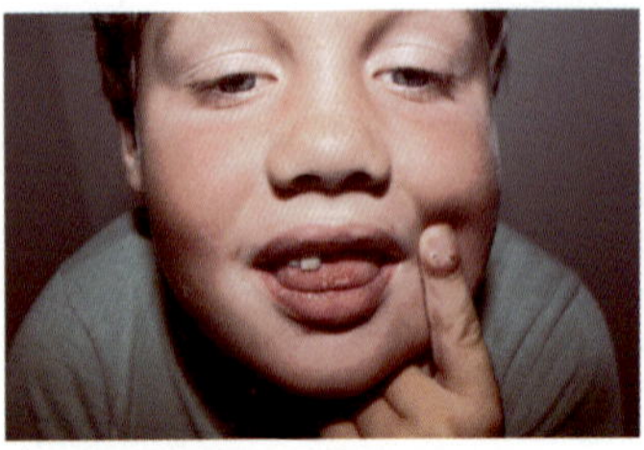

Figure 14.16 Herpetic Gingivostomatitis

Multiple oral vesicular lesions consistent with herpes gingivostomatitis. Vesicular lesions from autoinoculation are present on the finger (herpetic whitlow). (Courtesy of Michael J. Nowicki, MD.)

Associated Clinical Features

Urticaria is a localized, edematous skin reaction from histamine release that usually follows an infection, insect sting or bite, ingestion of certain foods, or medications. It is characterized by a sudden onset of pruritic, transient well circumscribed wheals scattered over the body. These are flat-topped and may vary from pinpoint size to several centimeters in diameter. They usually have a central clearing, peripheral extension, and can have tense edema (Fig. 14.17). Most urticarial reactions last 24 to 48 h; on rare occasions, they may take weeks to resolve. Rarely, there may be systemic reactions such as wheezing, stridor, or angioedema.

Differential Diagnosis

Erythema multiforme, arthropod bites, dermatographism, contact dermatitis, reactive erythemas, allergic vasculitis, juvenile rheumatoid arthritis, mastocytosis, and pityriasis rosea can all present with a similar-appearing rash.

ED Treatment and Disposition

Treatment is symptomatic. Oral antihistamines are useful in the control of pruritus. If a systemic reaction is also part of the initial presentation, epinephrine and steroids should be added to the therapy. In most cases it is very difficult to identify the etiologic factor. Unless there is evidence of acute angioedema, most cases can be discharged home on oral antihistamines.

Clinical Pearl

1. Erythema multiforme can be commonly mistaken for polycyclic urticaria (multiple red wheals of different sizes). Clinically these two entities can be differentiated by the duration and color of the lesions. In urticaria, the center is clear and each lesion usually lasts a few hours. In erythema multiforme, the center is dusky and the lesion remains in the same place for several days to weeks.

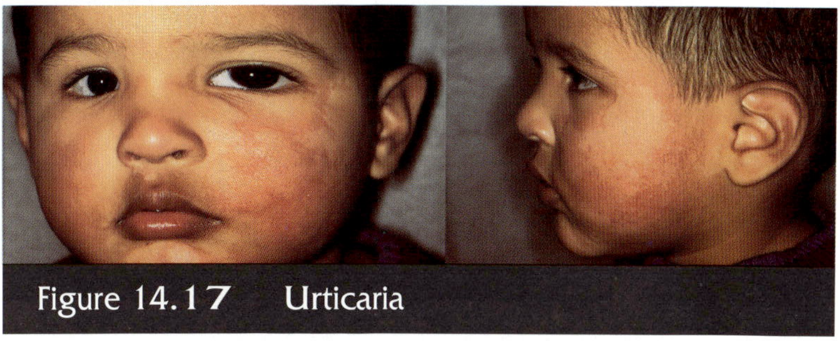

Figure 14.17 Urticaria

Preschool child with annular raised pruritic lesions with central clearing and tense edema of polycyclic urticaria. The lesions had completely disappeared after about 5 min. (Courtesy of Kevin J. Knoop, MD, MS.)

Associated Clinical Features

Scarlet fever manifests as erythematous macules and papules that result from an erythrogenic toxin produced by a group A streptococcus. The most common site for invasion by this organism is the pharynx and occasionally skin or perianal areas. The disease usually occurs in children (2 to 10 years of age) and less commonly in adults. The typical presentation of scarlet fever includes fever, headache, sore throat, and malaise followed by the scarlatiniform rash (Fig. 14.18). The rash is typically erythematous, blanches (in severe cases may include petechiae), and owing to the grouping of the fine papules gives to the skin a rough sandpaperlike texture (Fig. 14.19). On the tongue, a thick, white coat and swollen papillae gives the appearance of a strawberry ("strawberry tongue").

Differential Diagnosis

A similar syndrome is caused by staphylococci producing an exfoliative exotoxin which can be differentiated from the streptococcal infection because of the absence of pharyngitis, strawberry tongue, and negative cultures. Enteroviral infections, viral hepatitis, infectious mononucleosis, toxic shock syndrome, drug eruptions, rubella, mercury intoxication, and mucocutaneous lymph node syndrome should be considered.

ED Treatment and Disposition

Penicillin, either benzathine penicillin G or oral penicillin, to maintain levels for 10 days is the key to therapy. Alternatives include erythromycin, or clindamycin in penicillin-allergic patients.

Clinical Pearls

1. Petechiae (commonly found as part of the scarlatiniform eruption) in a linear pattern seen along the major skin folds in the axillae and antecubital fossa are known as "Pastia's lines."
2. In black skin, the rash may be difficult to differentiate and may consist only of punctate papular elevations called "goose flesh."

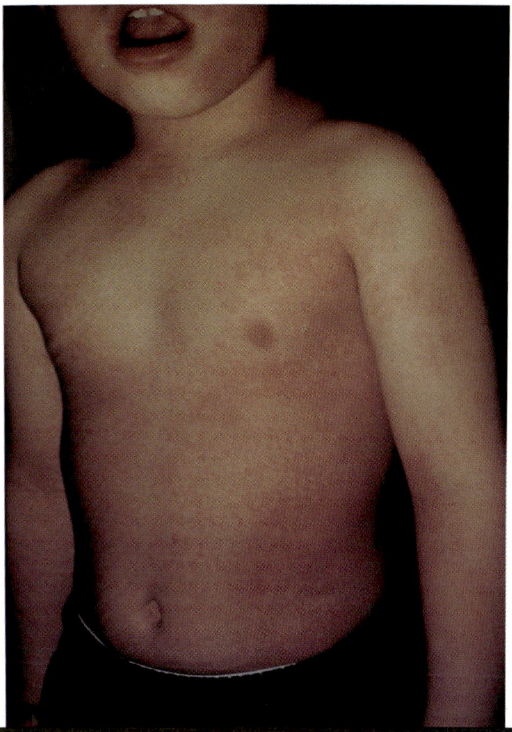

Figure 14.18 Scarlatina

Erythematous scarlatiniform rash of scarlet fever. (Courtesy of Lawrence B. Stack, MD.)

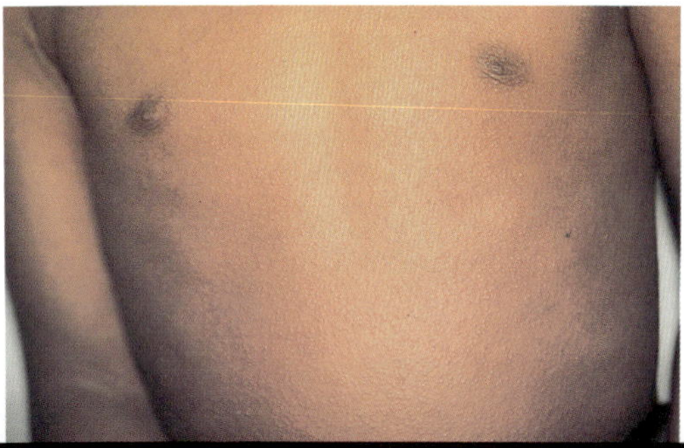

Figure 14.19 Sandpaper Rash

Typical sandpaper rash of scarlet fever. The grouping of the fine papules gives the skin a rough sandpaperlike texture. (Courtesy of Jeffery S. Gibson, MD.)

Associated Clinical Features

Strawberry hemangioma often appears as small telangiectatic papules or a patch surrounded by an area of pallor. These lesions grow and become vascularized during the first 2 months of life. The classic lesion is a raised gray to reddish nodule with defined borders (Fig. 14.20). They commonly regress in almost all patients by 2 to 3 years of age. In a few cases, very large vascular lesions can cause platelet trapping or high-output cardiac failure. Localized hemangiomas can affect the airway, eyes, or other areas on which they occur.

Differential Diagnosis

Malignant vascular tumors, pyogenic granulomas, and giant melanocytic birthmarks should be considered.

ED Treatment and Disposition

Most cases require no therapy because strawberry hemangiomas usually regress without residual lesion. Treatment is indicated when there is an obstruction of a vital orifice (i.e., airway, mouth, or nares) or vision (eyelids), or if hematologic or cardiovascular complications are present. Parental reassurance is important because there is great pressure to treat for cosmetic reasons. Steroids, liquid nitrogen, grenz ray therapy, and pulse dye laser are some of the different therapeutic modalities used in its treatment. In complex cases, dermatologic consultation is recommended.

Clinical Pearl

1. The diagnosis of strawberry hemangioma should always be considered in the presence of any purplish, red, raised, tumorlike lesion not present at birth which appears in the first month of life.

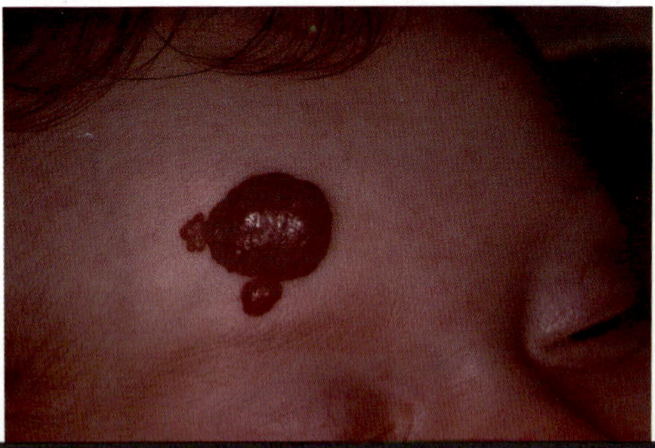

Figure 14.20 Strawberry Hemangioma

Raised umbilicated vascular lesion on the right forehead consistent with strawberry hemangioma. (Courtesy of Anne W. Lucky, MD.)

Associated Clinical Features

Orbital cellulitis is a serious bacterial infection characterized by painful, purple-red swelling of the eyelids, restriction of eye movement (Fig. 14.21), proptosis, and a variable degree of decreased visual acuity. It may begin with eye pain and low-grade temperature. In general it is caused by *Staphylococcus aureus, Haemophilus influenzae, Streptococcus,* or *Pneumococcus.* It usually follows an upper respiratory tract infection or sinusitis but can occur from local trauma. If not treated promptly, it can lead to abscess formation, blindness, or meningitis. Periorbital (preseptal) cellulitis usually presents with edema and erythema of the eyelids (Fig. 14.22), minimal pain of the affected area, and fever. Proptosis or ophthalmoplegia are not characteristic. Common organisms are *H. influenzae* type B or *Pneumococcus.* In cases of eyelid trauma, *S. aureus* and group A streptococcus are the most common pathogens.

Differential Diagnosis

Erysipelas, allergic reactions, trauma, sunburns, frostbite, chemical burns, subperiosteal abscess, and cavernous sinus thrombosis should be considered.

ED Treatment and Disposition

Parenteral antibiotic coverage with broad spectrum antistaphylococcal coverage, ophthalmologic consultation, and admission are indicated in cases of orbital cellulitis. Computerized tomography of the orbit is necessary in certain cases to rule out the possibility of an abscess that may require surgical drainage. In febrile or ill-appearing patients with periorbital cellulitis, admission is indicated with broad spectrum antibiotic therapy. This coverage can be adjusted once results of cultures are available. Mild cases of preseptal cellulitis (especially those with history of trauma, e.g., abrasion, insect sting) can be treated as outpatients with close follow-up. Adequate coverage for *Staphylococcus* and *Streptococcus* is necessary.

Clinical Pearls

1. Periorbital cellulitis presents with circumferential redness, edema, and tenderness in the febrile toddler. Orbital cellulitis must be considered if there is eye pain or globe motion limitation.
2. The conjunctiva is typically clear with periorbital cellulitis.

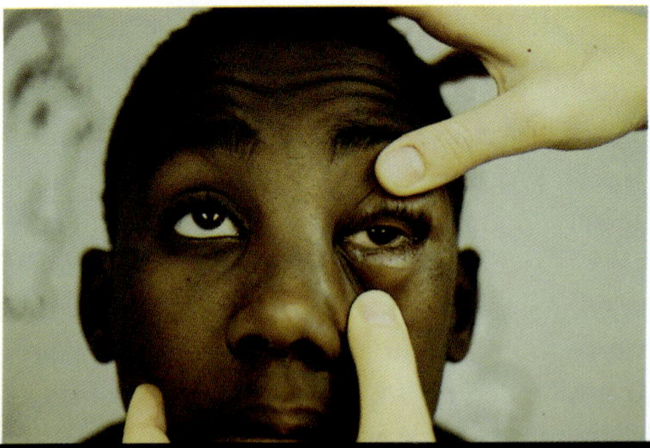

Figure 14.21 Orbital Cellulitis

Left orbital cellulitis with decreased range of motion secondary to edema. Note the infected conjunctiva. (Courtesy of Javier A. Gonzalez del Rey, MD.)

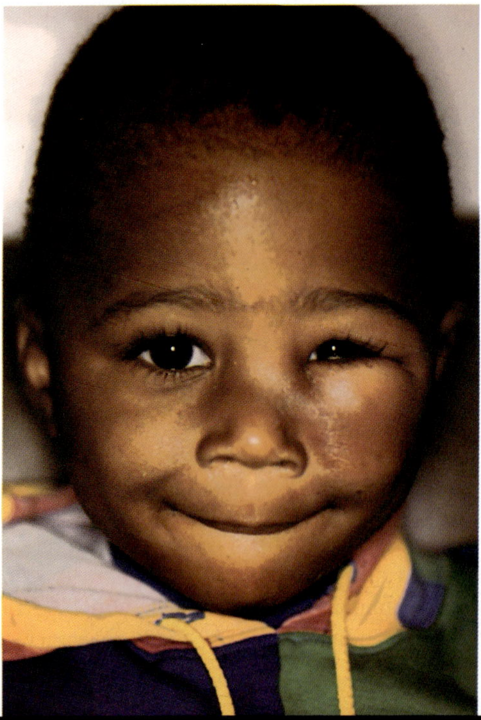

Figure 14.22 Periorbital Cellulitis

Left periorbital cellulitis with edema and erythema of the eyelids. Note that the conjunctiva is clear and not infected. (Courtesy of Kevin J. Knoop, MD, MS.)

Associated Clinical Features

Cat scratch disease is a benign self-limited condition that manifests with regional lymphadenopathy (Fig. 14.23) which usually follows (1 to 2 weeks) a skin papule at the presumed site of bacterial inoculation. A history of contact or scratch from a cat (Fig. 14.24 is usually present. Lymphadenopathy may persist for months, and in rare cases patients may develop complications such as encephalitis, osteolytic lesion, hepatitis, weight loss, fever, and fatigue. A skin test using cat scratch antigen can identify the etiology in suspected patients when confirmation of the diagnosis is needed.

Differential Diagnosis

Lymphogranuloma venereum, bacterial adenitis, sarcoidosis, infectious mononucleosis, tumors (benign or malignant), tuberculosis, tularemia, brucellosis, and histoplasmosis should be considered.

ED Treatment and Disposition

The disease is usually self-limited and management is primarily symptomatic. Parents and patients should be reassured that the nodes are benign and frequently resolve within 2 to 4 months. In cases of painful fluctuant nodes, needle aspiration may be necessary for relief of symptoms. Antibiotic therapy should be considered for acutely or severely ill patients. Several anecdotal reports have suggested that oral antibiotics such as rifampin, trimethoprim-sulfamethoxazole, and ciprofloxacin; or intravenous gentamicin, cefotaxime, and mezlocillin may be effective. Surgical excision of the affected nodes is generally unnecessary.

Clinical Pearl

1. Cat scratch disease is the most common cause of regional adenitis and should be considered in all children or adolescents with persistent lymphadenopathy.

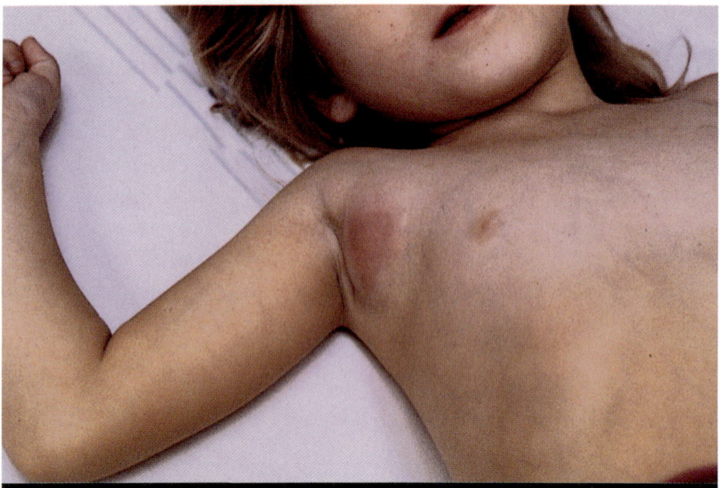

Figure 14.23 Cat Scratch Disease

An erythematous, tender, suppurative node is seen in a young febrile patient with a history of cat scratch on the extremity. The node required drainage 2 days later. (Courtesy of Kevin J. Knoop, MD, MS.)

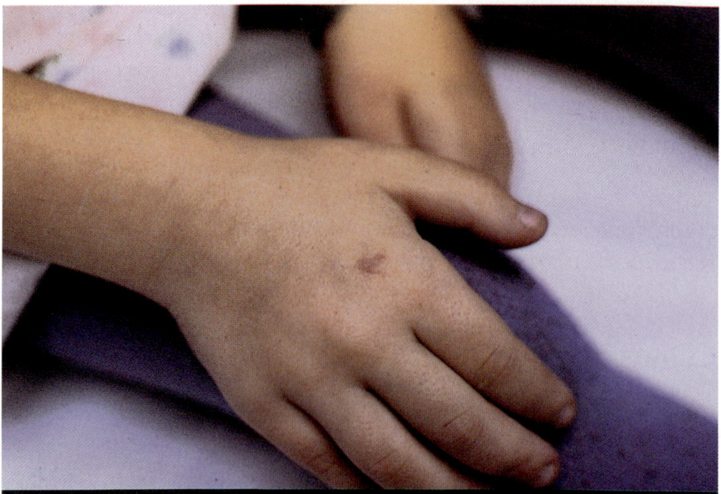

Figure 14.24 Cat Scratch Disease

The precipitating wound which caused the suppurative node in Fig. 14.23. (Courtesy of Kevin J. Knoop, MD, MS.)

Associated Clinical Features

There are several fractures unique to children. These include physeal fractures, torus fracture, green stick fractures, avulsion fractures, and bowing fractures or deformities. Physis fractures (growth plate fractures) are relatively common because of weakness of the germinal growth plate. The Salter-Harris (SH) classification was designed to describe each type of physeal fracture, its prognosis, and treatment (Fig. 14.25).

Differential Diagnosis

SH type I: Fracture that extends through the physis. It is a very difficult radiologic diagnosis since it may not be displaced. It is usually a clinical diagnosis, but occasionally there is a physeal widening observed on the x-ray.

SH type II: Oblique fracture extending through the metaphysis into the physis. It is the most common and the prognosis is good.

SH type III: This rare type of fracture goes along the growth plate, then extends through the epiphysis, ossification center, and articular cartilage into the joint.

SH type IV: Fracture that extends from the metaphysis, across the growth plate, and into the joint.

SH type V: Crushing injury to the growth plate.

ED Treatment and Disposition

Immobilization by splinting is the treatment of choice in types I and II (minimum of 3 weeks). In these cases, reduction is easy to achieve and maintain. Growth is unimpaired. Types III and IV may require open reduction to avoid later traumatic arthritis and in some cases growth arrest. Type V fractures are rare and require very close follow-up because of arrest of growth caused by the death of the germinal cells. Types III, IV, and V require immediate orthopedic consultation.

Clinical Pearl

1. After initial assessment and evaluation, always suspect SH type I if there is evidence of tenderness around the growth plate area despite negative x-rays.

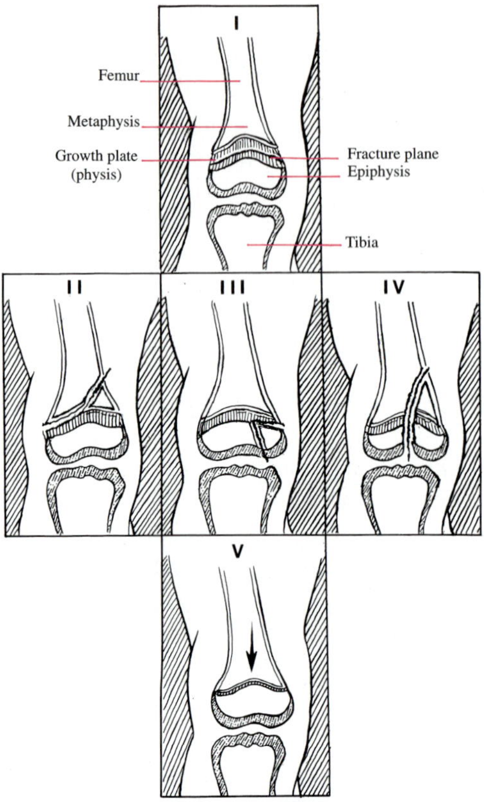

Figure 14.25 Salter-Harris Fracture Classification

Salter-Harris classification for epiphyseal plate fractures.

Associated Clinical Features

A single strand of hair or thread may encircle a finger, a toe, or the penis, leading to constriction (Fig. 14.26). Children in their first year of life are particularly at risk from inadvertent attachment of a parent's hair or loose thread. The digit appears edematous, erythematous, and painful. If not corrected vascular compromise or infection can ensue.

Differential Diagnosis

Insect bites, trauma, or cellulitis of the digit may have a similar appearance.

ED Treatment and Disposition

Visualization of the constricting material may be difficult. Edema, erythema, and periarticular skin folds may hide the hair or thread. It is imperative to carefully retract the skin around the proximal aspect of the edema. A magnifying lens may be helpful in identifying the band. Since the removal can be painful, consider local digital block prior to removal. Using a small hemostat, grasp a portion of the material and then cut it with a surgical blade. On occasions, depilatory agents have been used to remove hair fibers. Elevation of the involved digit after removal of the constricting agent provides resolution of the edema and erythema within 2 to 3 days. In some cases the digital blood supply may have been irreversibly compromised. Subspecialty consultation should be considered whenever neurovascular integrity is in question.

Clinical Pearl

1. In the vast majority of cases, a clear line of demarcation can usually be identified between the normal tissue and the affected area.

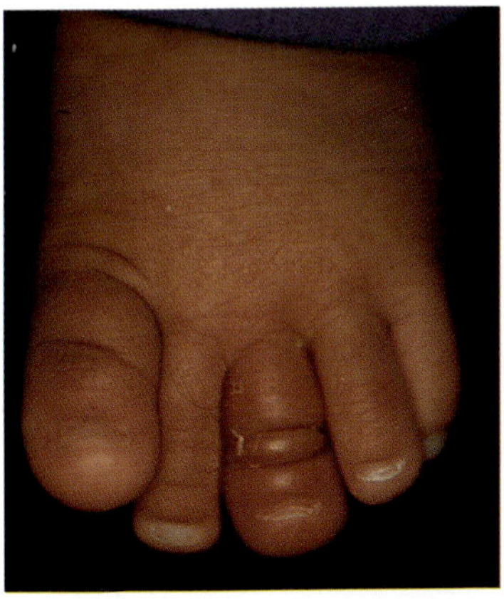

Figure 14.26
Hair Tourniquet

A strand of hair has encircled the middle toe in two places, causing erythema and swelling. (Courtesy of Kevin J. Knoop, MD, MS.)

Associated Clinical Features

Nursemaid's elbow is a condition that occurs commonly in children younger than 5 years of age whom are usually picked up or pulled by the arms while the arm is pronated. The children present unwilling to supinate or pronate the affected elbow (Fig. 14.27). Generally they keep the arm in a passive pronation and develop pain over the head of the radius. Radiographic studies should be considered only in patients with an unusual mechanism of injury or those who do not become rapidly asymptomatic after the reduction maneuvers.

Differential Diagnosis

Radial head fracture or complete dislocation, posterior elbow dislocation, condylar and supracondylar fractures of the distal humerus, or buckle fracture of radius or ulna should be considered.

ED Treatment and Disposition

Carefully palpate for tenderness at all points of the affected arm. (There is no tenderness found when not rotating the involved arm.) Orthopedic consultation is generally not indicated unless an underlying fracture is diagnosed. Reduction is usually achieved by supination of the forearm while applying pressure over the head of the radial head and flexing the elbow. Usually a palpable click can be felt over the area. The patient usually becomes asymptomatic after a few minutes (Fig. 14.28). When the injury has been present for several hours, reduction may be difficult and it may take several hours to recover full function of the elbow.

Clinical Pearls

1. In any child (usually between ages 1 to 5 years) who presents with sudden onset of elbow pain and immobility following a traction injury, the diagnosis of nursemaid's elbow should be strongly considered.
2. Nonjudgmental parental education about the mechanism should be an integral part of the visit.

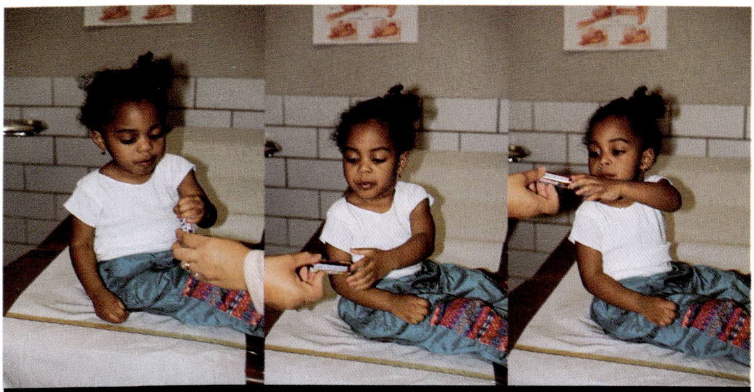

Figure 14.27 Nursemaid's Elbow

This child presents with pseudoparalysis of the right arm after a pulling injury. Note how she avoids use of the affected arm and preferentially uses the other arm. (Courtesy of Kevin J. Knoop, MD, MS.)

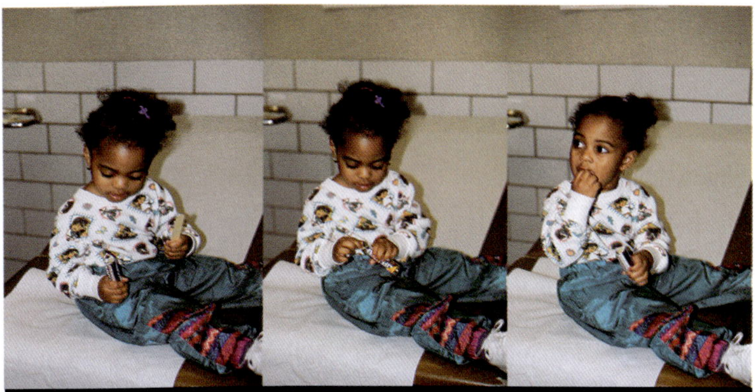

Figure 14.28 Nursemaid's Elbow—Reduced

After reduction, there is initial reluctance to use the injured arm. With distraction and encouragement, the patient demonstrates successful use of the extremity. (Courtesy of Kevin J. Knoop, MD, MS.)

Associated Clinical Features

Enterobius vermicularis is a 0.5-inch threadlike, white worm that infects the colon and causes intense pruritus of the perianal region where the adult gravid female migrates to deposit eggs (Fig. 14.29). In rare occasions it can cause vulvovaginitis. The diagnosis can be made by direct visualization of the nematode by the parents or by using a transparent adhesive tape touched to the perianal lesion (at night). This tape is then applied to a glass slide for microscopic examination under low power.

Differential Diagnosis

Perianal irritation, fissures, hemorrhoids, and contact dermatitis should be considered.

ED Treatment and Disposition

The treatment of choice is pyrantel pamoate or mebendazole. Either of these drugs is given as a single dose and repeated in 1 to 2 weeks (to treat secondary hatchings of the organism). Because of the high frequency of reinfections, families should be treated as a group.

Clinical Pearls

1. Reinfection from other infected individuals or autoinfection is necessary to maintain enterobiasis in the individual since these nematodes usually die after depositing the eggs in the perianal region. Good personal hygiene may reduce chances of infection.
2. If there is evidence of cellulitis, antibiotic coverage primarily against *Staphylococcus* is indicated.
3. If infection and point tenderness (in the absence of cellulitis) persist, antipseudomonal coverage should be considered.
4. Pinworms are the most common cause of pruritus in children.

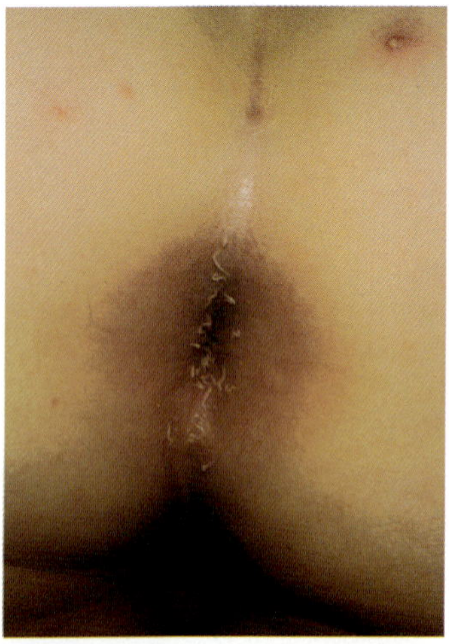

Figure 14.29
Pinworms

Multiple tiny pearly-white worms are seen at the anus. (Courtesy of Timothy D. McGuirk, DO.)

CHAPTER 15

CHILD ABUSE

Robert A. Shapiro
Charles J. Schubert

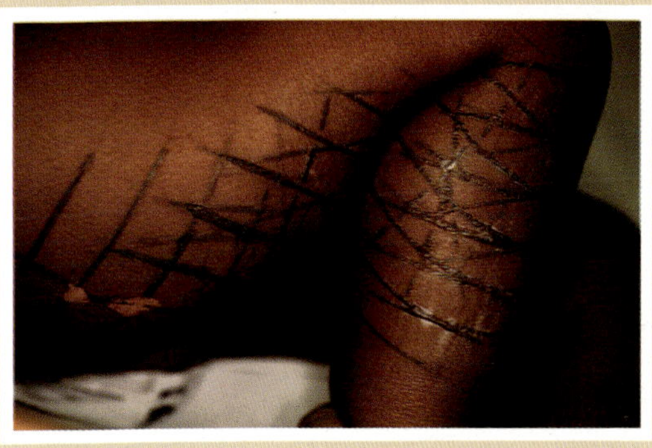

Associated Clinical Features

Burns in children are frequently the result of child abuse. The most common types of pediatric burns from abuse are immersion burns and contact burns. Certain clues may assist the physician in differentiating accidental burns from inflicted burns, but often considerable doubt remains even after a careful evaluation.

In an *immersion burn,* a thoughtful assessment of the pattern and location of the burns, as well as of the unaffected areas, helps to differentiate between accidental and inflicted burns. Postulate possible mechanisms for the injury, and correlate the assessment with the given history. A child who is held firmly and deliberately immersed has burn margins that are sharp and distinct. If the child has little opportunity to struggle, few, or no, burns from splashing liquid will occur. In contrast, a child who accidentally comes into contact with a hot liquid will move about in an attempt to escape further injury. This movement causes the burn margins to be less distinct and may result in additional small burns as hot liquid splashes onto the skin. Children who are "dipped" into a bath of hot water often show sparing of their feet and/or buttocks because they are held firmly against the tub's bottom (Fig. 15.1). A child who has a hand dipped and held into hot water may reflexively close the fingers, sparing the palm and fingertips.

Contact burns usually create a burn with a distinct and recognizable shape. Contact burn patterns most commonly associated with abuse include burns from curling irons, hair dryers, heater elements, and cigarettes (Figs. 15.2, 15.3, 15.4, and 15.5). A child who has multiple contact burns or who has burns to areas that are unlikely to come in contact with the hot object accidentally should be evaluated for abuse.

Differential Diagnosis

Some burn look-alikes may be confused with child abuse. Impetigo (Fig. 15.6) may be mistaken for healing cigarette burns, and bullous impetigo can resemble second-degree burns. Contact dermatitis and cellulitis may resemble first-degree burns.

ED Treatment and Disposition

Document thoroughly all burns that may be due to abuse. Draw sketches and take photographs of the injuries. Obtain a skeletal survey in children under the age of 2 years. Report any suspected abuse immediately to the local child protective agency before discharge from the ED. Provide standard burn therapy.

Clinical Pearls

1. Evaluate the alleged history carefully and obtain sufficient details before making any judgment. Assess whether the explanation and history that are given of the alleged episode are inconsistent with the injuries and/or with the child's developmental abilities. Suspect abuse if, without convincing explanation, the historian alters the initial history.
2. Maintain a high index of suspicion whenever caring for a pediatric burn patient. Look carefully for other signs of abuse, such as bruising, fractures, or signs of neglect.
3. Accidental burns from a cigarette are usually single, superficial, and not completely round. Common sites of accidental cigarette burns are the face, trunk, and hands.
4. Report suspicions to the mandated child protection agency whenever a burn may have been deliberately inflicted.
5. Injuries due to suspected child abuse may be photographed without parental consent in most states.

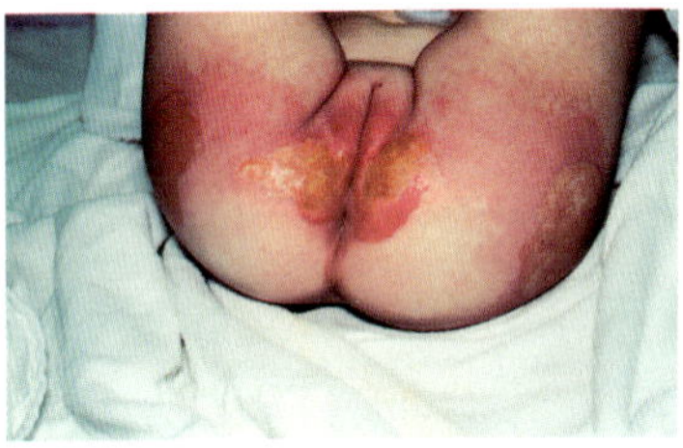

Figure 15.1 Immersion Burns

Immersion burns are often associated with toilet training accidents. This girl was plunged into hot water after soiling herself. She shows sparing of the buttocks, which contacted the surface of the bathtub and avoided being burned. (Courtesy of *The Visual Diagnosis of Child Physical Abuse,* American Academy of Pediatrics, 1994.)

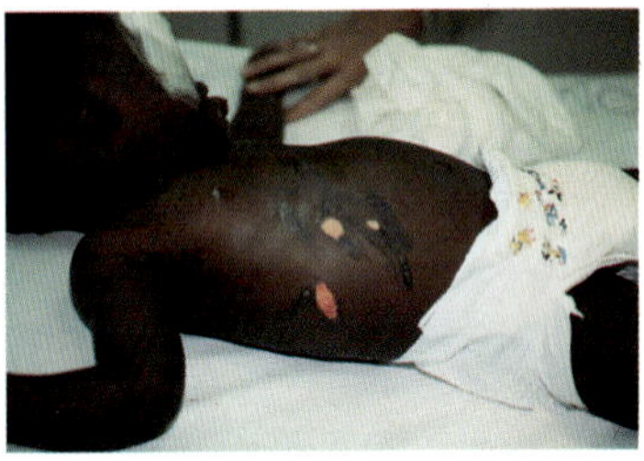

Figure 15.2 Contact Burn (Curling Iron)

Burns on the chest and abdomen from a curling iron. The burn pattern on the injured skin indicates multiple contact burns from an object the size and shape of a curling iron. Accidental curling iron burns occur, but because this infant has so many burns, the injury is suspicious for abuse. Child abuse should be suspected and reported unless the historian can provide a plausible explanation of how these burns occurred accidentally. (Courtesy of Robert A. Shapiro, MD.)

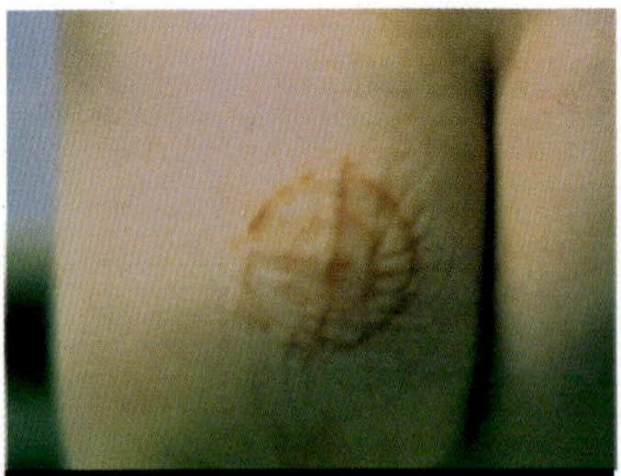

Figure 15.3 Contact Burn (Hair Dryer)

The heated grid from the end of a hair dryer caused this child's burns. The burn size and pattern marks of the burn matched exactly the hair dryer grid that was found in the child's home. The history of accidental injury was thought to be unlikely, and child abuse was suspected. (Courtesy of Robert A. Shapiro, MD.)

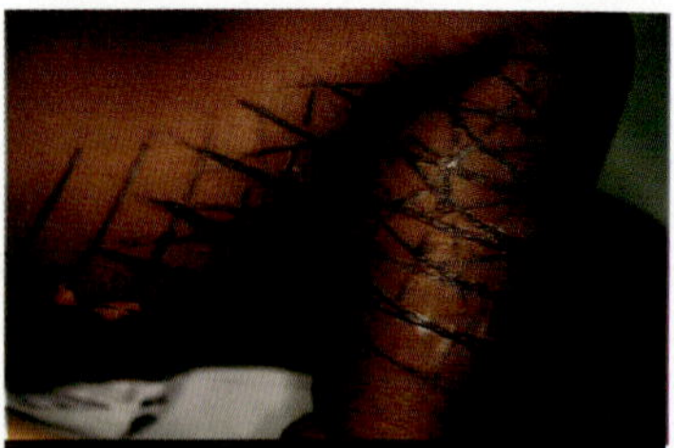

Figure 15.4 Contact Burn (Heater Grate)

This child was held against a heater grate. The pattern became more obvious with the child's knee flexed—the position of the leg at the time of the injury. (Courtesy of David W. Munter, MD.)

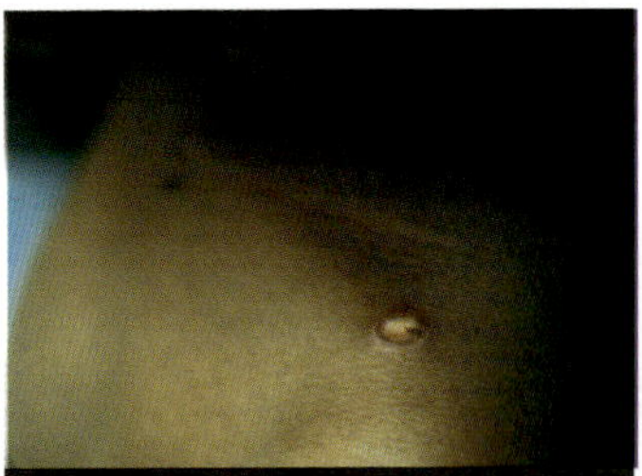

Figure 15.5 Contact Burn (Cigarette)

Cigarette burns are circular injuries with a diameter of about 8 mm. It can be difficult for the clinician to determine if the burn is from an accidental injury or from abuse. Children who accidentally run into a lit cigarette often have burns to the face or distal extremities. Accidental burns may be less distinct and deep compared with inflicted burns. A report of alleged child abuse should be made if there are multiple cigarette burns, burns to locations unlikely to come into contact with a cigarette accidentally, or other signs that suggest abuse. (Courtesy of Robert A. Shapiro, MD.)

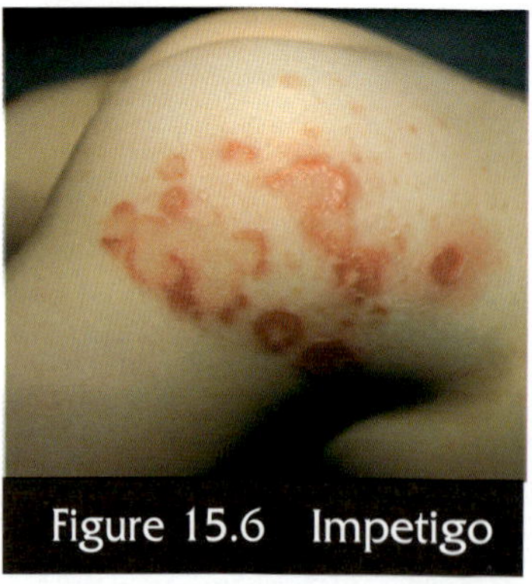

Figure 15.6 Impetigo

These circular lesions of impetigo resemble healing cigarette burns. (Courtesy of Michael J. Nowicki, MD.)

Associated Clinical Features

Bruises are the most common manifestation of physical child abuse. Child abuse should be suspected whenever bruises are: (1) over soft body areas, such as the thighs, buttocks, cheeks, abdomen, and genitalia, since common childhood activities do not commonly cause trauma to these areas; (2) more numerous than usual; (3) of different ages (suggests repeated episodes of abuse); (4) the shape of objects such as belts, cords, or hand prints (demonstrates that the injuries were inflicted) (Figs. 15.7, 15.8); or (5) noted in young, nonambulating children (infants are not capable of getting into accidents).

The color of the ecchymosis will change as healing progresses. New injuries are usually red and purple. They may also be tender and swollen. Within a few days, the bruise may turn blue, then green, then yellow, and finally brown. The shape and margins of the bruise become less distinct as it heals. The time period in which these color changes occur is variable. Some bruises resolve within a few days, whereas others resolve over weeks. The amount of time until resolution depends on factors such as the location, size, and depth of the injury.

Bite marks (Figs. 15.9, 15.10) have special forensic characteristics that should be recorded. The size, shape, and pattern of the injury can identify a specific perpetrator. Most human bite injuries are caused by children, not adults, but recognition of an adult bite is important because the injury represents abuse. Compared with an adult's, the shape of a child's bite is rounder. If the impressions from the canines are visible in the bite, the perpetrator's age can be estimated. Most children under 8 years of age have less than 3 cm between their canines. Some bites have saliva within the center of the bite, which also can be used to identify the perpetrator. Although some bite marks are immediately obvious during the initial inspection, others can be difficult to recognize. If an adult bite is suspected but unprovable because distinct impressions of the teeth are absent, reexamination of the injury a few days later may facilitate recognition and documentation.

Bites from animals are usually easy to distinguish from human bites. The size is usually smaller, and shape of the arch mark is narrower than a human's. Sharp animal canines often cause tearing of the skin instead of the crushing seen in human bites.

Differential Diagnosis

Bleeding disorders, such as idiopathic thrombocytopenic purpura (ITP), Henoch-Schönlein purpura, and leukemia, can mimic child abuse. Folk remedies, such as cupping and coining, may result in soft-tissue findings that are not reportable as abuse (see "Lesions Mistaken for Abuse").

ED Treatment and Disposition

Completely undress the child and look for all additional signs of abuse (Figs. 15.11 and 15.12). Obtain a complete history of all injuries. Sketch and photograph the injuries. Obtain a platelet count and bleeding studies [prothrombin time and partial thromboplastin time (PT and PTT)] to rule out a bleeding diathesis as the cause of the findings. For children under 2 or 3 years who have extensive injuries, obtain a skeletal survey, serum glutamic-oxaloacetic transaminase (SGOT), serum glutamic pyruvate transaminase (SGPT), amylase, and urinalysis.

If human bites are found or suspected, consider consultation with a forensic dentist. If appropriate, collect swabs for forensic analysis from the center of unwashed, fresh bites, which may contain saliva from the perpetrator.

Report suspected abuse to the legally mandated child protection agency before the child is discharged from the emergency department.

Clinical Pearls

1. Determination of the age of a bruise is imprecise. Bruises that are "fresh" ($<$ 48 h) are usually recognizable because they are tender, red, and swollen. Occasionally, bruises may not be visible for up to 48 h after an injury.
2. Children may deny abuse when questioned because of threats made to them. The child in Fig. 15.13 initially denied that he had been gagged. He told the examining physician that he had spilled some cleaning fluid onto his lips.
3. When a parent or caretaker inflicts an injury while disciplining a child, the incident must be reported to the local child protection agency. Even if corporal punishment is lawful in a given state, the infliction of an injury is never lawful.
4. Place a millimeter ruler or coin next to a pattern injury before taking photographs so that measurements can be made.
5. Consent is not required in most states to photograph injuries suspicious for child abuse.

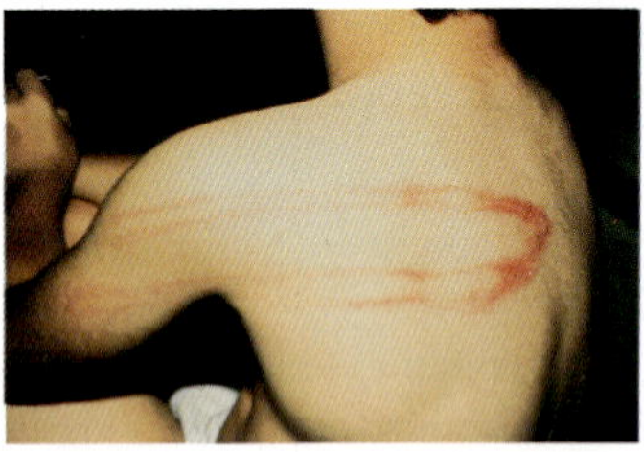

Figure 15.7 Looped Pattern Markings

Loop marks are clearly seen within the bruising on this child's back. The loop marks indicate that an extension cord, a belt, or some similar object was used to punish him. The color of the bruise is red, which indicates that the injury is only a few days old. (Courtesy of Robert A. Shapiro, MD.)

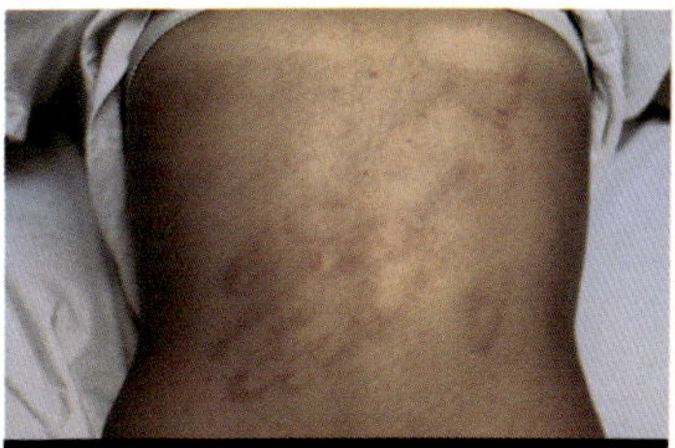

Figure 15.8
Hand Print Bruise

Bruise from a slap showing the outline of her father's hand is clearly seen on the back of this adolescent. (Courtesy of Robert A. Shapiro, MD.)

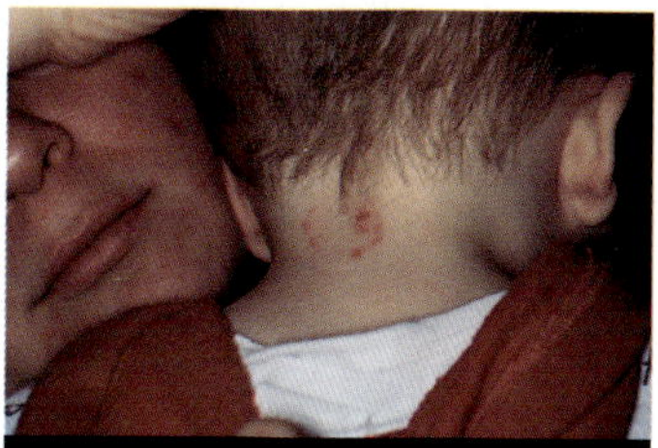

Figure 15.9
Bite Mark (Child)

Distinct impressions of teeth are seen in this injury. The shape of the injury outlines the upper and lower oral arches. Note the size of the mother's mouth in relationship to the size of the bite on the neck, making an adult mouth an unlikely source. (Courtesy of Kevin J. Knoop, MD, MS.)

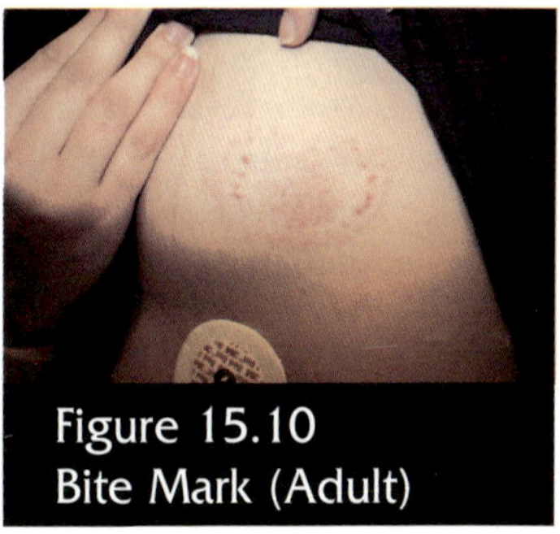

Figure 15.10
Bite Mark (Adult)

This bite mark is on a young girl's breast. Note the larger size of the wound, which is more consistent with an adult bite. (Courtesy of Robert A. Shapiro, MD.)

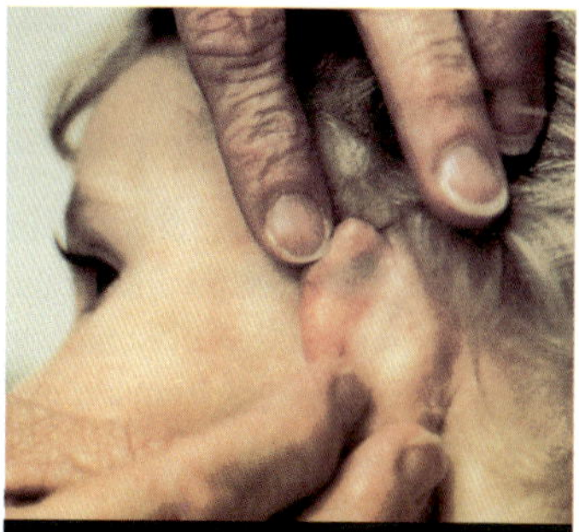

Figure 15.11 Pinch Marks on Pinna

Children may be pulled up or along by their ears, causing this injury. A child's ears should be inspected for this injury whenever abuse is suspected. (Courtesy of Robert A. Shapiro, MD.)

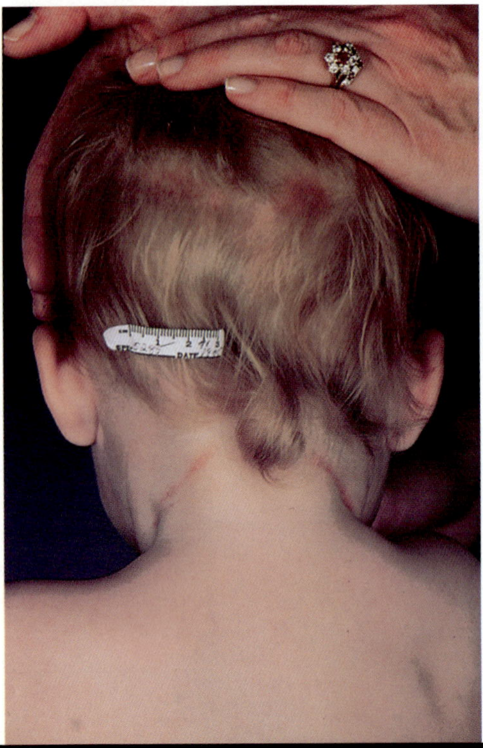

Figure 15.12 Strangulation Bruise

This child was beaten while at the sitter's and suffered circumferential linear neck abrasions consistent with attempted strangulation. There is also occipital ecchymosis from the abuse. (Courtesy of Barbara R. Craig, MD.)

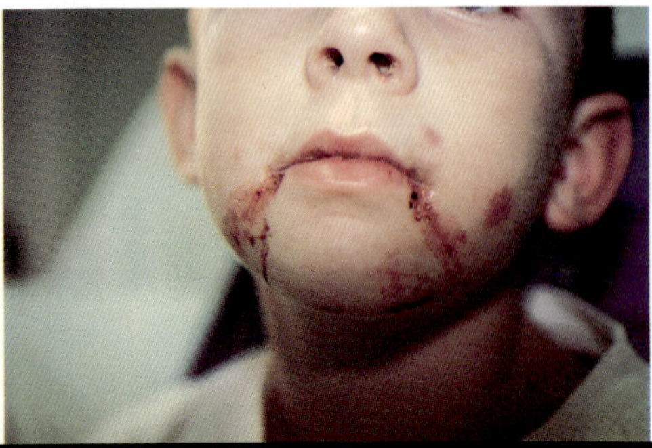

Figure 15.13 Gagging Bruise

This child had a sock stuffed into his mouth and tied around his head. The bruises in the corners of the child's mouth are indicative of gagging. Additionally, there are circular bruises on his left and right cheeks caused from the perpetrator's fingers as he held the child still to insert the sock. Pattern markings within the bruises match the fabric pattern of the sock. Photographs of these patterns should be obtained and provided to the police. The red color of the bruises and the fresh facial excoriations indicate that the injuries are recent. (Courtesy of Robert A. Shapiro, MD.)

Associated Clinical Features

Whenever bruising is excessive, is not associated with a compatible history, or occurs in an unusual distribution, seek a specific etiology. It may be appropriate to suspect and report child abuse when these conditions exist, but also consider other diagnoses.

Common Childhood Bruising

Accidental trauma can result in a bruise to any part of the body, but the forehead and the extensor surfaces of the tibia, elbow, and knee are the most common locations. When other areas of the body are bruised, etiologies other than accidental bruising should be considered.

Mongolian Spots

Mongolian spots are bluish, sacral or truncal lesions, most often seen in non-Caucasian infants and young children. They may be mistaken for bruises. Mongolian spots may be limited to only a few lesions, or they may extend up the back and shoulders of the child (Fig. 15.14).

Cupping, Coining, and Moxibustion

Asian families sometimes practice traditional cures with their children, such as cupping, coining, and moxibustion. Each of these practices leaves markings on the child's skin, which may be interpreted as child abuse. In cupping, a flammable object is ignited and placed into a cup. After the flames have extinguished, the cup is inverted and placed onto the child's skin. As the warm air within the cup cools, a vacuum is produced. This "cure" leaves circular suction markings on the child's skin but should not be painful to the child. Coining (Fig. 15.15) is done by rubbing a coin up and down the child's back, just lateral to the spine. This results in bilateral ecchymosis and chronic skin changes on the back. Coining should also not be painful to the child. Neither of these practices should be reported as child abuse. In moxibustion, a flammable object, such as a thread, is ignited on or near the child's skin. Moxibustion may cause superficial burns. Whether moxibustion is reported as child abuse would depend on the physical findings and the judgment of the physician.

Henoch-Schönlein Purpura

Henoch-Schönlein purpura (HSP) is a vasculitis of the small blood vessels. The skin lesions are usually small, symmetric, palpable purpuras. They may appear in a linear pattern and are often confined to the lower extremities (Fig. 15.16). Associated symptoms may include joint and abdominal pain.

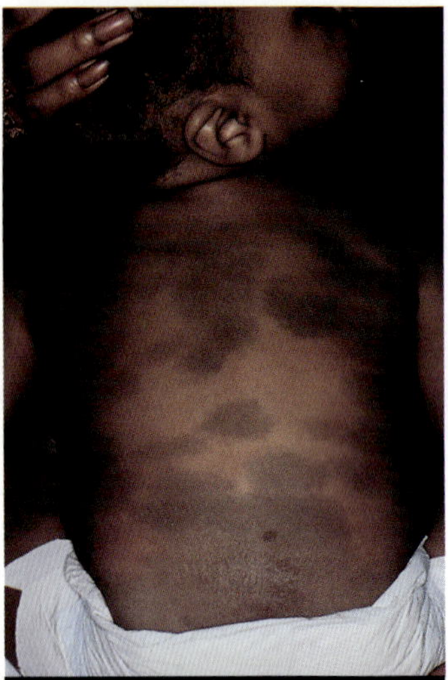

Figure 15.14 Mongolian Spots

Numerous mongolian spots on this youngster extend up the back and shoulders. (Courtesy of Douglas R. Landry, MD.)

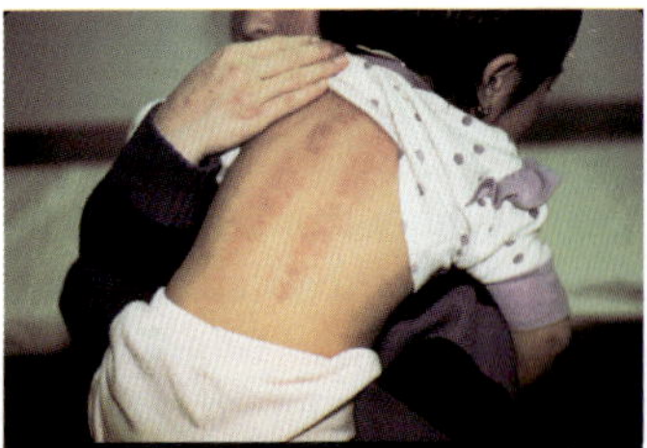

Figure 15.15 Coining (Cheut Sah or Cao Gio)

This child has petechiae and bruising along her spine. Her parents were practicing the Southeast Asian practice of coining, a healing remedy, in which a coin is rubbed along the spine to heal an illness. Coining should not be painful and is not considered abusive. (Courtesy of Robert A. Shapiro, MD.)

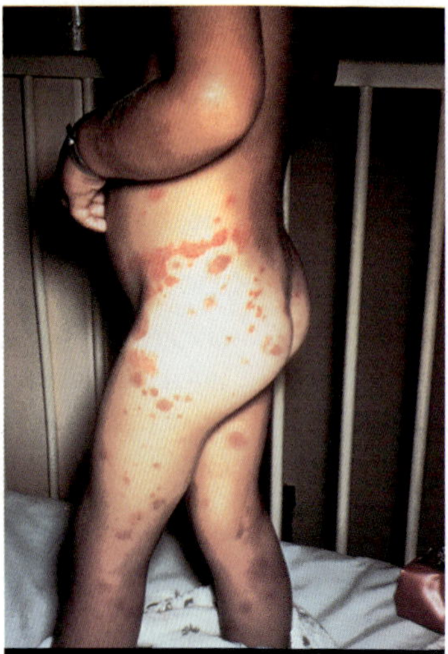

Figure 15.16 Henoch-Schönlein Purpura (HSP)

This child has palpable purpura on the extensor surfaces of the legs. HSP should be considered whenever there is symmetric ecchymosis along the extensor surfaces of the extremities and buttocks. The illness is most often seen in school-age children. Migratory arthritis and abdominal pain may be present. (Courtesy of Ralph A. Gruppo, MD.)

Idiopathic Thrombocytopenic Purpura

Idiopathic thrombocytopenic purpura (ITP) is an acquired platelet disorder which results in abnormal bleeding. It is most common in 1- to 4-year-old children. The presenting complaint is most often abnormal bruising. The bruises can appear anywhere on the body and are numerous, mimicking child abuse (Fig. 15.17). The child may also have epistaxis, hematuria, or other bleeding.

Hemophilia

Hemophilia is usually diagnosed soon after birth because of abnormal bleeding. The ecchymosis and soft-tissue swelling are greater than would be expected given the history of trauma (Fig. 15.18).

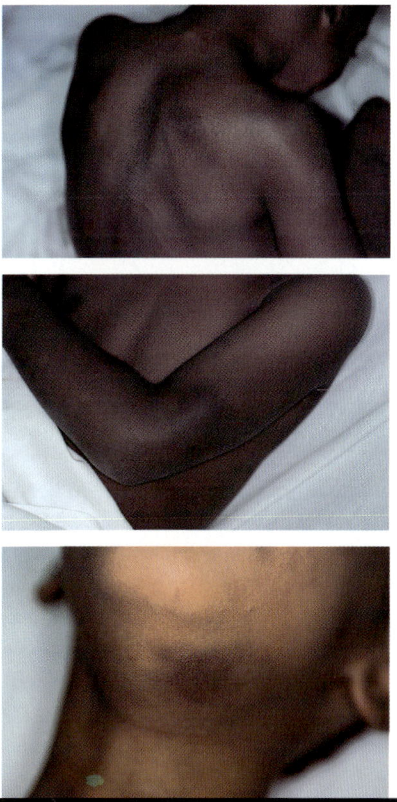

Figure 15.17
Idiopathic Thrombocytopenic Pupura (ITP)

This child has many areas of ecchymoses that appear to be in random areas of his body (back, arm, chin). The child's parent could provide no explanation for the bruising and was concerned that something was wrong with the child. ITP should be suspected in any pre-school-age child who has multiple, unexplained bruises. A platelet count will diagnose ITP. (Courtesy of Kevin J. Knoop, MD, MS.)

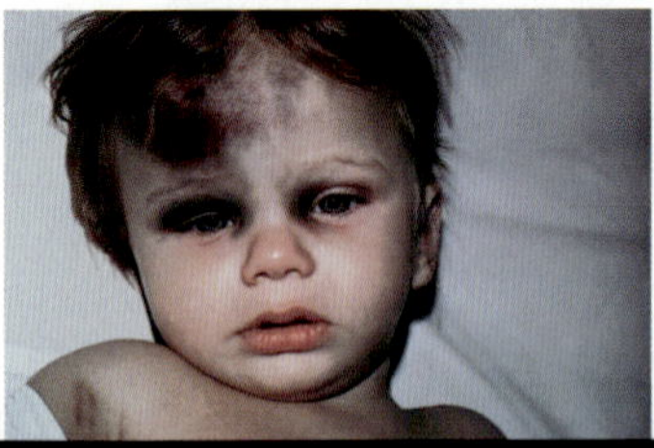

Figure 15.18 Hemophiliac with Bruising

This child's bruising is due to factor VIII deficiency. The degree of bleeding within the ecchymosis is more extensive than that seen in children without coagulopathies. A history of other abnormal bleeding episodes or a history that the child suffers from a coagulopathy is most often obtained at the time of presentation. (Courtesy of Ralph A. Gruppo, MD.)

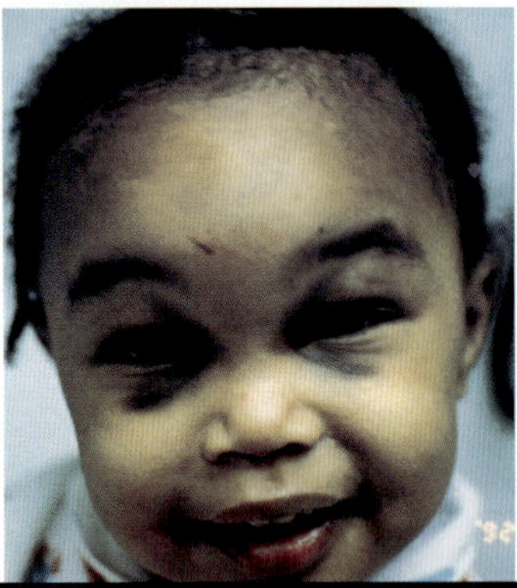

Figure 15.19 Raccoon Eyes, or Black Eyes

The etiology of this child's raccoon eyes was a forehead hematoma. He fell onto his forehead a few days earlier and developed a hematoma, a common accidental injury. As the hematoma healed, blood from the hematoma tracked down along the facial soft tissues and settled under his eyes. The resulting ecchymosis suggests that he was punched, leaving him with two black eyes. The absence of other trauma about the eyes, such as lacerations, abrasions, soft-tissue swelling, or eye injury should cause the examiner to consider a diagnosis other than direct trauma. Observation or palpation of forehead soft-tissue swelling results in the correct diagnosis. (Courtesy of Robert A. Shapiro, MD.)

ifferential Diagnosis

iagnostic suspicion and awareness of the above conditions is the ost important step leading to the correct diagnosis. HSP, mongoan spots, and cultural practices such as moxibustion and cupping re diagnosed clinically. If ITP or other thrombocytopenic disorers are suspected, a platelet count is diagnostic. Newborns and inants with significant bleeding should have PT, PTT, and bleeding ime tests to rule out a coagulopathy.

ED Treatment and Disposition

A hematologist should be consulted for children with platelet disorders and coagulopathies. HSP requires supportive care and close follow-up. The most serious complication of HSP is bowel obstruction from intussusception.

Clinical Pearls

1. Mongolian spots are noted first in the newborn period.
2. Consider HSP in school-age children with purpura of the lower extremities.
3. Consider ITP in preschool children who have multiple ecchymosis and petechiae without other signs or indications of abuse.
4. Vitamin K deficiency is a cause of bleeding in infancy.
5. Trauma to the forehead may cause bilateral eye ecchymosis (Fig. 15.19) within a few days and can be mistaken for eye trauma.

Associated Clinical Features

Certain fractures should always raise a suspicion of child abuse such as metaphyseal corner fracture, rib fractures, fractures in a nonambulating child, and untreated healing fractures. Fractures incompatible with the history and those for which no explanation is available are also suspicious of child abuse (Figs. 15.20 to 15.24).

Differential Diagnosis

Normal pediatric radiographic variants, periosteal changes caused by conditions other than healing fractures, and illnesses that cause fragile bones may all be mistaken for fractures due to child abuse. A pediatric radiologist should be consulted if any doubt exists about the radiographic interpretation. Specific disorders that can be mistaken for child abuse include osteogenesis imperfecta, copper deficiency, osteopetrosis, rickets, scurvy, hypervitaminosis A, osteomyelitis, tumors, leukemia, prostaglandin E overdose, and Caffey's infantile cortical hyperostosis.

Conditions that cause "brittle bones" must be considered when unexpected fractures are discovered, even though such cases are rare. The most frequently discussed brittle bone disorder is osteogenesis imperfecta (OI), a rare inherited connective-tissue disorder. Associated features seen in some children with OI include blue sclerae, wormian bones (seen on the skull x-ray), and osteopenia. A family history of bone fragility, hearing loss, and short stature is often present. In rare instances, children with OI lack these associated features.

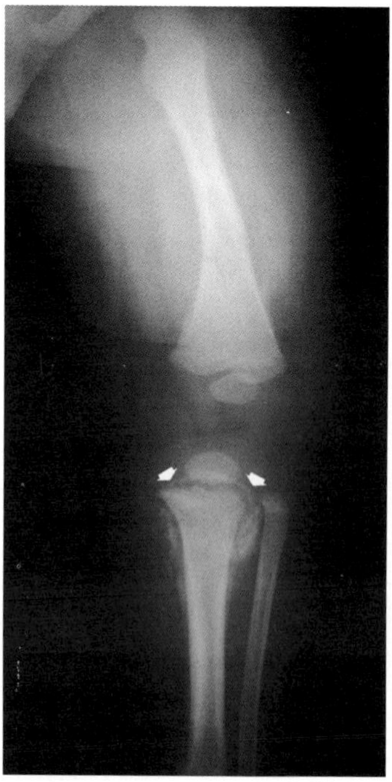

Figure 15.20 Healing Corner Fracture

This radiograph shows a healing metaphyseal corner fracture of the proximal tibia, sometimes referred to as a bucket handle fracture. Arrows point to the impressive periosteal elevation, causing the bucket handle appearance. This fracture is most often seen in children who have been the victims of child abuse, the result of shaking or pulling. (Courtesy of Alan E. Oestreich, MD.)

ED Treatment and Disposition

If abuse is suspected in a child under 2 or 3 years of age, obtain a skeletal survey. The skeletal survey should include at least one view of each extremity and single views of the chest, abdomen, entire lateral spine, anteroposterior (AP) spine, and lateral skull. Consider a head CT or MRI in infants with skull fractures, if abuse is suspected. Suspected abuse must be reported immediately to the appropriate child protection agency. Fractures should be managed appropriately.

Clinical Pearls

1. Suspect abuse when a child has multiple fractures, fractures of different ages, unsuspected (occult) fractures, fractures without a consistent trauma history.
2. Accidental trauma that includes rotational forces can result in a spiral fracture.
3. Obtain a skeletal survey in any child under 2 years of age who has injuries suspicious of abuse.
4. Radiographic signs of healing are typically first seen 10 days after a fracture.
5. Fractures that are not immobilized have a larger callous compared with immobilized fractures.

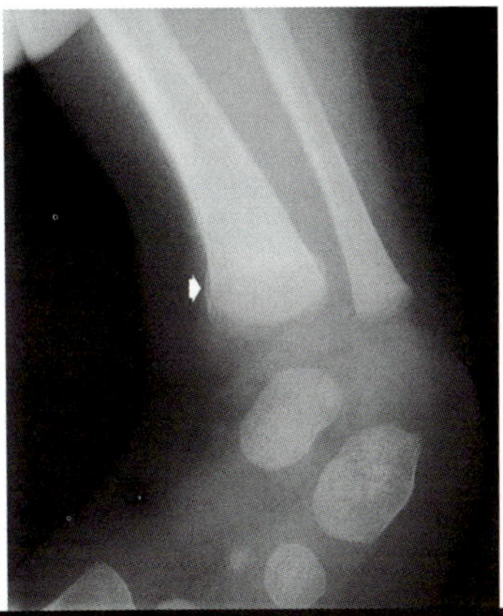

Figure 15.21 Healing Corner Fracture

Periosteal reaction (arrow) of the distal tibia from a corner fracture. (Courtesy of Alan E. Oestreich, MD.)

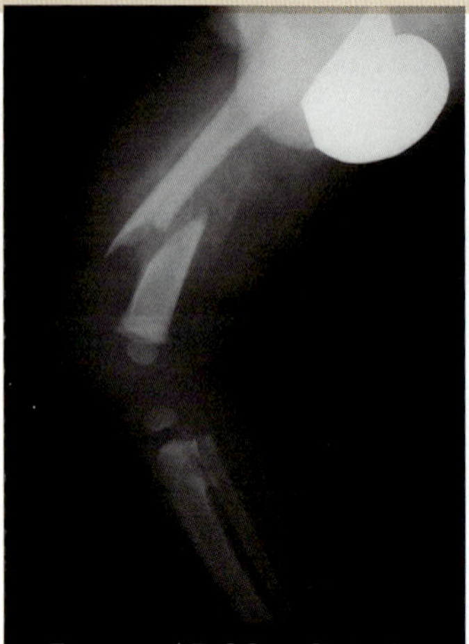

Figure 15.22 Spiral Femur and Proximal Tibia Fracture

This radiograph shows a displaced spiral femur fracture with faint callus formation. The age of the fracture is just over 10 days. There is also periosteal reaction of the proximal tibia, which is more solid and therefore older than the femur fracture. Spiral femur fractures are caused by trauma that includes a twisting, rotational force to the bone. Accidental falls can result in spiral fractures if the child's foot is fixed while his or her body is rotating. Spiral fractures from abuse are often caused by an angry adult who twists the leg of the child. The radiographic finding in this photograph is almost certainly indicative of child abuse because there are two injuries which occurred at different times and no treatment was obtained when the injuries occurred. (Courtesy of Alan E. Oestreich, MD.)

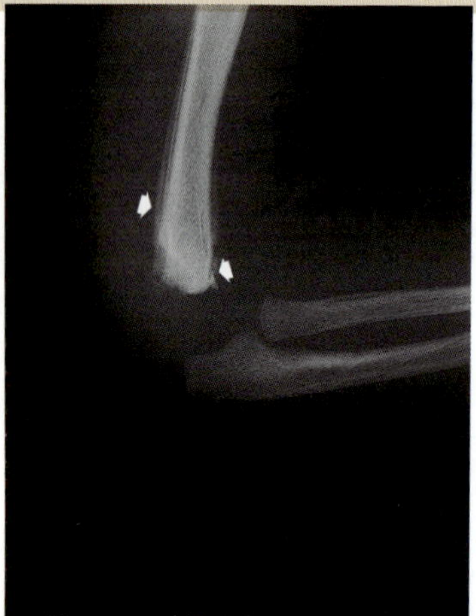

Figure 15.23 Healing Fracture of the Distal Humerus

The periosteal reaction along the distal humerus dates this fracture as older than 10 days. No treatment was obtained for the acute injury. (Courtesy of Alan E. Oestreich, MD.)

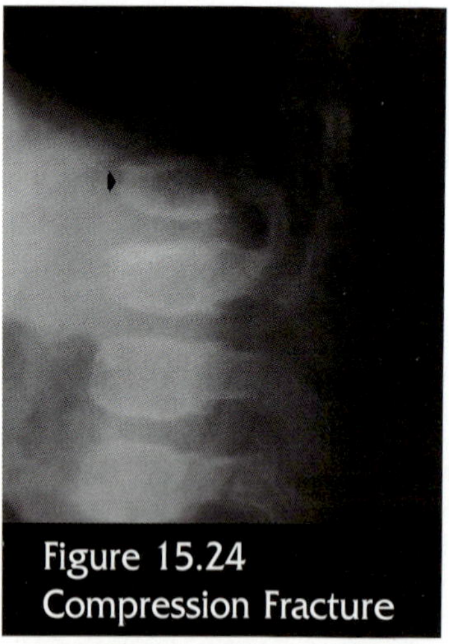

Figure 15.24 Compression Fracture

The wedging of T-12 (arrow) and probably L-1 indicates vertebral compression fractures. These fractures are the result of significant forces applied to the spinal column and are often indicative of child abuse. (Courtesy of Alan E. Oestreich, MD.)

Associated Clinical Features

Straddle injuries are a frequent cause of genital trauma and most often result in unilateral abrasions, bruising, and hematomas of the labia majora and clitoral hood (Fig. 15.25). A clear history describing the straddle injury should be given by the caretaker.

Differential Diagnosis

Sexual abuse must be considered in all children with genital injuries. Injuries involving the hymen are not typical of straddle injuries and are usually the result of sexual abuse or assault.

ED Treatment and Disposition

Check for urethral injury. Sitz baths and Polysporin ointment promote healing and minimize discomfort. If the child has difficulty voiding, she should be encouraged to void in a bath of warm water.

Clinical Pearls

1. Straddle injuries usually present with a clear mechanism of injury and a physical examination that supports the history.
2. Straddle injuries rarely involve the hymen or internal vaginal mucosa.

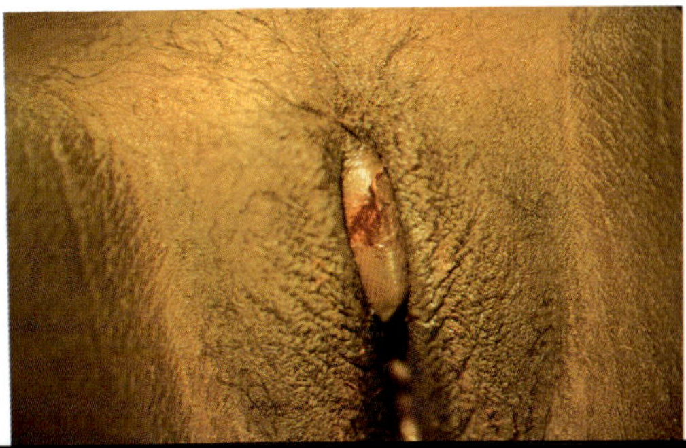

Figure 15.25 Straddle Injury

Laceration of the clitoral hood resulted after a fall onto the bar of a bicycle. (Courtesy of Robert A. Shapiro, MD.)

Associated Clinical Features

Adhesions of the labia minora occur in young girls and may persist until puberty. A thin translucent line is seen where the labia meet (Fig. 15.26). The extent of the adhesions vary from child to child. Involvement is often limited to the posterior portion of the labia, but some children have more extensive adhesions completely obscuring the introitus. It is postulated that vulvar irritation and poor hygiene contribute to the etiology of labial adhesions.

Differential Diagnosis

The hymen and introitus may be obscured by the adhesions. If the adhesions are unrecognized, a diagnosis of hymenal trauma and "gaping" introitus may be incorrectly made. Adhesions may be mistaken for vaginal scars.

ED Treatment and Disposition

Prescribe estrogen creme (Premarin) to be applied gently over the adhesions twice daily for 2 to 4 weeks. Recurrence is not uncommon.

Clinical Pearls

1. Adhesions may be congenital or acquired.
2. It is possible that vulvar irritation from sexual abuse may cause labial adhesions, but clear supporting evidence is lacking.

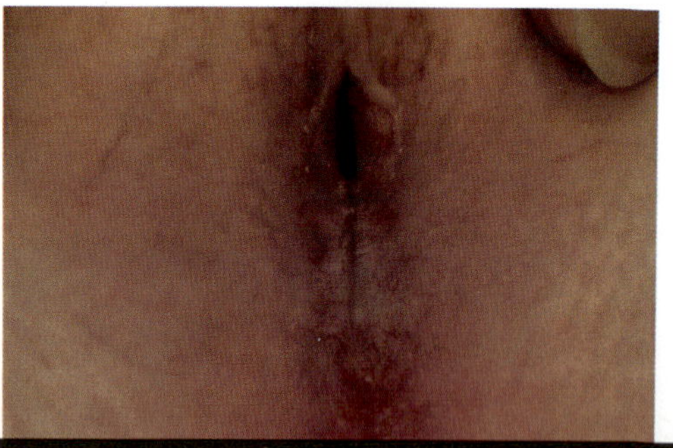

Figure 15.26 Labial Adhesions

Labial adhesions obscure the hymen in this prepubertal girl. (Courtesy of Robert A. Shapiro, MD.)

Associated Clinical Features

Prepubertal girls with urethral prolapse present with vaginal bleeding, vaginal mass, or urinary complaints. On examination, an annular, erythematous vaginal mass is seen (Fig. 15.27). Upon close examination, the mass can be seen to originate from the urethra. If necrotic, the mass is friable.

Differential Diagnosis

Urethral prolapse may be mistaken for vaginal injury, sexual abuse, or vaginal mass.

ED Treatment and Disposition

The prolapse may resolve within a few weeks with conservative medical management consisting of daily sitz baths and topical antibiotics. Topical estrogen cream and oral antibiotic therapy have also been used with some success. Surgical repair is usually not required but may be indicated if necrosis is present or conservative management fails.

Clinical Pearls

1. Urethral prolapse often presents with painless genital bleeding of unknown etiology.
2. Prolapse is more common in African American girls.

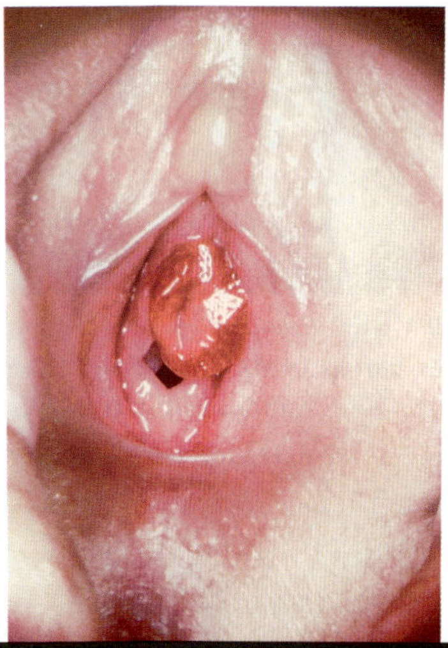

Figure 15.27 Urethral Prolapse

A round reddish-purple mass is seen in this child's introitus. Careful examination reveals the mass originates from the urethra. (Courtesy of Michael P. Poirier, MD.)

Associated Clinical Features

Acute bruising to the glans and corona of the penis can occur if the toilet seat falls onto the penis during voiding, trapping the penis between the seat and toilet bowl (Fig. 15.28). This injury is not uncommon in boys of about 3 years of age who are both inexperienced at voiding while standing and are short enough for this injury to occur.

Differential Diagnosis

Genital trauma is always suspicious for sexual abuse. The mechanism of injury may be difficult to determine if the injury was unwitnessed.

ED Treatment and Disposition

No specific treatment is needed unless the child is unable to void. If the child cannot void, a retrograde urethrogram and urologic consult are indicated.

Clinical Pearl

1. Genital injuries are suspicious of sexual abuse if no appropriate history of accidental trauma is given.

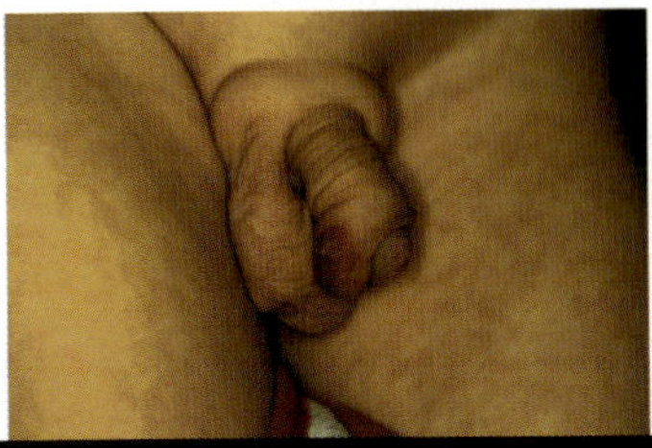

Figure 15.28 Toilet Bowl Injury

This toddler presented with a straightforward history of the toilet seat falling onto his penis during voiding. Despite the swelling and ecchymosis, he was able to void without difficulty. (Courtesy of Kevin J. Knoop, MD, MS.)

Associated Clinical Features

Presenting complaints are often rectal pain, itching, bleeding, and rash. Symptoms may be present for months prior to the diagnosis. The child may be constipated because of stool retention and may have recently been given laxatives because of these symptoms. Systemic symptoms are absent. The perianal area is erythematous and tender (Fig. 15.29). The involved area is well demarcated from the uninfected skin. Anal fissures and bleeding may be seen.

Differential Diagnosis

Sexual abuse is often misdiagnosed because of the child's complaints of rectal pain and bleeding and the above findings on examination. This infection can also be mistaken for poor hygiene, dermatitis, nonspecific irritation, and constipation.

ED Treatment and Disposition

Culture or obtain direct antigen studies for group A beta-hemolytic streptococci. Treat with oral penicillin for 10 days. Substitute erythromycin for patients allergic to penicillin. Treatment failures should be treated with IM penicillin and/or oral clindamycin.

Clinical Pearls

1. Direct antigen studies are sensitive (89%) and specific (100%) for perianal group A streptococci infection.
2. Examine the pharynx for streptococcal infection when considering perianal strep infection.
3. Infection is unusual in children older than 10 years.

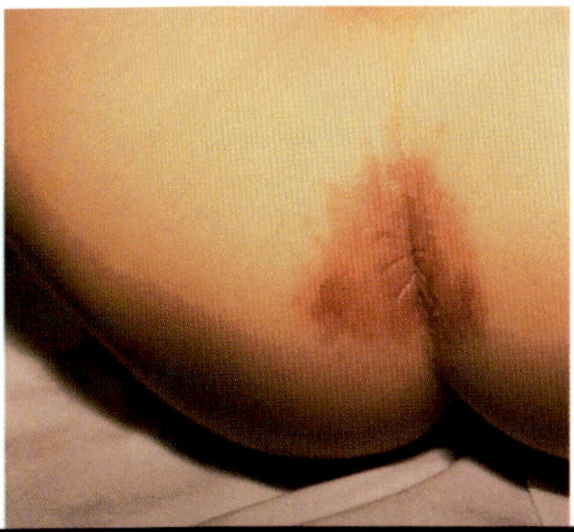

Figure 15.29 Perianal Streptococcal Infection

Intense erythema around the anus consistent with perianal streptococcal infection. (Courtesy of Raymond C. Baker, MD.)

Associated Clinical Features

Lichen sclerosus atrophicus (LSA) is an unusual dermatitis which affects the anogenital area. The diagnosis should be suspected whenever an area of hypopigmentation in the shape of an hourglass is seen around the child's anus and genitalia. The hypopigmented area is caused by small white or yellowish papules which coalesce into large plaques. The affected skin is atrophic and bleeds easily after minor trauma. The hemorrhagic form of LSA includes subepithelial hemorrhagic lesions to the labia and affected skin, which can be mistaken for traumatic lesions (Fig. 15.30). Children may complain of pruritus and dysuria.

Differential Diagnosis

The findings of hemorrhage around the genitalia and rectum are often mistaken for signs of sexual abuse.

ED Treatment and Disposition

Use symptomatic treatment if needed; 1% hydrocortisone cream can be prescribed. Refer to dermatologist for treatment.

Clinical Pearl

1. Lichen sclerosus atrophicus is the most common dermatitis mistaken for sexual abuse.

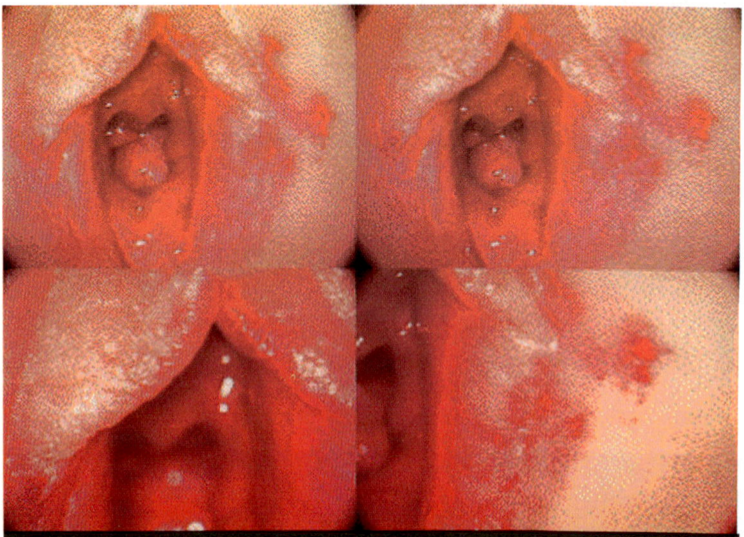

Figure 15.30 Lichen Sclerosus Atrophicus

The perineum surrounding the vagina has a bruised appearance. Atrophic skin is also evident. (Courtesy of Robert A. Shapiro, MD.)

CHAPTER 16

ENVIRONMENTAL CONDITIONS

Ken Zafren, Alan B. Storrow,
Joseph C. Schmidt, Lawrence B. Stack

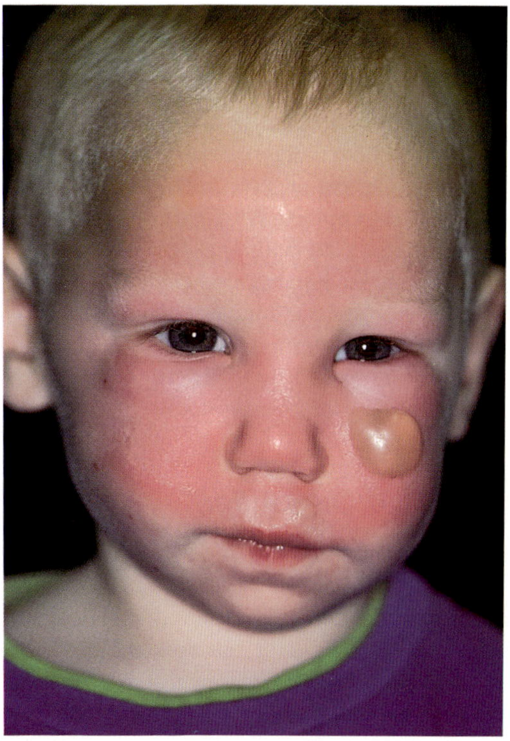

Associated Clinical Features

Ultraviolet (UV) radiation causes both acute and chronic skin changes. Sunburn is a partial-thickness burn (Fig. 16.1), which may become full thickness if infected. "Sun poisoning" is a severe systemic reaction to UV radiation. Patients complain of nausea, vomiting, headache, fever, chills, and prostration. Excessive UV radiation may cause injury to the cornea and conjunctiva, termed ultraviolet keratitis (photokeratitis, snow blindness).

Photosensitivity reactions (photodermatoses) are of several types. Phototoxic reactions are an abnormal response to UV radiation caused by a substance that is ingested (prescription or over-the-counter medications) or applied to the skin (even seemingly innocuous perfumes or shampoos); there is a direct relation between the amount of UV exposure and severity. Photoallergic reactions are clinically similar to contact dermatitis and, like phototoxic reactions, may be precipitated by ingested or applied drugs. Unlike phototoxic reactions, photoallergies may be precipitated by a small amount of light. Phytophotodermatitis is precipitated by skin contact with certain plants followed by exposure to UV radiation. It can resemble either phototoxic or photoallergic reactions.

Differential Diagnosis

Phototoxicity should be suspected in any patient with a severe or exaggerated sunburn. Photoallergy is easily misdiagnosed as allergic eczema or contact dermatitis, especially since onset is often delayed up to 2 days after exposure. Phytophotodermatitis may mimic severe sunburn or contact dermatitis, especially rhus (poison ivy, sumac, or oak) dermatitis. Endogenous photosensitizers (endogenous photodermatoses) include solar urticaria, porphyria cutanea tarda, polymorphous light eruption, and systemic lupus erythematosus. These may be provoked by visible light as well as by UV radiation.

ED Treatment and Disposition

Treatment of sunburn and sun poisoning involves standard burn and supportive care. Sunburn is usually a self-limited problem. Cool compresses and nonsteroidal anti-inflammatory drugs may be beneficial. Steroids may be useful for sun poisoning. Ultraviolet keratitis is treated with mydriatic-cycloplegic eyedrops to decrease pain. Severe cases may require bilateral eye patches with antibiotic ointment, and patients may also need narcotic analgesics. These patients require 24- to 48-hour follow up, and ophthalmology referral is indicated to rule out retinal damage.

Treatment of photosensitivity reaction has two components: treatment of the sunburn and recognition of the sensitizing agent or endogenous medical condition. Topical steroids and oral analgesics and antipruritics may be helpful. Systemic steroids may be re-

Patients with tick paralysis may require supportive care, including mechanical ventilation. Most patients likely require admission. Patients with tick-borne illnesses may require admission for supportive care or intensive antibiotic treatment.

Clinical Pearls

1. In North America, tick paralysis resolves rapidly after removal of the tick, with improvement in hours and complete recovery in days; in Australia, progression may continue for 48 h after tick removal, and recovery may be prolonged.
2. A pruritic eschar may form at the site of the tick bite in relapsing fever, but is usually gone by the time symptoms appear.
3. A clear history of tick bite is present in less than one-third of Lyme disease cases.
4. Unusual neurologic presentations, particularly bilateral peripheral seventh-nerve palsies, should prompt consideration of Lyme disease.

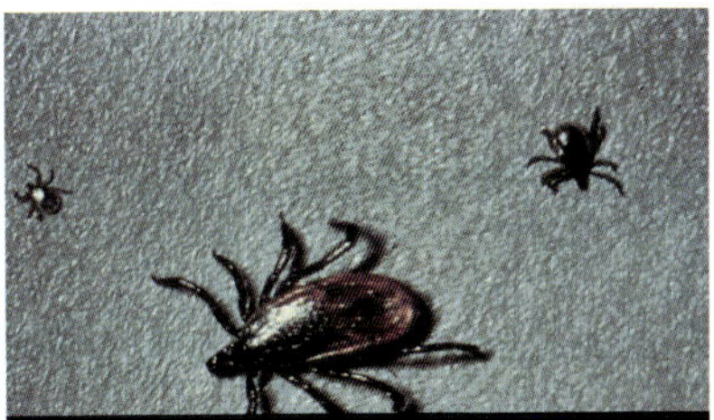

Figure 16.3
Deer Tick

Ixodes dammini, the deer tick, is a vector of Lyme disease and babesiosis. (Courtesy of the Centers for Disease Control and Prevention, Atlanta, GA.)

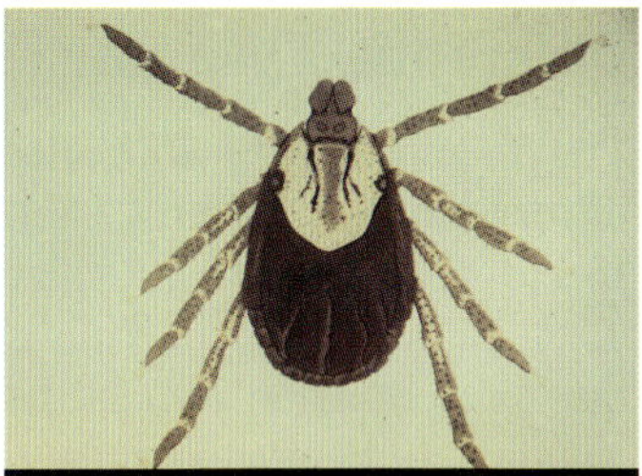

Figure 16.4
Wood Tick

Dermacentor andersonii, the wood tick, is a vector of Rocky Mountain spotted fever and Colorado tick fever. (Courtesy of the Centers for Disease Control and Prevention, Atlanta, GA.)

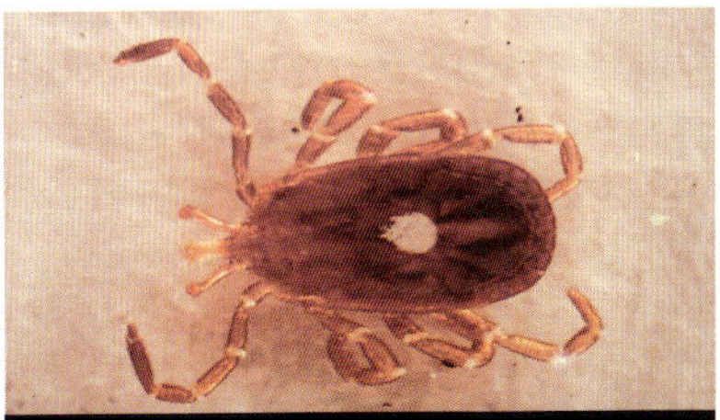

Figure 16.5
Lone Star Tick

Amblyomma americanum, the Lone Star tick, has been implicated as a vector in Lyme disease. (Courtesy of Sherman Minton, MD.)

Associated Clinical Features

The brown recluse spider (*Loxosceles reclusa*) is the prototypical member of the genus *Loxosceles,* which as a group can produce the typical necrotic arachnidism following envenomation. These spiders have a worldwide distribution and are identified by the striking fiddle-shaped markings on their anterodorsal cephalothorax (Fig. 16.6). Initial envenomation may be painful, although patients often report no recollection of being bitten. Initial stinging gives way to aching and pruritus. The wound then becomes edematous with an erythematous halo surrounding a violaceous center (Fig. 16.7). The erythematous margin often spreads in a pattern influenced by gravity, leaving the necrotic center near the top of the lesion (Fig. 16.8). Bullae may erupt, and over a period of 2 to 5 weeks the eschar sloughs, leaving a deep, poorly healing ulcer (Fig. 16.9). In unusual cases systemic symptoms (loxoscelism) may present with hemolytic anemia as a predominant feature. Children are at higher risk of systemic disease. Other symptoms include fever, chills, nausea, vomiting, rash, arthralgia, weakness, and leukocytosis.

Differential Diagnosis

The diagnosis of brown recluse envenomation is based on typical history, clinical features, and possible exposure to the offending species. The local wound can be confused with cellulitis, decubitus ulcer, burns, and pyoderma gangrenosum. Systemic involvement may present as an isolated hemolytic anemia, thrombocytopenia, jaundice, or hemoglobinuria.

ED Treatment and Disposition

Most cutaneous lesions secondary to brown recluse bites can be managed with cold compresses, elevation, loose immobilization, and attention to tetanus immunization. Severe lesions may require reconstructive plastic surgery several weeks after wound stabilization. The use of dapsone to prevent lesion progression is controversial. Any systemic reaction with evidence of hemolysis, hemoglobinuria, or coagulopathy should prompt admission. Hyperbaric oxygen (HBO) therapy and antivenin have been suggested as possible adjuncts, but no clear consensus of preferred treatment has been established.

Associated Clinical Features

Poison ivy, oak, and sumac (Figs. 16.12 and 16.13) cause more cases of allergic contact dermatitis than all other allergens combined. At least 70% of the U.S. population is sensitive to the *Toxicodendron* species.

The dermatitis begins as pruritus and redness (Fig. 16.14), usually within 2 days of exposure in susceptible persons. The degree of dermatitis depends on the patient's degree of sensitivity, amount of allergen exposed, and the reactivity of the skin at the exposed body location. The dermatitis may vary from erythema, to erythema with papules, to erythema with vesicles and bullae. A linear distribution of the cutaneous lesions is strongly suggestive of toxicodendron dermatitis. This distribution occurs from contaminated fingernails scratching the skin or plant parts rubbing against the skin.

Differential Diagnosis

Medical problems which may appear like a *Toxicodendron* rash include photodermatitis, cellulitis, thermal burns, and other causes of contact dermatitis.

ED Treatment and Disposition

If symptoms are limited to erythema and papules and a small surface area, calamine lotion or topical steroid sprays provide adequate symptomatic relief. Pruritus can be treated with antihistamines. Vesicles and bullae require Domeboro compresses (for 60 min, three times daily) to help dry these lesions and relieve pruritus. Systemic corticosteroids tapered over 3 weeks are used in severe reactions. Secondary infection should be treated with systemic antibiotics against staphylococcal and streptococcal species.

Clinical Pearls

1. Fluid from the vesicles or bullae does not contain any allergen.
2. Removal of the allergen from the skin within 30 min of exposure may prevent dermatitis.
3. Deliberate removal of allergen from under the fingernails may prevent dermatitis spread.
4. Treatment with systemic steroids for less than 2 or 3 weeks may result in rebound exacerbations of the dermatitis.

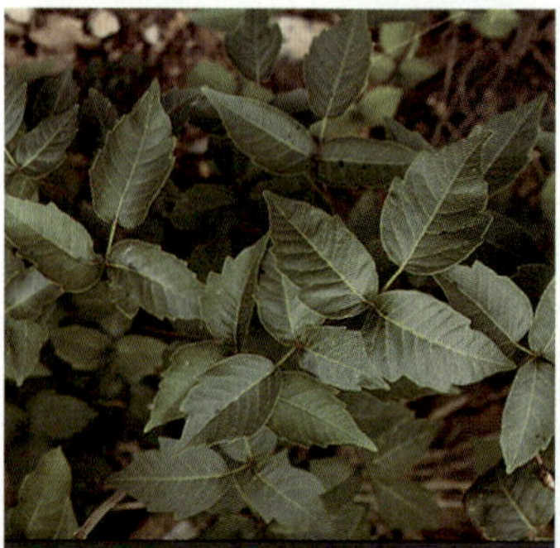

Figure 16.12
Poison Ivy

Toxicodendron radicans (poison ivy—shrub or climbing vine). Note that the leaves of poison ivy have three leaflets. Poison ivy occurs throughout the United States. (Courtesy of Lawrence B. Stack, MD.)

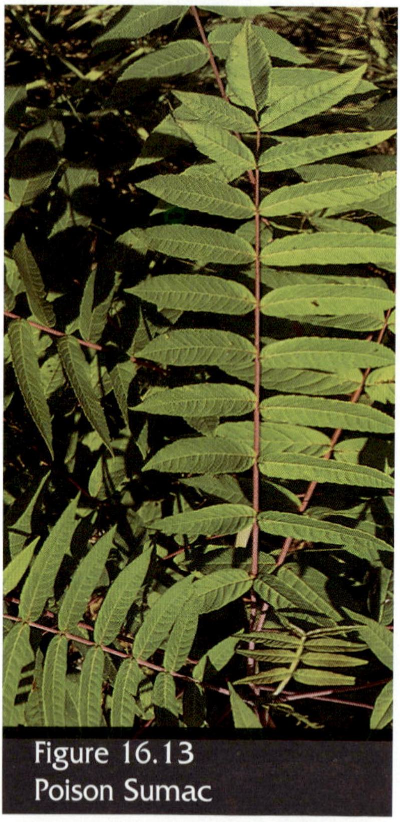

Figure 16.13
Poison Sumac

Toxicodendron vernix (poison sumac). Note that the leaves of poison sumac have 7 to 13 leaflets. It grows as a tree or woody coarse shrub. Only one species of poison sumac is found in the United States. (Courtesy of Lawrence B. Stack, MD.)

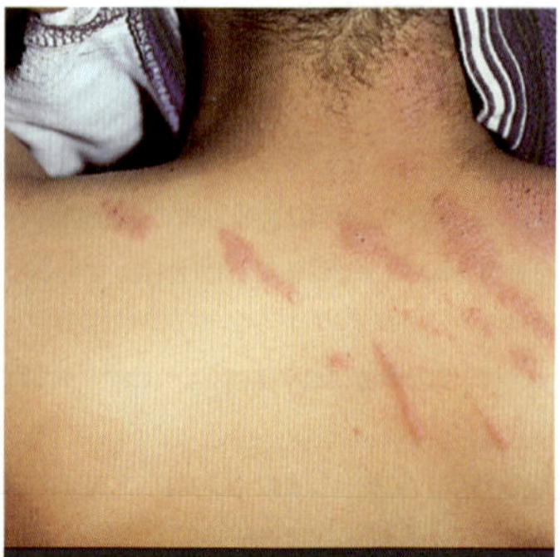

Figure 16.14 Poison Ivy Exposure

Erythematous papules and vesicles in a linear distribution consistent with *Toxicodendron* dermatitis. (Courtesy of Alan B. Storrow, MD.)

CHAPTER 17

MICROSCOPIC FINDINGS

Diane M. Birnbaumer

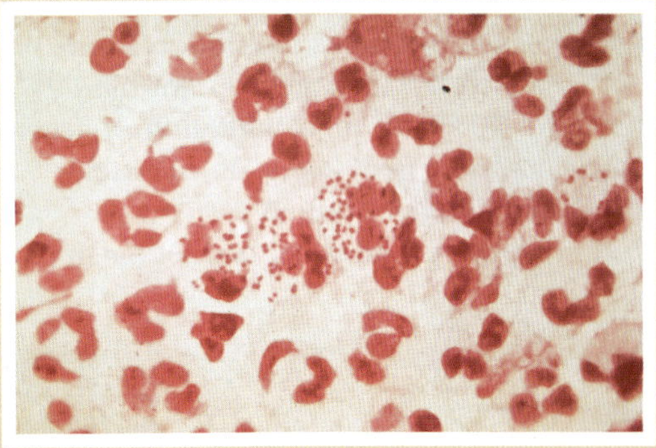

Uses

To determine adequacy of specimen (e.g., sputum); to determine the morphology of predominant organisms in a specimen. See Figs. 17.1 to 17.4.

Materials

Freshly collected specimen to be examined, glass microscope slide, crystal violet, Gram's iodine, acetone-alcohol (acetone, 30 mL, and 95% alcohol, 70 mL), safranin, Bunsen burner.

Method

1. Put specimen on dry, clean glass microscope slide and allow to air dry.
2. Heat fix specimen by gently passing over flame.
3. Cover specimen with crystal violet for 1 min.
4. Rinse off completely with water; do not blot.
5. Cover specimen with Gram's iodine for 1 min.
6. Rinse off completely with water; do not blot.
7. Decolorize for 30 s with gentle agitation in acetone-alcohol.
8. Rinse off completely with water; do not blot.
9. Cover with safranin for 10 to 20 s.
10. Rinse off completely with water and let air dry.

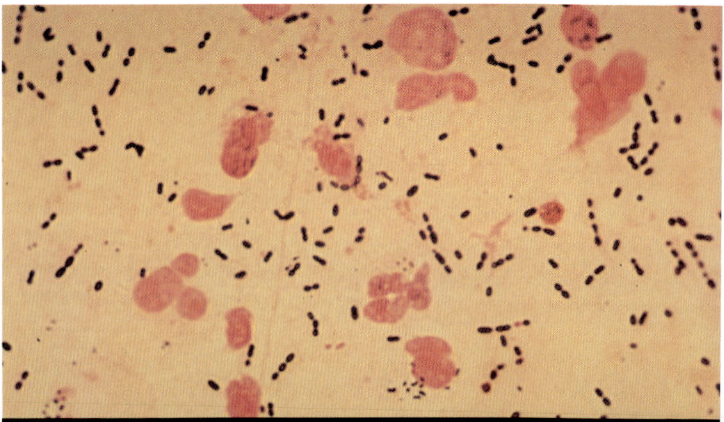

Figure 17.1 Gram's Stain—Streptococcus pneumoniae

Gram-positive, kidney-shaped diplococci of *S. pneumoniae*. (Courtesy of Roche Laboratories, Division of Hoffman-LaRoche Inc. Nutley, NJ.)

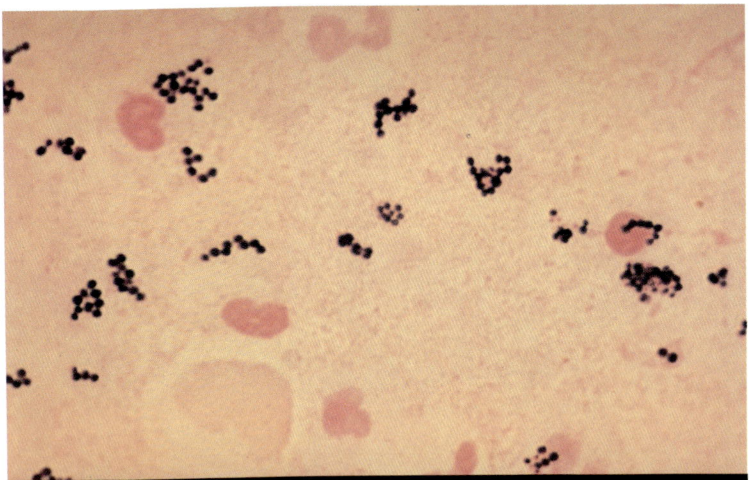

Figure 17.2 Gram's Stain—Staphylococcus aureus

Small clusters of gram-positive cocci seen in *S. aureus* infection. (Courtesy of Roche Laboratories, Division of Hoffman-LaRoche Inc. Nutley, NJ.)

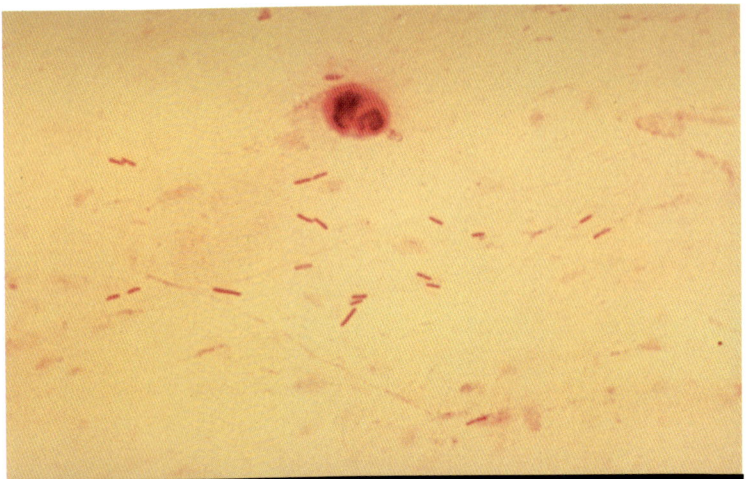

Figure 17.3 Gram's Stain—Gram-Negative Rods

Gram-negative rods of *Pseudomonas aeruginosa.* (Courtesy of Roche Laboratories, Division of Hoffman-LaRoche Inc. Nutley, NJ.)

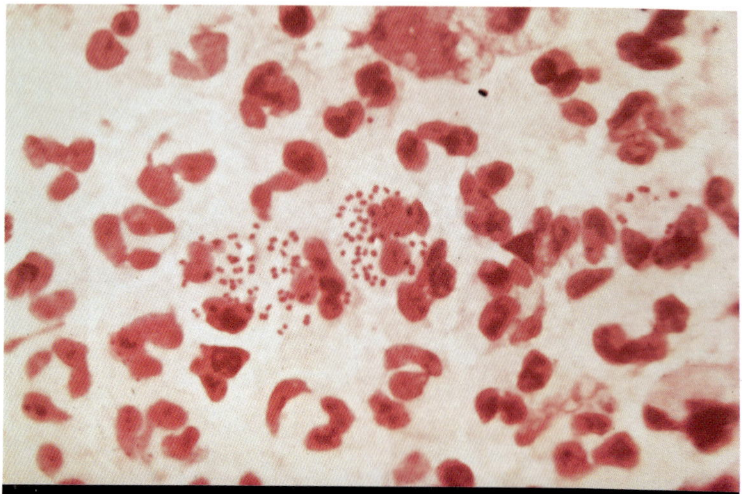

Figure 17.4 Gram's Stain—Neisseria gonorrhoeae

Multiple gram-negative, intracellular diplococci from a patient with *N. gonorrhoeae.* (Courtesy of Morse, Moreland, Thompson: *Atlas of Sexually Transmitted Diseases*. London, Mosby-Wolfe, 1990.)

Uses

To examine for clue cells, *Trichomonas,* and sperm. See Figs. 17.5 to 17.7.

Materials

Aqueous sodium chloride, glass microscope slide, coverslip.

Method

1. Place a drop of saline onto the middle of the glass slide. (Alternative Method: Place several drops of saline in a small glass test tube and place the swab in the tube. The swab can then be wiped onto a slide at a later time.)
2. Mix a small amount of vaginal fluid to be examined into the saline drop.
3. Overlay a coverslip.
4. Examine directly through microscope at 40 × and 100 × (oil immersion).

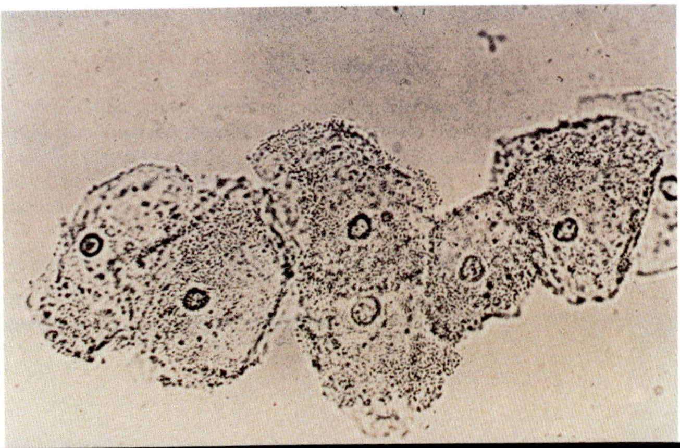

Figure 17.5 Clue Cells

"Glitter cell," or "clue cell": Epithelial cell covered with adherent bacteria in a wet mount of a vaginal specimen from a patient with *Gardinerella vaginalis* (also known as nonspecific vaginitis or bacterial vaginosis). Note the refractile appearance, indistinct borders, and ragged edges of the epithelial clue cell. (Courtesy of Curatek Pharmaceuticals.)

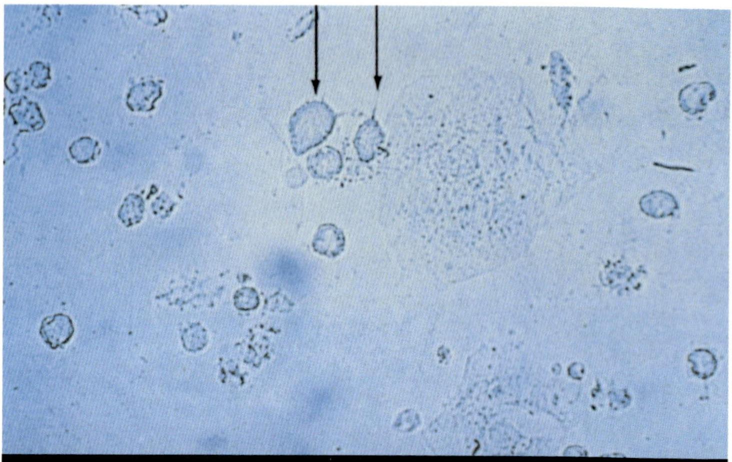

Figure 17.6 Trichomonas

Saline wet mount demonstrating oval-bodied, flagellated trichomonads. They are similar in size to leukocytes and can be distinguished from them by their motility and presence of flagella. (Courtesy of H. Hunter Hansfield: *Atlas of Sexually Transmitted Diseases*. New York, McGraw-Hill, 1992.)

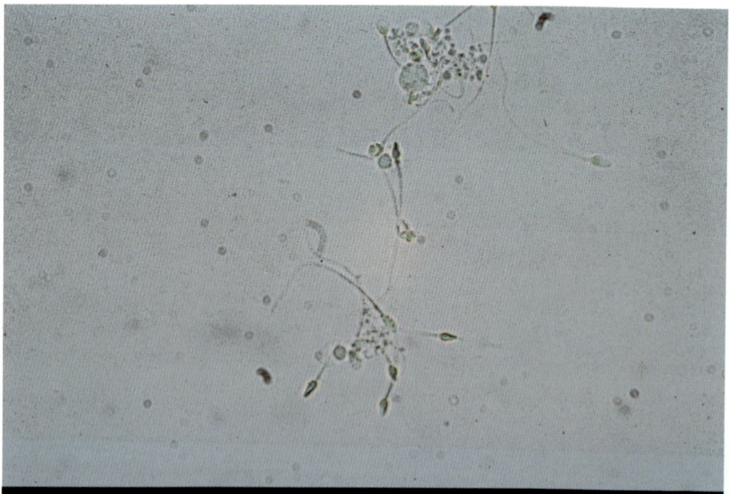

Figure 17.7 Spermatozoa

Spermatozoa may be motile or immotile. (From Susan K. Strasinger: *Urinalysis and Body Fluids*, ed. 3, F. A. Davis, 1994.)

Uses

To examine for yeast and fungus. See Fig. 17.8.

Materials

Ten percent aqueous potassium hydroxide (KOH), glass microscope slide, coverslip.

Method

1. Place a drop of KOH onto the middle of the glass slide.
2. Suspend a small amount of vaginal fluid into the drop of KOH.
3. Overlay a coverslip.
4. Let sit at room temperature for 30 min; as an alternative, gently heat the slide over a Bunsen burner but do not boil.
5. Examine under microscope for hyphae and spores.

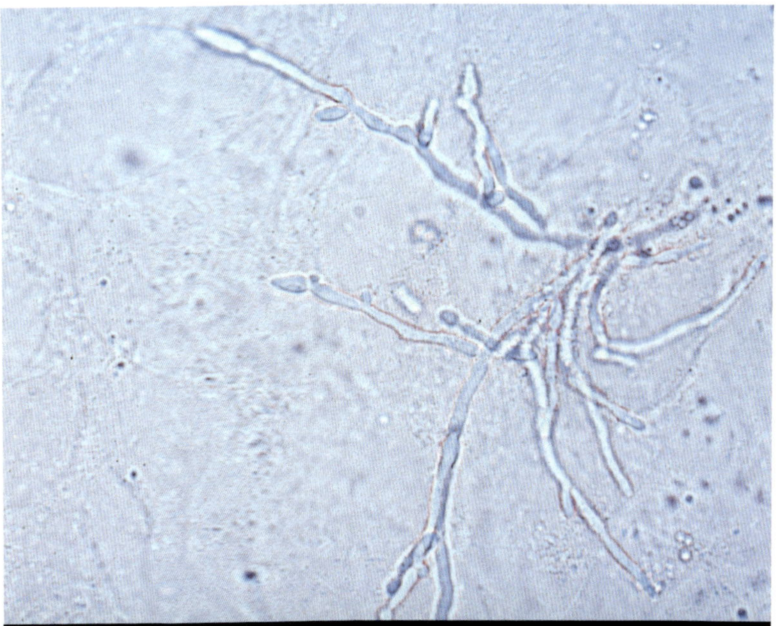

Figure 17.8 Candida albicans

Potassium hydroxide preparation of vaginal secretions from a patient with vaginal candidiasis due to *Candida albicans*. Note the pseudohyphae characteristic of this organism. (Courtesy of H. Hunter Hansfield: *Atlas of Sexually Transmitted Diseases*. New York, McGraw-Hill, 1992.)

Uses

To evaluate a patient for the presence of fecal leukocytes. See Fig. 17.9.

Materials

Freshly collected liquid stool specimen, glass microscope slide, coverslip, methylene blue.

Method

1. Place a drop of liquid stool onto the glass slide.
2. Add two drops of methylene blue to the stool specimen.
3. Mix thoroughly.
4. Overlay with a coverslip.
5. Place the edge of a piece of filter paper adjacent to the coverslip to absorb any excess methylene blue.
6. Examine using 10 × objective to scan specimen and 40 × and 100 × to identify specific leukocytes.

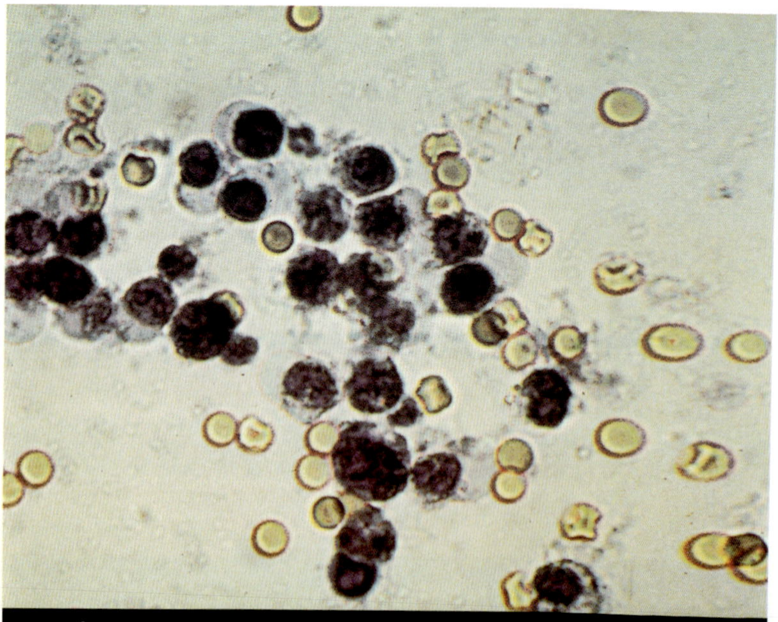

Figure 17.9 Fecal Leukocytes

Multiple white cells in the stool specimen from a patient with bacterial diarrhea. (Courtesy of Herbert L. DuPont, MD.)

Uses

To determine fungal dermatoses or skin infestations. See Figs. 17.10 to 17.13.

Materials

Fresh skin scraping, glass microscope slide, coverslip, potassium hydroxide (10%).

Method

1. Specimen collection:
   a. Gently scrape skin lesion with edge of a 15-blade scalpel.
2. Slide preparation:
   a. Place a drop of KOH onto the middle of the glass slide.
   b. Suspend a small smount of skin scraping into the drop of KOH.
   c. Overlay a coverslip.
   d. Let sit at room temperature for 30 min; as an alternative, gently heat the slide over a Bunsen burner but do not boil.
   e. Examine under microscope for hyphae, spores, or infestations.

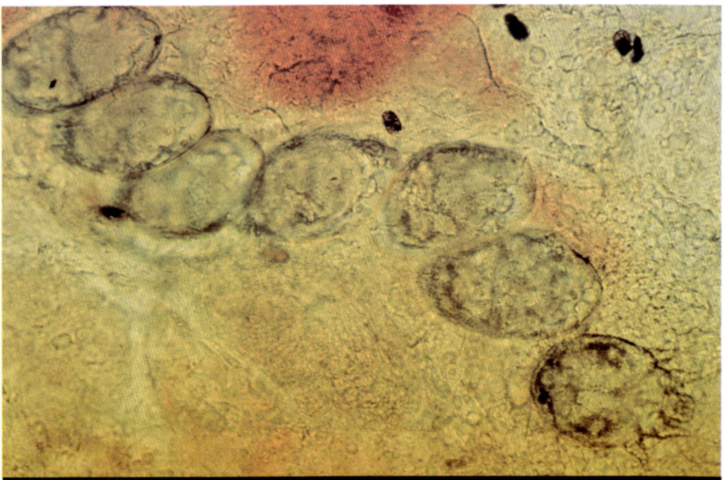

Figure 17.10 Scabies

Skin scraping from a patient with scabies. Note the intact mite at the lower right of the photograph, and the ova and fecal pellets. (Courtesy of Dept. of Dermatology, Naval Medical Center, Portsmouth, VA.)

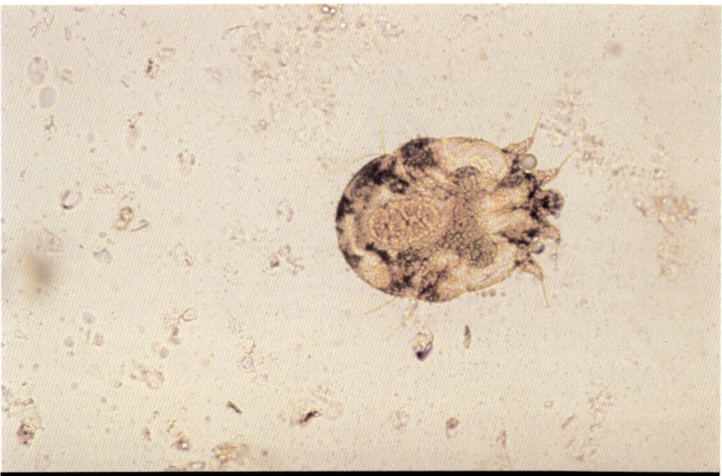

Figure 17.11 Scabies

Adult female scabies mite. (Courtesy of Morse, Moreland, Thompson: *Atlas of Sexually Transmitted Diseases*. London, Mosby-Wolfe, 1990.)

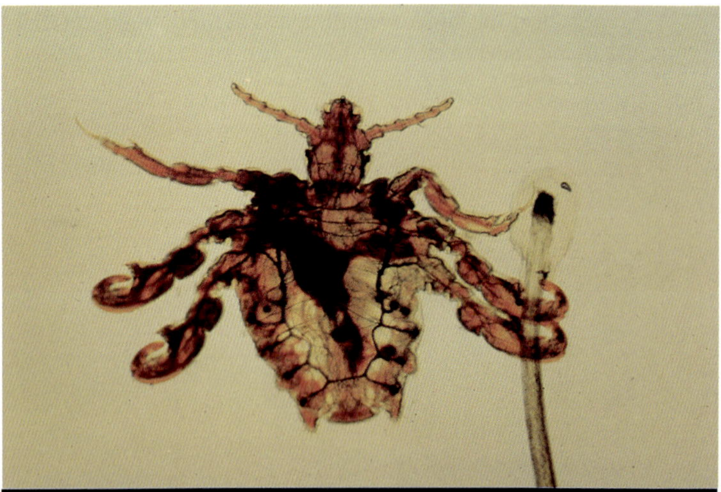

Figure 17.12 Pediculosis

Phthirus pubis, the crab louse. Note the short body and clawlike legs, which are ideally suited for clinging to the hair shaft. (Courtesy of Dept. of Dermatology, Naval Medical Center, Portsmouth, VA.)